Local Foods Meet Global Foodways

I0887319

This book explores the intersection of food and foodways from global and local perspectives. The collection contributes to interdisciplinary debates about the role and movement of commodities in the historical and contemporary world. The expert contributions collectively address a fundamental tension in the emerging scholarly terrain of food studies, namely theorizing the relationship between foodstuff production and cuisine patterns. They explore a wide variety of topics, including curry, bread, sugar, coffee, milk, pulque, Virginia ham, fast-food, obesity, and US ethnic restaurants.

Local Foods Meet Global Foodways considers movements in context, and, in doing so, complicates the notions that food 'shapes' culture as it crosses borders or that culture 'adapts' foods to its neo-local or global contexts. By analysing the dynamics of contact between mobile foods and/or people and the specific cultures of consumption they provoke, these case studies reveal the process whereby local foods become global, or global foods become local, to be a dynamic, co-creative development jointly facilitated by humans and nature.

This volume explores a vast expanse of global regions, such as North and Central America, Europe, China, East Asia and the Pacific, India, sub-Saharan Africa, the Atlantic Ocean, and the USSR/Russia. It includes a foreword by the eminent food scholar Carole Counihan, and an afterword by noted theorist of cuisine Rachel Laudan, and will be of great interest to students and researchers of history, anthropology, geography, cultural studies and American studies.

This book is based on a special issue of *Food and Foodways*.

Benjamin N. Lawrance is the Barber B. Conable, Jr. Endowed Chair of International Studies at the Rochester Institute of Technology, USA. He is the author of *Trafficking in Slavery's Wake: Law and the Experience of Women and Children in Africa* (2012), *Locality, Mobility, and 'Nation'* (2007), *Interpreters, Intermediaries and Clerks* (2006), and *The Ewe of Togo and Benin* (2006).

Carolyn de la Peña is Professor of American Studies and Director of the Humanities Institute at the University of California at Davis, USA. Her most recent book is *Empty Pleasures: The Story of Artificial Sweeteners from Saccharin to Splenda* (2010).

Local Foods Meet Global Foodways

Tasting History

Edited by
Benjamin N. Lawrance and Carolyn de la Peña

Routledge
Taylor & Francis Group
LONDON AND NEW YORK

First published 2012
by Routledge
2 Park Square, Milton Park, Abingdon, Oxon, OX14 4RN

Simultaneously published in the USA and Canada
by Routledge
711 Third Avenue, New York, NY 10017

Routledge is an imprint of the Taylor & Francis Group, an informa business

First issued in paperback 2012

This book is partly based on volume 19, issues 1-2, of *Food and Foodways,* and includes new material and additional essays from other issues of *Foods and Foodways*. The Publisher requests that those authors who may cite this book, also cite the bibliographical details of the issue, where appropriate.

British Library Cataloguing in Publication Data
A catalogue record for this book is available from the British Library

ISBN13: 978-0-415-69773-0 (hbk)
ISBN13: 978-0-415-82995-3 (pbk)

Typeset in Garamond
by Taylor & Francis Books

Disclaimer
The publisher would like to make readers aware that the chapters in this book are referred to as articles as they had been in the special issue. The publisher accepts responsibility for any inconsistencies that may have arisen in the course of preparing this volume for print.

Contents

Notes on Contributors

Aaron Bobrow-Strain is Associate Professor of Politics at Whitman College, USA. He is the author of *White Bread: A Social History of the Store-Bought Loaf* (2012) and *Intimate Enemies: Landowners, Power, and Violence in Chiapas* (2007), as well as many articles on agriculture, food, and politics in the United States and Mexico.

Carole Counihan is Professor of Anthropology at Millersville University, USA. She is author of *The Anthropology of Food and Body: Gender, Meaning, and Power, Around the Tuscan Table: Food, Family and Gender in Twentieth Century Florence*, and *A Tortilla Is Like Life: Food and Culture in the San Luis Valley of Colorado*. She is editor of *Food in the USA*, with Penny Van Esterik of *Food and Culture*, and with Psyche Williams-Forson of *Taking Food Public: Redefining Foodways in a Changing World*. She is editor of *Food and Foodways*.

Carolyn de la Peña is Professor of American Studies and Director of the Humanities Institute at the University of California, Davis, USA. She is the author of *Empty Pleasures: The Story of Artificial Sweeteners from Saccharin to Splenda* (2010), *The Body Electric: How Strange Machines Built the Modern American* (2003) and *Rewiring the Nation: The Place of Technology in American Studies* with Siva Vaidahyanathan (2007).

Megan E. Edwards studied at The College of William and Mary, USA, where her interest in anthropology, historical archaeology and food took root. She has an M.A. in Archaeology from the Queen's University of Belfast, with a dissertation on the medieval butchery trade in Scotland. She is currently in the Department of Anthropology at the University of Chicago, USA, where she is researching the impact of colonial initiatives and post-medieval social change on whiskey in early modern Ireland.

Jenny Elaine Goldstein is a Ph.D. candidate in Geography at the University of California, Los Angeles, USA. Her research interests include food production and distribution, agricultural policy, and environmental conservation in East Africa, Indonesia, and the United States. She holds an M.A. in Geography from UCLA and a B.A. from Barnard College.

G. Roger Knight teaches in the School of History and Politics at the University of Adelaide, Australia. He writes about sugar and the industries that produce it, with special reference to Indonesia. He is co-editor of *Sugarlandia Revisited: Sugar and Colonialism in Asia and the Americas, 1800 to 1940* (2007). He is presently working on aspects of colonial society in the erstwhile Netherlands Indies, and his monograph on the history of the Java sugar industry from the 1820s to the 1980s is forthcoming.

Benjamin N. Lawrance is the Barber B. Conable, Jr. Endowed Professor of International Studies at the Rochester Institute of Technology, USA, and teaches in the Department of Sociology and Anthropology. He is author with Richard L. Roberts of the forthcoming *Trafficking in Slavery's Wake: Law and the Experience of Women and Children in Africa* (2012), *Locality, Mobility, and 'Nation'* (2007), *Interpreters, Intermediaries and Clerks* (2006) with Richard Roberts and Emily Osborn, and *The Ewe of Togo and Benin* (2005). He is currently writing a book on anti-trafficking in sub-Saharan Africa with a fellowship from the NEH.

Rachel Laudan, raised on an English farm, morphed from a geologist to an academic historian of science. Winning the Julia Child/Jane Grigson Prize of the International Association of Culinary Professionals for the *Food of Paradise: Exploring Hawaii's Culinary History* (1996) prompted her to write freelance. She has since won the Sophie Coe Prize of the Oxford Symposium on Food and Cookery, been Scholar-in-Residence for the International Association of Culinary Professionals, and keynote speaker for many academic and culinary conferences. Her book *Cuisine and Empire* is forthcoming with the University of California Press. She lives in Mexico City.

Stephanie R. Maroney is a Ph.D. student in the Cultural Studies program at the versity of California, Davis, USA. Her research examines the way that cookbooks, recipes, and foodstuffs reflect particular notions of race, class, and gender. Stephanie is interested in how discourses of food and eating construct group identities within cultural and colonial encounters.

Ty Matejowsky is Associate Professor of Anthropology at the University of Central Florida, USA. He received his Ph.D. in anthropology from Texas A&M University (2001). His ongoing research in the Philippines examines a number of issues related to globalization, including fast food, urban development, disaster responses, and international migration. Publications include "Like a 'Whopper Virgin': Anthropological Reflections on Burger King's Controversial Ad Campaign" (2010) in *Studies in Popular Culture* and "Jolly Dogs and McSpaghetti: Anthropological Reflections on Global/Local Fast Food Competition in the Philippines" (2008) in *Journal of Asia-Pacific Business*.

Daniel Nemser is Assistant Professor of Spanish in the Department of Romance Languages and Literatures at the University of Michigan, USA, and is the author of several articles on Spanish colonialism, law, and race in the Americas. His current project examines the roots of *mestizaje* discourse in the construction of categories of mixing and purity in colonial Latin America.

Audrey Russek is Assistant Professor of History at Gustavus Adolphus College, USA. Her research focuses on sensory history, material culture, and women's studies, and she is currently writing a book on the cultural history of restaurants in the United States.

Andrea S. Wiley is Professor of Anthropology and Director of the Human Biology Program at Indiana University, Bloomington, USA. Her research explores the relationship between cow milk consumption and child growth and development, human biological variation in relation to milk consumption and policies promoting milk. She is author of three books, including *Re-Imagining Milk* (2011). She is currently completing, *Cultures of Milk: Dairy Consumption in India and the United States* (forthcoming with Harvard University Press).

Foreword

Carole Counihan

This book emerged from a special double issue of the journal *Food and Foodways* co-edited by Carolyn de la Peña and Benjamin Lawrance. In my capacity as editor-in-chief of the journal, I worked with Carolyn and Benjamin on this project over a period of several months from the inception of the idea of a special issue in early 2009 to its publication in March 2011. I was excited about this project from the beginning and I was never disappointed, for Carolyn and Benjamin held to the highest standards of editorial and intellectual excellence throughout the process. The resultant papers are outstanding in their exploration of diverse historical periods, geographic locations, and fascinating insights surrounding the longstanding global movement of foods, peoples, and cultures. In this book, two additional articles (published in earlier issues of *Food and Foodways*) complement the original seven articles from the special journal issue and expand its coverage.

Articles are united by a concern with the complex dynamic of foodways mobility – of local foods going global and becoming relocalized as they penetrate new peoples and cultures. Foods move through diverse processes including colonization, migration, capitalist expansion, imperialism, war, and the globalization of fast food. Approaching these issues from the perspectives of anthropology, cultural studies, geography, history, and sociology, articles ponder the relationship between taste, value, meaning, and availability of specific foods in specific places and historical moments. Articles look at colonization through several case studies, including the creation of a creolized New World ham in seventeenth- and eighteenth-century Virginia, the conflicting meanings of *pulque blanco* and *pulque mezclado* in colonial Mexico City, the creation of curry in eighteenth-century India by the British East India company and its relocalization in England, and the meanings surrounding sugar, particularly its "whiteness," in 1930s-1950s Dutch-colonized Indonesia. Articles look at accessibility, taste and meaning in the twentieth century, movement and transformation of foods through studies of white bread and Greek restaurants in post-WW II United States, of contemporary milk in China and India, of coffee in Rwanda, and of fast food in the Philippines. Articles share a common interest in how diverse foods, cuisine, beliefs and eating behaviors adapt, change, and take on new values as they are localized in diverse settings and come to signify inclusion and exclusion, status, shifting identities, and power relations.

This volume is timely because food access is an increasingly salient political issue. The articles make important contributions to understanding how and why foods move, under what conditions they are accepted or rejected, and how they are transformed in both substance and meaning as they navigate the globe. They offer original empirical data and innovative thinking about the crucial contemporary issue of how to maintain sufficient access, global diversity, local sovereignty, and cross-cultural communication around food.

INTRODUCTION

Foodways, 'Foodism,' or Foodscapes? Navigating the Local/Global and Food/Culture Divides

Carolyn de la Peña and Benjamin N. Lawrance

The term *foodways* has emerged from the intersection of popular and scholarly literature about cuisine to account for everything about eating, including what we consume, how we acquire it, who prepares it, and who is at the table.[1] In the words of Patricia Harris, David Lyon, and Sue McLaughlin, foodways, as a concept, summons to mind "[o]ur attitudes, practices, and rituals around food" and offers a "window onto our most basic beliefs about the world and ourselves."[2] Robert Blair St. George has described foodways as a form of vernacular expression with autoethnographic dimensions.[3] Other recent characterizations of the term foodways have focused on the procurement, preparation, and consumption of food.[4] Foodways has invigorated food studies and done much to awaken readers to the profound impact foods have on culture, politics, and industrial practices.[5]

This volume — which on a practical level emerged from a conference at the Robert Mondavi Institute for Wine and Food Science at the University of California, Davis, and a subsequent special issue of *Food and Foodways* exploring food globality and foodways localities[6] — uses the term "foodways" primarily as a critical lens to explore trans-cultural, trans-national, and trans-regional mobility, locality, and local embeddedness of foodstuffs. Our focus on *global* foodways explores local dynamics of global food and drink production, consumption, and mobility via a trans-locational lens. The chapters address issues of migration, settlement, colonization, imperialism, race and identity, consumption, distribution, governmentality, and globalization. Sites and processes include the transplanting and importation of food crops and animals from one region of the world to another; the hybridization of foodstuffs; the dissemination of technologies of food production; the creation of recipes and beverages for local and global markets; the shift in consumption patterns as echoes of modernity and post-modernity; and the relationship between food, drink, and political change.

Here in this anthology, nature and culture converge to create desirable, or undesirable, food and drink. We see this as a logical next step in the expanding domain of food and cuisine studies, the contours of which have recently been articulated by Carole Counihan and Penny Van Esterik. In the second edition of their now-standard reader, they ponder the mushrooming of the sub-field, and in particular how "food has permeated almost every scholarly field and become a widely accepted research topic."

Whereas when they embarked on their careers, food was "marginalized as a scholarly focus," by the late 2000s, the proliferation in food, drink and cuisine research extends deeply into historical studies, anthropology, geography, ethnic studies, and sociology, and is also making significant inroads into human biology, archaeology, political science and economics.[7]

As an intellectual project, this volume emerged from an ongoing conversation about food, drink, and globalization between two scholars – one seeking to write a book about the history of a foodstuff and its attendant foodways; and the other exploring how to teach the emergence of food and cuisine within a global historical context as a vehicle for the examination of geopolitical change and social history.[8] This book represents a concerted effort to ground our common interests in the narratives of things within the dynamic "global" communities that produce, transport, and consume them. Alexander Nützenadel and Frank Trentmann have forthrightly observed that although food and globalization "are inseparable," financial markets, migration narratives, communication concerns and trans-national political contingencies have often overshadowed the contours of food globalization.[9] Popular histories of commodities and luxuries have done little to undercut this, however. Whereas we accept the generalized proposition that "things" can "talk," we continue as scholars to struggle to listen to them within their complex local *and global* contexts.[10] This volume offers numerous instances of that struggle, across disciplines and periods. Here anthropologists and geographers join cultural studies scholars, sociologists and historians, each offering a unique framework (some disciplinary, others interdisciplinary) to explore the intersection of dynamic communities and globalized commodity paths.

We are particularly interested in the relationship between the pieces in this anthology and two types of food research that have proven remarkably popular with academic and lay readers alike in recent years. The first are commodity histories: books that focus on one particular food object (salt, cod, the banana, et cetera) and trace its journey across time and space as a means to understand shifts in eating patterns as well as plant and human history.[11] The second are books and films (e.g. *The Omnivore's Dilemma*, or "Super Size Me") that trace the environmental and health consequences of particular modes of American/North American food harvesting and eating. There are, of course, numerous reasons why readers—academic and non-academic alike—are drawn to these texts. Yet at their core, what often makes them so compelling is their ability to render food into a glue that connects us, intimately, to broader social, political, and historical concerns. For Martin Spurlock, eating at McDonald's is not just a personal choice, it constitutes participation in a complex system that can both facilitate ill health and generate immense corporate profit.[12] For Michael Pollan, cheap corn is not only a consumer product, it is also—and most importantly—a byproduct of a system of intentional overproduction that helps certain people and harms others.[13] At the hands of skilled writers, single commodity studies reveal our supermarket shelves to be full of micro histories. Individual products we often take for granted come alive, and our personal purchases are revealed to be enabled by historical actors long silenced. In all of these books, the buying and eating of food becomes something far more than a personal experience. It is a means of participation in a dynamic system to which we are conjoined (or not) through ingestion.

Yet there are important elements of this interconnectivity that are difficult to explore with these approaches. For instance, in single-commodity studies, stories about bananas, potatoes, tea, and cod have enthralled lay readers and scholars alike with tales of intrigue, happenstance, and opportunity. At the same time, their close focus on the movement of a particular commodity or luxury good has, on occasion, obscured the pre-conditions of cultural, political, and economic change that enable a particular traveling food to be accepted (or rejected). Single commodity foci can also easily neglect instances where cuisine—or ideas of cuisine—impact individual and community food and drink choices. They may leave little room for stories wherein individuals are valued or devalued by others because of their consumption (or non-consumption) or particular foods. Projects tightly focused on the social and political practices of industrialized food production in the United States have their own challenges. While they shine a powerful light on the practices of subsidies, trade policies, agribusiness, and fast food, they can obscure the myriad ways in which foods move across borders, especially those not of the United States. Aesthetics-driven frameworks, including "foodscapes" and "foodism," mire us in the present, limiting our ability to see how people across time and societies have dealt with the cultural and dietary changes that accompany shifts in food supplies.[14] And they concretize particular terms, like "local" and "global" in ways that while perhaps true of the present, within an American context, are more flexible elsewhere, particularly in the past.[15]

We believe that the perspectives taken by authors in this anthology have much to offer readers who are interested how particular food choices (or non-choices) bind us as individuals to complex, external social systems. At the same time, because their perspectives are historical, and global, they are able to offer evidence about just how these relationships are formed across boundaries, and over time, that can be of use to us in the present. While each is concerned with a particular site (from Rwandan coffee production, and milk in China, to sugar in Indonesia, and a Greek restaurant in New York City), a number of overlapping questions bind them to one another and offer insights beyond the sum of their parts into the broader field of global foodways. As readers move through diverse terrains from colonial Mesoamerica and contemporary Philippines, to tidewater Virginia and imperial Britain, we suggest that three sets of questions be kept uppermost in mind. These sets of questions comprise many of the core research concerns and pedagogical interests of scholars and teachers in cuisine, food, drink and nutrition today.

The first set of questions includes: How or in what contexts do food and drink become tasty and the object of desire (or otherwise)? Are the sensory experiences of taste and preferences for certain taste sensations the same across all of humanity? Or are these experiences and preferences more cultural than biological? Is this determined by political forces, cultural values, or both? Building on taste, the second broad set of questions concerns value, and how value is produced as plant and animal products move along chains of production and process. Do consumers, or producers, or both create value? How do they know and meet the interests and demands of the other? Can small groups of consumers have an impact on large producers, and even local markets? Is this impact easier, or harder, when products emerge from local versus global systems of production? A third set of concerns expands on taste and value and deploys foodways to destabilize the traditionally linear relationship between local and global, with respect to both production and consumption. In different ways, the authors ask: How can a product be perceived of as global when production and consumption appears to remain entirely local? Conversely, when a food or drink appears to be only discovered or encountered by new communities as a consequence of global flows, possibly colonial, imperial, or neo-colonial, what happens to our comprehension of foodways when evidence for the local is prioritized? Although there are no definitive answers to these expansive questions, in differing ways the authors attempt answers to one or several of them.

Notwithstanding the fact that the general questions above in various ways guided the authors in their respective research, we also observe responsive and thematic commonalities productive of interdisciplinary collaboration. To this end, we encourage readers to consider the collection as a whole. Interdisciplinarity in food and drink studies operates on the individual and collective level.[16] The anthology responds *collectively* to the themes of the original conference and synthesizes broad perspectives, knowledge, interconnections, and epistemologies of the relationship between food, drink, nutrition, and mobility. As the Afterword by cuisine scholar Rachel Laudan affirms, the chapters herein enable us to see that an interdisciplinary global foodways approach that holds in tension the local/global and nature/culture divides has three important things to offer the study of food and culture—themes, if you like, rather than definitive answers to the sets of questions asked above.

First, the interdisciplinarity of the global foodways rubric returns a needed sense of exchange and dynamism to the study of food flows. Second, it problematizes any designation of "local" food as determined by geography alone. And third, it takes us beyond the "McDonaldization of Everything" explanation of the culinary contours of globalization. Below we expand on each of these further.

COMMODITY "TRACING" IS DECEPTIVE

Whereas tracing commodities privileges particular socioeconomic sectors and can naturalize the "laws" of finance and monetarism, considering jointly the movement of foods and the reception of human actors opens up the field of influence and places rules and regulations on the table. By jointly considering mobile foods and their human communities (at points of origin and consumption), we break free from notions that commodities have had their truest, or most profound, influence when they remain single objects moving through space unencumbered by the impact of humans. Instead of focusing on where a food comes from and where it goes, several authors in this volume ask how it is instead that moving foods and drinks become desirable (or not).

In many respects sugar represents the *sine qua non* of commodity tracing for food historians, anthropologists, and others; and even before Sidney Mintz drew together what previously appeared to be competing narratives about labor, race, capital, consumption and production, it occupied the center-stage of narratives of global food and cuisine connectivity. Mintz and his followers emphasized commodities as vehicles whereby one may explore the dialectical processes of contradictory forces. The commercialization of sugar products had lasting effects in Europe and beyond, from facilitating the resource base of the industrial revolution, to transforming entire foodways and revolutionizing European tastes and consumer behaviors.[17] Historian Roger Knight extends these analytical insights in his examination of the transformation in taste in the decolonializing Dutch East Indies/Indonesia, and in particular the growth in demand for white factory-made sugar.

Over several decades from the 1930s, Indonesians began to abandon brown sugar forms in favor of white, as they began to associate white sugar with everything that was "up-to-date, fashionable, and desirable." But rather than pursuing the movement and consumption of sugar in a linear producer-consumer narrative characteristic of many popular commodity tracing monographs, Knight reveals the shift to white sweeteners to be highly contested and part of a broader set of struggles about market share, government patronage, and the embracing of modernity by decolonizing elites. What Knights sees as the "victory" of white sugar domestic cultural preferences is revealed to be tightly bound up with and dependent upon, the political economy of the local production of white sugar.

So-called commodities are often not quite what they seem; some food items masquerade as commodities, while others attain the status of commodity through a complex set of culturally determined processes. As cultural studies scholar, Stephanie Maroney, demonstrates, "curry powder" from its earliest date of invention (possibly the mid-seventeenth century), was constructed as a spice, treated as a commodity, and funneled into the Asian-European spice market for transport to Europe. Rather than being a locally produced and consumed spice, such as fenugreek or cardamom, the mixture was processed in India, but only for the purposes of export to the United Kingdom. Furthermore, the rapid popularization of all things Indian in metropolitan Britain via the publication of accessible, simple, and imitable recipes and cookbooks, "turned India's local food culture into a commodity constructed through colonialism."

Indeed the limits of commodity tracing are further illustrated in contrasting chapters on colonial Mexico, post genocide Rwanda, and twentieth century United States. Spanish language and literature scholar, Daniel Nemser, demonstrates how *pulque* (a traditional alcoholic drink of the indigenous population) emerged as a global product in spite of the fact that it was produced and consumed in what might otherwise have been considered an entirely local context, Mexico City. In seventeenth-century reports written by New Spain's colonial elite about the role of *pulque* in the June 8, 1692, Mexico City rebellion, Nemser finds a transnational biopolitical project enacted at the local level. *Pulque blanco* was recognized across New Spain as beneficial, but mixing other materials into it transformed *pulque blanco* into *pulque mezclada*, a completely different substance, credited with the propagation of all manner of "evil." Evidenced in the linguistic and conceptual slippage between *pulque mezclado* (mixed *pulque*) and *plebe mezclada* (mixed plebian masses), Nemser identifies a biopolitics aimed at purifying New Spain (socially, spiritually, and biologically), first through the purification of bodies and then through their spatial segregation. As Nemser states, "It was not just the salvation of the Indians' souls that mattered to these ecclesiastical authors; it was their belief that the threat of mixing was not contained in the metaphorical mug of *pulque mezclado* but overflowed, penetrating both the blood of the individual and the physiology of the social body." The ambiguity inherent in the notion of mixture, one that metaphorically connected the "impurification" of a beverage with the impurification of Spanish blood, proved mixing to be a threat to colonial order. The international politics of the colonial world thus played out in these local concerns about *pulque*.

International development programs and the politics of taste are on full display in geographer Jennifer Goldstein's analysis of boutique coffee production in Rwanda. Whereas sugar has anchored commodity-tracing scholarship, coffee production resides at the heart of contemporary programs and popular political action with respect sourcing so-called "fair-trade" consumer products. Goldstein's analysis problematizes the free trade/fair-trade dichotomy currently gripping coffee production and consumption that extends into almost every Western household via supermarket chains and so-called "ethical purchasing" at Starbucks.[18] Post-genocide Rwanda is the site of a new experiment eclipsing this binary, but one that attends directly to the taste buds of American caffeine aficionados in particular. Coffee-harvesters, many of whom have no desire to consume the beverage, are actively cultivating their palates to recognize flavors they would never encounter in tropical central Africa, such as blueberry, cherry and caramel.

Focusing specifically on the interwar years, American Studies scholar and historian Audrey Russek argues that, recent immigrants, and those native-born Americans seeking "authentic" foreign experiences were the most frequent patrons of U.S. ethnic restaurants at the turn of the century. Immigration restrictions after World War I, however, required ethnic restaurateurs to cultivate broader markets. These new "ethnic" restaurants were more foreign-themed than authentically foreign. Interiors often featured romantic visions of faraway places, complete with costumed serving staff and fanciful menus. Foods combined ethnic and American tastes. It would be easy to dismiss these sites as kitsch, offering little of value to what might be construed as local ethnic communities. Russek's analysis, however, reveals that proprietors frequently used their dining rooms as a means of emphasizing the value of their "local" cultural heritage and cuisine even while their own recipe and ambience choices effectively "Americanized" both.

With the food rationing and importation bans of World War II, foreign recipes prepared with American techniques and local foods became a ubiquitous part of American national cuisine. So much so, that by the 1950s many considered a particular kind of cosmopolitan palate as a sign of American identity, whereas immigrants who exclusively practiced the foodways of their homelands were characterized as requiring Americanization. By focusing on the context in which foods and beverages were consumed, Russek, Goldstein, Knight, Maroney, and Nemser, and others in this volume, reveal the complex interplay between local foods and globalized cultural environments that might be obscured were we to focus exclusively on the movement of commodities across time and space.

BEYOND "LOCAVORES"

A second contribution of a renewed attention to the relationship between substance and location is the way that global foodways problematizes any easy designation of "local" food as determined by geography alone. Locality and the particulars of the local have maintained a powerful hold on scholars of food, cuisine and nutrition since Mintz and others pushed back against world-systems theory in the 1970s. It was Mintz who observed that, "the postulation of a world-system forces us frequently to lift our eyes from the particulars of local history, which I would consider salutary. But equally salutary is the constant revisiting of events 'on the ground,' so that the architecture of the world-system can be laid bare."[19] Nemser's analysis of *pulque* attends to this antagonism intuitively, insofar as he reveals that the international colonial context of the struggle over an indigenous beverage was deeply interwoven with local concerns with pollution and *mestizaje*. Knight's examination of local sugar consumption patterns connects preference to political and social mobility in the tense years prior to and after decolonization in Indonesia. For her part, Russek's exploration of the origins of the "local" American ethnic restaurant in the early-to-mid twentieth century reveals that locality operates on two levels: first as a dining space for single working-class (often immigrant) males; and second, as a site for serving specialized "reproductions of global cultures and foodways," not "actual foreign dishes."

The increasingly popular term "locavore," coined circa 2005, describes an individual who promotes the practice of eating a diet consisting of food harvested from within a "local" area, most commonly considered a 100-mile (160 km) radius. The concept has gained such traction that the *New Oxford American Dictionary* selected "locavore" as its word of the year in 2007.[20] Some locavores adhere to *The 100-Mile Diet: A Year of Local Eating* (2007) or other provocative texts, such as Barbara Kingsolver's *Animal, Vegetable, Miracle: A Year of Food Life* (2007). Other "locavores" are devotees of farmers' markets, community-supported agriculture, and community gardens. Yet it is also interesting to consider the way that communities make "local" even the most distant of goods. While human agency moves commodities, and products may navigate global foodways, decisions about what constitutes food and drink—curry, bread, coffee, and so forth—are always produced locally.

Anthropologist Andrea Wiley's fieldwork on the meanings of milk in China, India, and the United States reveals that while milk is exported to China with American messages of strong bones and child growth, it is only consumed after local meanings of well-being have been attached. While Indians and Americans have traditionally included milk in their diets, the Chinese have long viewed milk with revulsion. In all three countries, however, milk is now consumed in significant amounts. Wiley argues that milk has grown popular in India and China while maintaining relevance in the United States by being positioned as a food that enhances well-being, which is defined differently in each context. In China and India, this well-being is achieved through milk's association with child growth, which becomes a symbol of national development and strength. In the United States, however, the association between milk and growth is not likely to resonate with an aging population concerned about obesity and disease. There, milk promotions have associated the commodity with weight loss and disease prevention. Within each context (the United States, India, and China), milk undergoes particular transformations (e.g., lactose-free, dry, pasteurized) in order to enable it to be viewed as a health-enhancing product. Thus, even as the global spread of "nutritionism" could impose a uniform discourse about milk, local contexts rework this concept (and the milk itself) so as to incorporate it into unique histories and desires.

And even products that seem fundamentally "from nowhere," such as white bread, are discovered to be local in origin, especially when we stretch our analysis to move from nature to culture. Sociologist and professor of government, Aaron Bobrow-Strain, turns to history to transform our local starch of choice—"American" white bread—into a commodity deeply enmeshed in global politics. Focusing on the early Cold War period, Bobrow-Strain discusses what he terms U.S. "white bread imperialism," a set of practices that cemented American foodways with American national security in the minds of policymakers and the general public. Instead of atoms, he argues, it was bread grains that were "the strategic particles" of the Cold War.

But the power of bread as an indicator of "white" progress and American democracy was drawn in large part from its local affiliations within the United States (in spite of its industrial production). This local meaning was enhanced by bread's performance abroad, such as in Japan, where occupying forces, convinced of the superiority of white bread, worked with great determination to displace rice with it. The absence of bread, a ubiquitous topic in the American media, characterized Soviet life as rife with suffering, while affirming the superiority of American values and democracy. Even after the

European bread crisis waned and the United States lost ground to the Soviets militarily, technologically, and educationally, Americans proudly held tight to the notion that (at least) their bread was superior, if not in taste, then in nutritional value. Wiley and Bobrow-Strain remind us that global foods, through the eyes of consumers, are often understood in particularly local contexts.

By expanding our definition of "local" from one of bio-region to one of culture-region, scholars in this collection imagine a more robust definition of food locality that co-considers where food is grown and where it attaches. But as the case studies of milk, bread and the expansion of the fast food industry in the Philippines underscore, nutrition standards and changing dietary desires are equally powerful concepts for investigating the allure of the local. Anthropologist Ty Matejowsky examines the perception of diet and fast food among young Filipinos and uncovers startling information about the global obesity pandemic. As corporate chain restaurants that promote diets rich in calories, saturated fat, salt, and sugar expand rapidly around the globe, urban populations throughout Africa, Asia, Latin America, and elsewhere are experiencing significant increases in obesity, cardiovascular disease, hypertension, and type two diabetes mellitus. Matejowsky identifies "rapid nutrition transition" as a core factor in the expansion of Filipino girth, but rather than viewing this simply as another narrative of globalization and modernization, he ties it to local values and concerns, "especially the indigenization of corporate fast food's standardized menu and service format to better accommodate local tastes and preferences."

Indigenization provides an excellent metaphor for a more rigorous understanding of local and locality, and indeed a healthy critique of locavore. Virginia ham, for example, celebrated throughout the U.S. and beyond as a uniquely local blend of Tidewater culinary skill and cuisine knowledge, is revealed by anthropologist Megan Edwards to be a rich imbrication of European, African and indigenous American methods and endemic fauna and flora. Edwards upends the contemporary image of Smithfield hams and their porcine kin as "location-specific *terroir* foods" and "islands of time" standing in defiance of the "crush of global modernity." Instead, she argues "the grande dame of globalizing forces" — trans-Atlantic colonialism — descended in the seventeenth and eighteenth centuries on the Chesapeake Bay to act as "midwife" in the birth of this unique local and indigenous food.

No less so that those frequenting farmers markets and slow food restaurants in Western bourgeois bohemian enclaves, twenty-something Filipinos desirous of new brands, indigenous-named foodstuffs, and adaptations of local cuisine, facilitate new consumer expectations about appropriate dietary choices at the local level. Counter-intuitively, *perceived* nutritional qualities of Western fast food hold the key to understanding the original allure of standardized prepared chain restaurant fare. Matejowsky argues that the "efficiency and regimentation" of the culinary approach associated with American-style fast food, including advanced kitchen technology, reinforced Filipino notions that it was generally superior to indigenous cuisine as it was designed scientifically. But over time, fast food forms have returned to local cuisines and indigenous standards in their battle to attract brand-savvy and urban consumers. The obesity epidemic is thereby revealed to be only the underbelly of local manifestations of shifting ideas of social status, material affluence, and modern taste. Thus in this and other ways, Matejowsky, Russek, Edwards, Wiley, Bobrow-Strain, among others redirect our attention toward the cultural contours of the local.

PROBLEMATIZING McDONALDIZATION

Finally, the collection reveals how the concept of global foodways takes us beyond the seductive McDonaldization of Everything narrative.[21] Many of us may lament the proliferation of mega-food purveyors, from Walmart to McDonald's, and the attendant struggles of local food producers and consumers to sustain markets in the face of such competition. Michael Pollan's hugely successful *Omnivore's Dilemma* and Robert Kenner's documentary film "Food, Inc." (2008) thrust the American family into the center of one aspect of this debate, specifically the dependence of the modern American cuisine and economy on corn/maize.[22] Yet if we are going to successfully address the problems with global food "creep," it is important that we understand fully the reasons why individuals embrace food and drink practices from beyond their borders. Food, nutrition, and taste provide rich vehicles for the interrogation of changes in attitudes and policy, from industrial white bread as a Cold War weapon to coffee as tool for imagined economic uplift. As chapters in this collection reveal, adopting global foodways is, in many instances, a way for people within localities to enhance their own status, and they speak to ideas of self as much as other.

There is a complex story told here wherein local values coincide with practices that may, in fact, make it more difficult for local food practices to survive (or for their local origins to be known). As Maroney reveals, members of the British East India Company enjoyed the flavors of curry they encountered while stationed in India. Upon returning home, many wanted to create a curry market for themselves. Their tendency to call any saucy Indian dish a "curry," however, combined with the desire of many to profit by creating ready-made curry powder for consumer purchase, enabled a British curry to emerge with little resemblance to the local dish. Examining references to the consumption of curry in novels and cookbooks, Maroney shows the importance of these local actors in shifting "curry" from the colonial margins to the colonial center.

With Virginia ham, the story turns more on the desire of producers to hide the locality of a regional dish in favor of more cosmopolitan (if inaccurate) origins. Rather than drawing attention to its indigenous smoking techniques, inventive curing practices due to trade shortages, and smart adaptations to its geographical location, Virginia ham producers instead claimed that it was indistinguishable from its European cured meat ancestors. Edwards carefully traces several factors that influenced the development of this well-known foodstuff, including the advantages and limitations of the climate and colonial location, the existing techniques for curing meats in Europe, shortages of curing ingredients due to trade and warfare, the use of indigenous smoking techniques, and the fashion of European elites consuming foods from exotic colonial locations while also resurrecting the food practices of ancient Greece and Rome. If these origins are unfamiliar to aficionados of Virginia ham, it is in part because Virginian elites' efforts to prop up their threatened identities as Englishmen worked to eliminate knowledge of these influences, focusing instead on how they were emulating the foodways of European elites.

Matejowsky demonstrates that the allure of fast food does not necessarily translate into the success of McDonald's in the Philippines. Whereas the underperformance of McDonald's is a source of embarrassment for the international conglomerate, "homegrown outfits" like Chinese fast food purveyor Chowking, Greenwich Pizza, and, especially, Jollibee, demonstrate that local foods, even "fast" ones compete and win when they aggressively market "Filipino-influenced menus." If McDonaldization remains a useful metaphor for the globalization of cuisine and markets, it is perhaps most effective as an analytical tool for interrogating nutritional changes in tandem with dietary trends. For whereas the golden arches may not dominate the East Asia/Pacific physical landscape as they do the United States, the implications of the shift in consumption patterns are certainly emulated in the dramatic shifts in public health indices.

If dietary and nutrition shifts are a cause for concern in the Philippines, the awareness of and co-optation of Western tastes about coffee are source of pride for Rwanda's coffee doctors. "Cuppers," or expert coffee tasters, according to Goldstein, demonstrate the systematic training which enables them to grade coffee varieties in a way nearly indistinguishable from Americans and Europeans as a means of career elevation. One could argue, of course, that such techniques reproduce the same kinds of palate monocultures within African markets that have taken hold elsewhere. Goldstein's examination of Rwandan specialty coffee, however, complicates this analysis by looking at local motivations for a globalized product. Cuppers, the tasters trained by international coffee buyers who serve American and European markets, claim that these skills, in fact, improve the quality of their own local products. Goldstein explains the systematic training cuppers undergo, and notes the benefits, in a local context, of these methods of discernment that lead to fairly stable product distinction across regions and traditions and, therein, greater economic return to local farmers. Yet the leveling of "taste" difference in Rwanda, while profitable when that taste is calibrated to American and European markets, may not serve locals well with Japan emerging as a potentially lucrative market for specialty coffee.

Goldstein's fieldwork raises questions about how "value" is best determined for local markets when those goods must meet global markets where consumers—and tastes—change. But it is equally powerful as a story about U.S. foreign policy goals in stabilizing post-genocide Rwanda, and sheds important light on American perceptions of their role in the post-Cold War global landscape. Rather than opting for a "fair-trade" or "shade-grown" model that would bring Rwandan coffee into direct competition with its neighbors, the U.S.A.I.D.-sponsored project promoted a *terroir* approach, with a nod to the regional specializations usually associated with French viticulture.

Goldstein's discovery, however, is only one of many such interventions. From subsidized California rice "aid" to North Korea, to trademark infringement lawsuits directed at small-scale farmers in the Global South, U.S. political realities blaze their own powerful foodways abroad and at home. Brobow-Strain reveals the industrial enterprise behind American white bread to be tool for post-war reconstruction reifying American capitalism and liberalism as the embodiment of "strength, stability, choice, and abundance." But just as we must move away from the flattening of McDonaldization narratives, Brobow-Strain shows that Americans' understandings of diet and place in the world and their strong confidence in the "choiceworthiness of American industrial foodways and industrial food production system" were the flipside of postwar food imperialism. In this way, the authors in this volume, including Goldstein, Bobrow-Strain, Matejowsky, Edwards, Maroney and others, turn the corner on McDonaldization by focusing attention on food and drink choice, desire and taste, and their attendant politics.

CONCLUSION

We offer this collection to stimulate further teaching and thinking about the history of traveling foods, the politics of food locality and the culture of global foodways. Their authors suggest that foods "travel" without necessarily moving across time, space, and culture. They reveal that food and drink does not have to come from where we are in order for it to be local. And they argue that the "global" functions not only as a particular geographic site from which foods emerge, but also as a cultural imaginary with which individuals can affiliate for enhanced prestige by altering consumption. It is our hope that these chapters may enhance the stories currently told about food and better connect our understanding of food as object, to our lived experiences of food as culture, in a world that, while intensely globalized, remains in many ways, profoundly local.[23]

We agree with Counihan and Van Esterik that the growing sense of the politicization of food, and social movements tied to consumption and production, from "fair trade" to anti-fast food initiatives in public schools, is at the root of currently immensely popular books, films and social media campaigns. Because it concerns, at once, production and consumption, material and taste, object and self, food and drink offers scholars "limitless grist" for exploring the personal and political, the material and symbolic, the self and other and the body and soul.[24] At the same time, we believe the essays in this volume illustrate that an emphasis on global foodways provides a rich and rewarding intellectual framework for the expansion of food and cuisine studies. It serves not only as an antidote to the presentism pervading many popular accounts of food, diet and culture, but as Rachel Laudan observes in her Afterword, it also returns us to the core tension between geography and culture wherein resides cuisine. Indeed, we see the convergence of taste, desire, and foodways in a globalized context as the next wave of a profoundly insightful and interdisciplinary *terroir*.

Ultimately, the value of this collection is in the opportunities it provides to consider, in one place, divergent stories across time and place held together by one common thread: the collision between human actors and food products that occurs when one, or both, are in transit. We hope that these pieces, when considered alongside a number of previously published essays in *Food and Foodways* on global and local foods, provide a resource for those interested in theorizing the local, ferreting out the global, and detangling the exchanges and flows embedded in any story that transforms food, and eaters, into cuisine.[25]

Notes

1. Among the earliest deployments was S. L. Oliver, Saltwater Foodways: New Englanders and Their Food in the 19th Century (1970).
2. P. Harris, D. Lyon, and S. McLaughlin, The Meaning of Food (2005), pp. viii-ix.
3. R. B. St. George, ed., Possible Pasts: Becoming Colonial in Early America (2000), 26. For auto-ethnography, see Mary Louise Pratt, "Arts of the Contact Zone," Profession 91 (1991): 33-40.
4. For example, A. Bower, African American Foodways: Explorations of History and Culture (2008); H. A. Diner, Hungering for America: Italian, Irish, and Jewish Foodways in the Age of Migration (2003); E. C. Rath and S. Assmann, Japanese Foodways, Past and Present (2010).
5. For example, J. Staller and M. Carrasco, Pre-Columbian Foodways: Interdisciplinary Approaches to Food, Culture, and Markets in Ancient Mesoamerica (2009); P. B. Lewicka, Food and Foodways of Medieval Cairenes: Aspects of Life in an Islamic Metropolis of the Eastern Mediterranean (2011). For general approaches, see recently Jeffrey Pilcher, *Food in World History* (Routledge, 2005) and B.W. Higman, *How Food Made History* (Wiley-Blackwell, 2011).

6. The authors would like to thank Clare Hasler, director of the RMI, Barry Klein, former Vice Chancellor of Research at UC Davis, the UC Davis Humanities Institute, and the University of California Multi-Campus Research Groups in World History and Food and the Body for support for this event and research on food and culture, as well as Ami Sommariva and Kelley Gove for research assistance. See Food and Foodways 19.1-2 (2011). Benjamin Lawrance also wishes to acknowledge the generous support of the Dean's Office in the College of Liberal Arts, at the Rochester Institute of Technology and the Conable Endowment in International Studies, which provided funding for a second conference exploring "cuisine studies" and planning this volume, held at R.I.T. in April 2011.
7. C. Counihan and P. Van Esterik, "Introduction to the Second Edition," in Counihan and Esterik (eds.), Food and Culture: A Reader 2nd Edition (2008), 1.
8. C. de la Peña, Empty Pleasures: The Story of Artificial Sweeteners from Saccharin to Splenda (2010); Benjamin Lawrance teaches a course entitled "A World of Things." Syllabus available upon request.
9. A. Nützenadel and F. Trentmann, "Mapping Food and Globalization," in Nützenadel and Trentmann (eds.), Food and Globalization, 1.
10. L. Daston, ed., Things That Talk: Object Lessons From Art and Science (2007); "Focus: Thick Things," Isis 98 (2007): 80-142; S. Mintz, Sweetness and Power: The Place of Sugar in Modern History (1986); M. Adas, Machines as the Measure of Men (1990).
11. A non-exhaustive list might include, for example (in alphabetical order): K. Albala, Beans: A History (2007); S. Allen, The Devil's Cup: A History of the World According to Coffee (2003); M. Booth, Opium, A History (1998); M. Booth, Cannabis: A History (2004); S. & M. Coe, The True History of Chocolate (1996); I. Gately, Tobacco: A Cultural History of How an Exotic Plant Seduced Civilization (2002); B. Hodgson, Opium: A Portrait of the Heavenly Demon (1999); D. Koeppel, Banana: The Fate of the Fruit That Changed the World (2008); M. Kurlansky, Cod (1997); M. Kurlansky, Salt: A World History (2002); P. Laszlo, Citrus: A History (2007); P. Macinnis, Bittersweet: The Story of Sugar (2002); L. Martin, Tea: The Drink That Changed the World (2007); R. Moxham, Tea: Addiction, Exploitation, and Empire (2003); A. Pavord, Uncommon Grounds: The History of Coffee and How It Transformed Our World (1999); R. Phillips, A Short History of Wine (2000); P. Rain, Vanilla: The Cultural History of the World's Favorite Flavor and Fragrance (2004); J. Turner, Spice: The History of a Temptation (2004); J. Warner, Craze: Gin and Debauchery in an Age of Reason (2002); A. Wild, Coffee: A Dark History (2005); S. Yafa, The Potato: How the Humble Spud Rescued the Western World (2006).
12. "Super Size Me" by Martin Spurlock, 2004.
13. M. Pollan, The Omnivore's Dilemma: A Natural History of Four Meals (2006).
14. The humanist, Raymond Tallis, argues that "foodism" emerges as an explicit engagement with and hunger for the hedonistic pleasure encumbered in the consumption of food. R. Tallis, Hunger (2008), 35. J. Johnston and S. Bauman, "Introduction: The World of Foodies," in Johnston and Bauman (eds.), Democracy and Distinction in the Gourmet Foodscape (2010), 3, deploy "foodscape" to describe the "cultural spaces" of "gourmet food." For a critique, see F. Davolio and R. Sassatelli, "Comment on Josée Johnston and Shyon Baumann/1: Foodies Aesthetics and their Reconciliatory View of Food Politics," Sociologica 1/2009, doi: 10.2383/29566. For "critical consumption" see R. Sassatelli, "Virtue, Responsibility and Consumer Choice. Framing Critical Consumerism," in J. Brewer and F. Trentmann (eds.), Consuming Cultures, Global Perspectives (2006), 219-250.
15. For a critique of local, see J. Pratt, "Food Values: The Local and the Authentic," Critique of Anthropology 27 (2007): 285-300. Also, R. Sassatelli, "The Political Morality of Food: Discourses, contestation and alternative consumption," in M. Harvey, A. McMeeckin, and A. Warde (eds.), Qualities of Food: Alternative Theoretical and Empirical Approaches (2004), 176-91.
16. W. H. Newell, "A theory of interdisciplinary studies." Issues in Integrative Studies 19 (2001): 1-25; J. Moran, Interdisciplinarity (2002); T. Augsburg, Becoming Interdisciplinary: An Introduction to Interdisciplinary Studies (2005).
17. S. W. Mintz, Tasting Food, Tasting Freedom: Excursions into Eating, Culture, and the Past (1996).
18. http://www.starbucks.com/responsibility/learn-more/goals-and-progress/coffee-purchasing [accessed July 20, 2011].
19. S. W. Mintz, "The So-Called World-System: Local Initiative and Local Response," Dialectical Anthropology 2.2 (1977): 253-270.

20. http://en.wikipedia.org/wiki/Local_food [accessed August 5, 2010].
21. G. Ritzer, The McDonaldization of Society (1993).
22. See http://michaelpollan.com/books/the-omnivores-dilemma/ [accessed July 20, 2011]. For a conservative critique, see B. Hurst, "The Omnivore's Delusion: Against the Agri-intellectuals," (July, 2009 edition of The American, the journal of the conservative think tank American Enterprise Institute).
23. J. Carney & R. N. Rossomoff, In the Shadow of Slavery: Africa's Botanical Legacy in the Atlantic World (2010).
24. Counihan and Van Esterik, "Introduction," 2.
25. 13. K. J. Cwierta, "From Ethnic to Hip: Circuits of Japanese Cuisine in Europe." Food and Foodways 13 (2005): 241-272; K. Elwert-Kretschmer, "Culinary Innovation, Love, and the Social Organization of Learning in a West African City," Food and Foodways 9 (2001): 205-233; B. M. Forrest and A. L. Najjaj, "Is Sipping Sin Breaking Fast? The Catholic Chocolate Controversy and the Changing World of Early Modern Spain." Food and Foodways 15 (2007): 31-52; R. Launay, "Tasting the World: Food in Early European Travel Narratives." Food and Foodways 11 (2003): 27-47; E. Searles, "Food and the Making of Modern Inuit Identities." Food and Foodways 10 (2002): 55-78; A. Suranyi, "Seventeenth-Century English Travel Literature and the Significance of Foreign Foodways." Food and Foodways 14 (2006): 123-149.

Milk for "Growth": Global and Local Meanings of Milk Consumption in China, India, and the United States

ANDREA S. WILEY

Department of Anthropology, Indiana University, Bloomington, Indiana, USA

Whereas milk production and consumption and the genes that allow for milk digestion throughout life are strongly variable across populations, historically only a minority of human groups valued milk as an important component of local foodways. By the early 21st century, however, milk consumption has become globally normative, and a spectacular rise in intake has been documented in countries such as China and India. Meanwhile, in the United States, consumption has declined markedly, especially among children. In this article, I argue that milk has been able to succeed in India and China by being positioned as a food with special qualities that enhance physical growth, which in turn serves as a powerful metaphor for individual and national power and wealth. Simultaneously, milk is being repackaged as a salve for the problems of modernity in the United States. Milk's unique history in each country provides an interpretive framework within which these meanings emerge, and milk's current success in local foodways depends on traditional modes of processing.

The late anthropologist Marvin Harris once divided up human societies into the "lactophiles" and "lactophobes" (Harris 1985), arguing that the fondness or disdain of mammalian milk was a profound delineator of cultural difference. The lactophiles were definitely in the minority, localized to areas populated by peoples of northern European descent, pastoralists of east and west Africa, and some middle Eastern and central Asian populations, all with long histories of dairying. The centrality of milk to their foodways was evident in milk's economic and cultural valuation as well as high frequencies of the genetic alteration that allows for digestion of the milk sugar lactose throughout life (i.e., *lactase persistence*; Durham 1991). However, over the past decades, global patterns of milk production and consumption have shifted markedly, and this essentialized differentiation between lactophobic and lactophilic foodways has become an inadequate descriptor of contemporary dietary practices. Global trade in dairy products is at an all time high, as is the overall volume of milk production and consumption, a trend especially evident in East, South, and Southeast Asia and to a lesser extent in Latin America.

With a rise in per capita incomes, many developing countries are said to be on the cusp of a "livestock revolution," manifesting as increased demand for milk and other animal-source foods (C. L. Delgado 2003). A 2007 *New York Times* article noted that in countries with emerging economies: "It turns out that, along with zippy cars and flat-panel TVs, milk is the mark of new money, a significant source of protein that factors into much of any affluent person's diet" (Arnold 2007). The question arises as to why people in such countries have embraced *milk* as a key symbol of their economic success. How does this particular commodity, now described as "wholesome" or "old-fashioned" by the U.S. dairy industry, become symbolically aligned with these high-tech trappings of modernity? Despite these nostalgic descriptors, widespread consumption of fresh milk in the United States (as well as in Europe) was, in fact, closely tied to modernizing processes that are now playing out across the globe (Atkins and Bowler 2001; DuPuis 2002).

Milk seems to be a surprising food to attain a strong presence in the global marketplace, especially in its fluid form. Milk's historically local roots are in part a function of its short shelf-life, which can only be extended by mechanized pasteurization. It is also bulky and heavy and hence expensive to transport, and currently only about 7% of total fluid milk production is traded internationally (Knips 2005). Furthermore, unlike other drinks such as Coca-Cola, which have been aggressively marketed across the globe, milk has no single brand or logo to support its marketing. While there may be recognition of multinational corporate names such as Nestlé, most fluid milk is consumed from local processors with indigenous brands.

India and China are good examples of the global ascendance of milk drinking, and given their size and growing affluence, they have attracted the attention of the international dairy industry. A comparison of contemporary practices surrounding milk in these two countries and the United States, each of which has a quite distinct history with milk, provides insights into the malleability of milk's local meanings and how these intersect with globalizing processes that attempt to impose uniformity on views of milk. I argue that milk has been able to achieve its status in India and China and maintain relevance in the United States by being positioned as a "special" food with properties that enable its consumers to achieve a variety of social and personal goals. The "specialness" of milk can be attributed to its "natural" qualities as a mammalian food but also the technological manipulations that transform it into a commercial commodity. As Peter Atkins writes in his recent book on milk's materiality, "food quality, more broadly, even when defined in physical or organoleptic terms, has taken many forms and . . . is best understood as part of a dynamic social process that was strongly influenced by the properties of the material" (Atkins 2010: xx).

One claim for milk's uniqueness as a food is that it enhances physical growth, with the latter marking not only the physical size of a country's citizenry, but also national and individual strength and power. In India and China (and the late nineteenth-century United States, when milk consumption likewise surged), where child growth may be stunted from undernutrition and infectious disease, evidence of enhanced physical growth provides confirmation of economic and social development and a thriving family. The fact that politically and economically powerful nations tend to have the highest levels of milk consumption and the tallest citizens creates a package of meanings that allows milk consumption to be an essential "mark of new money" in countries such as India and China. Ironically, fluid milk consumption has been sliding in countries such as the United States since the 1940s, and while the milk–growth linkage has continued salience there, it may not be sufficient to sell milk to an aging population, and concerns about "excess growth," rising rates of obesity, and chronic disease have required a reworking of the milk message to address these "diseases of modernity" (Cordain et al. 2005).

But in both India and China, milk had indigenous meanings that would seem to pose additional challenges to widespread adoption of milk as a marker of modernity. In China, milk was long reviled as a food of the "barbarian" Mongols, and ethnographers have commented on the absence of milch animals and widespread abhorrence of milk and its products there. In addition, most Chinese are *lactase impersistent*: they do not produce the enzyme lactase, which breaks down the milk sugar lactose in the small intestine, in adulthood. Lactase impersistence is an underlying cause of lactose intolerance, a cluster of uncomfortable gastrointestinal symptoms that may occur after consuming milk. India has low rates of lactase impersistence in the north and west, but notably higher rates in the south and east (Tandon et al. 1981). In various forms, milk has long been an integral part of local foodways, and there are strong political, economic, and cultural supports for milk and cows. Thus milk consumption would seem to be an odd part of a package that included sophisticated technological consumer durables.

Against these historical backdrops, milk consumption has skyrocketed in both countries. China's citizens now consume an average of 12 liters per year (up 1700 percent since 1970), while in India, per capita consumption has increased to 39 liters per year, a 240 percent increase from 1970 (see Table 1). Both are still modest in comparison to the 95 liters per year drunk in the United States and suggest the tremendous potential growth of the market for milk in the largest of the world's countries. Milk production

TABLE 1 Annual per capita consumption of fluid milk, 1970 and 2008 (liters)

	1970	2008	Change (ltrs)	% change
India	16.4	39.3	22.9	240%
China	0.7	11.9	11.2	1700%
U.S.	125.1	95.2	−29.9	76%

Source: United States Department of Agriculture, 2008.

is also a rapidly growing part of their agricultural economies. India now produces over twenty percent more milk than the United States, and China's production, which was negligible until 2000, has quintupled such that it is now around forty percent of U.S. levels and exceeds the output of Australia and New Zealand combined (United States Department of Agriculture 2008).

Meanwhile, in the United States, where milk was an icon of modernity in the early twentieth century (DuPuis 2002), "America's drink" struggles to maintain a place in contemporary diets despite a strong dairy industry, governmental support for milk, and overall low (but variable) rates of lactase impersistence. U.S. per capita intake of fluid milk has been declining steadily since it peaked in the 1940s and is about 76% of what it was in 1970 (see Table 1) and much lower than it was at the beginning of the twentieth century.

In subsequent sections, I outline the ways that milk has been promoted in India, China, and the United States, tracing the local meanings of milk and how these have been transformed during the recent escalation (in India and China) and decline (in the U.S.) of consumption. I focus on how milk's link to growth is elaborated in each country and the significance attached to child growth particularly in height, touching on the evidence that may support such claims. Next, I describe the ways that milk must be technologically transformed to achieve its "modern" status and how it is positioned in relation to modernity in the three countries. Last, I consider how the spread of milk consumption articulates with high rates of lactase impersistence, and how traditional modes of food processing may be deployed to help establish or maintain dairy products in local diets. Evidence suggests that fluid milk's ascendance may be historically delimited in all three countries, as these modes are invoked to maintain dairy intake.

PROMOTING MILK THROUGH GROWTH

The historical record documents milk's longstanding valuation in Europe (and subsequently areas fully colonized by Europeans) and India (albeit with relatively low levels of production and consumption) and its notable absence in China (Mendelson 2008), yet by the early twenty-first century, milk consumption—especially among children—has become globally normative (Wiley 2011). This has been achieved through promotional efforts by the dairy industry, governments, and health officials, dieticians, and nutritionists. Government, NGO, and corporate-subsidized school milk feeding programs have existed since the 1920s in the United States; China established one in 1999 (Chen 2003b), and long-standing school milk initiatives have continually expanded in India. Providing school milk serves the twin goals of enhancing students' educational success and establishing a market for local and multinational dairy companies. Milk's privileged position in such programs is justified by its presence in governmental dietary advice. The Dietary Guidelines for Americans and the pictorial version, the food pyramid, highlight the essential role for milk in the diet, recommending three cups of milk or equivalent dairy products per day (United States Department of Health and Human Services and United States Department of Agriculture 2005). Milk is now listed in China's food guide pagoda with the instructions "Eat milk and legumes and their products every day" (Ge, Jia, and Liu 2007) and is recommended in the Dietary Guidelines for Indians (National Institute of Nutrition 2006).

The health benefits of milk and dairy products are most often attributed to their high calcium and protein content. Although there are many plant and animal foods that provide protein, bovine milk is the richest source of calcium on a per serving basis, and milk seems to "own" this mineral. The Dietary Guidelines for Indians state: "Milk that provides good-quality proteins and calcium must be an essential item of the diet, particularly for infants, children, and women" (National Institute of Nutrition 2006). Milk's inclusion in China's food pagoda is justified as "products made with milk provide protein, vitamins, and minerals, especially calcium." The U.S. Dietary Guidelines likewise feature calcium as the justification for milk's strong presence there (United States Department of Health and Human Services and United States Department of Agriculture 2005). The association of calcium with milk appears in U.S. advertisements as early as the 1930s, but these became more explicit starting in the 1960s, emphasizing milk's ability to promote growth in height and "strong bones" because of its calcium.

The homogeneity of these messages reflects the global spread of scientific "nutritionism," the privileging of nutrients as descriptors and markers of food value (Pollan 2008). The connection between milk consumption and child growth, usually considered to be mediated by milk's calcium and/or protein, is a related message that appears to have global currency. Milk "makes sense" as a food that would promote growth. After all, mammalian mothers produce milk to support the growth and development of their infants, and cow's milk has its commercial roots as a breast milk substitute (DuPuis 2002). That milk (albeit from another species) might likewise promote growth among older children seems intuitive. It is worth noting that embedded in the milk–child growth connection are two distinct, though often conflated, concepts: growth in size (height) and strength ("strong bones"). These are different aspects of bone biology, but both can serve as powerful symbols for individual and national stature. In each country, the meanings attached to child growth—and how milk might contribute to it—reflect local histories and contemporary goals for personal and national well-being.

UNITED STATES

Articulation of the association of milk consumption with child growth was established by the early twentieth century in the United States in tandem with the emergence of a commercial dairy industry with strong ties to the U.S. Department of Agriculture (USDA). Cow's milk production dates back to the colonial period when it was introduced by European settlers, but remained a small-scale domestic enterprise until the mid-nineteenth century when large-scale production and distribution were initiated to serve growing urban populations (DuPuis 2002). Fresh milk as not widely consumed prior to the mid-nineteenth century, as milk was transformed into products that were less vulnerable to spoilage (e.g., cheese or fermented buttermilk; Mendelson 2008). Milk from nineteenth-century urban dairies was often contaminated due to the unhygienic and overall poor conditions in which the cows in peri-urban dairies were kept and spoilage during distribution, making it difficult to advertise as especially salubrious for children. However, with pasteurization and refrigerated transport, milk consumption became more widespread, and promoted as a particularly good food for children (Crumbine and Tobey 1929; DuPuis 2002).

A special relationship between milk and child growth was seized on by the U.S. National Dairy Council (NDC) when it was established in 1916, and with support from the USDA, the NDC began to advance milk as the ideal health- and growth-promoting food for children (DuPuis 2002). This message resonated well with an emergent middle-class public that had become preoccupied with the physical growth and feeding of children (Levenstein 1988) and was supported by experimental studies done by Elmer V. McCollum (the "father" of nutrition) and others in the early twentieth century demonstrating that rats and mice supplemented with milk grew at faster rates and to larger sizes than those fed different foods (Becker 1983 and McCollum 1957 provide historical reviews of this research). A widely cited set of studies in Great Britain in the 1920s (Leighton and Clark 1929; Orr 1928) demonstrated a similar effect in school children. These studies led many scientists to interpret the rise in milk consumption as a cause of increases in height over the twentieth century in the United States and Europe. For example, Stuart Patton, a well-known physiologist of mammalian lactation, writes: "While many factors have contributed to this increase [in height] it is obvious that calcium in the diet would be essential, and that products of the expanding American dairy industry would be the logical source of the calcium enabling this growth" (Patton 2004: 115).

Milk advertisements up through the late twentieth century generally featured European-American robust children, highlighted milk's contributions to their height or strength, and had a mix of individual and public health messages about the benefits of milk. For example, a 1947 advertisement sponsored by the National Dairy Products Association featured two generations of female basketball players, announcing:

> There've been some changes, all right, in the past generation . . . For one thing—Betsy Co-ed's grown a good bit *taller* since mother played center on the team! . . . This doesn't mean we're raising a race of Amazons . . . But it does mean younger folk have better *foods* to "grow on" than their parents ever did . . . Many of them are developments of National Dairy Laboratories . . . that milk, nature's most nearly perfect food, offers virtually all the raw materials of modern nutritional research . . . (*Journal of the American Dietetic Association* 1947)

One particularly explicit recent advertisement states, "Got Milk? Get Tall" (Milk Processor Education Program, n.d.-b). In another, Carson Daly pronounces, "Hey, everybody! Want to grow? About 15% of your height is added during your teen years and milk can help make the most of it" (Milk Processor Education Program, n.d.-a).

These recent promotions have existed amidst a downward trend in per capita milk intake over the second half of the century. This has occurred across all age groups, but has been especially precipitous among children (Enns, Goldman, and Cook 1997; Enns, Mickle, and Goldman 2002, 2003). In part, this trend is related to an unprecedented rise in bottled soft drinks, juices, and waters, which have made significant inroads into the beverage market such that U.S. adults now drink almost eight times more soda or fruit drinks than milk (Popkin et al. 2006). But the "drink milk and grow" message may not play as well as it did in the early and mid-twentieth century. Concerns about child obesity and "excess growth" are widely expressed by public health officials, clinicians, and parents.

Milk promotions met this new challenge with a new strategy designed to address these concerns about the U.S. population's physical condition. In 2004, Dr. Phil (McGraw) announced that "drinking milk can help you lose weight." and slogans such as "Milk your diet; lose weight! Including 24 ounces of lowfat or fat-free milk every 24 hours in a reduced-calorie diet provides calcium and protein to support healthy weight loss" were suddenly in wide circulation. This new portrayal of milk seemed poised to reinvigorate milk sales among perennially dieting but ever-fatter Americans. The promotion was pulled in 2007 when the FTC cited a lack of scientific support for the claim that milk consumption contributed to weight loss, but while the explicit statements about milk and weight loss are gone, among the current Got Milk? celebrities are winners of "The Biggest Loser" weight loss competition show.

CHINA

The Chinese government has made increasing milk production and consumption a national priority. Chinese Premier Wen Jiabao was quoted in 2006 as saying, "I have a dream to provide every Chinese, especially children, sufficient milk each day" (British Broadcasting Corporation 2007). Rhetoric in support of the domestic milk industry emphasizes its benefits to population health. As Jun Jing notes, "The Chinese government has tried to educate the public to heed the officially identified need to improve the country's 'population quality' *(renkou sushi)*" (Jing 2000: 12). Education about proper child nutrition and promotion of milk—using motifs drawn from U.S. nutrition discourse—is part of this effort, and encouraging milk consumption among children is a core component.

Marketing includes the use of patriotic slogans such as "One cup of milk can strengthen a nation" (Chen 2003a) and famous athletes such as Tian Liang, the Chinese Olympian diver, Liu Xiang, the Olympian hurdler, and triumphant Chinese astronauts fresh from their first successful spacewalk in 2008. China's most internationally visible athlete, seven-foot, five-inch tall National Basketball Association (NBA) player Yao Ming was featured as the Western Conference "Got Milk? Rookie of the Month" in 2001 wearing a milk mustache. In January 2007, China's Mengnui Dairy took this linkage one step further by entering into a partnership with the NBA, and acquiring the rights to promote their products in association with the NBA's activities in China and other countries. What sport to better illustrate the milk–height relationship than basketball?

The use of successful, internationally known, and powerful Chinese icons in advertisements highlights milk's relationship to strength and size and serves contemporary nationalist, family, and individual goals. It also addresses local concerns about Chinese "size deficits" perceived as problematic in light of the country's economic successes. Various Chinese officials articulate the view that the Chinese can "catch up" in size to Western populations by drinking more milk. The vice director of the Ministry of Agriculture only half-jokingly attributes China's soccer players' lack of international success to the fact that "they don't drink enough milk" (Chen 2003b). Based on her work on changing diets in China, Susan Brownell observed, "Dairy products are not a typical part of the Chinese diet. The emphasis on them for athletes is a result of an awareness that they form a large part of the Western diet, the assumption being that they explain the greater size and musculature of Western athletes" (Brownell 2005:254). A spokeswoman for Shanghai Bright Dairy and Food Company contends that consuming more milk will lead to more rapid physical growth among China's citizens and help make its men taller.

Such a claim may have its foundation in increases in height experienced by the Japanese in the post-World War II period, when average height rose markedly. In his analysis of the cause of this surge, Eiji Takahashi claimed that the addition of milk to the diet would have been "the most effective food for stimulating growth in height. . . . The short stature of Japanese in the past may be mainly caused by this low-calcium diet" (Takahashi 1966: 125). Hopes for an increase in physical growth among a new generation of Chinese children who drink milk was bolstered by a recent study demonstrating the positive effects of a school milk intervention on growth in height among Chinese girls ages 10–12 years with low baseline dairy and calcium intakes (Du et al. 2004). The girls, who were given 330 ml calcium-fortified milk five days each week for over two years, grew significantly more (0.7 cm) than a matched group given no supplementary food. Unfortunately, there was no control group that received a caloric supplement equivalent to that of the milk, and the milk was fortified with calcium, so it is impossible to conclude that milk has special effects on growth in height. Whether milk (as opposed to other dietary changes) will contribute to the growth of Chinese children remains to be seen.

It is ironic that milk has come to serve pronationalist goals in China. Cow's milk historically played a limited role in the Chinese diet. Most Chinese did not encounter milk after weaning, and the mutation conferring continued production of lactase, the enzyme that digests lactose, the sugar in milk, had no opportunity to spread (Huang 2002). The absence of milking traditions appears to have co-occurred with an aversion to milk. Robert Lowie marveled at the "astonishing fact that eastern Asiatics, such as the Chinese, Japanese, Koreans, and Indo-Chinese have an inveterate aversion to the use of milk" (Harris 1985: 130). Milking was practiced by nomadic peoples in the north and west but after the Mongol dynasty ended in the fourteenth century, use of milk products dwindled (Huang 2002). Eugene Anderson suggests that this outcome was part of a nationalist agenda of the Ming to denigrate foods associated with the foreign "barbarian" Mongols (Anderson 1987).

With China's rapid ascendance in the global economy, milk has become the means by which it effectively competes with historically powerful populations who happened to have dairying histories. The Chinese have responded to government and dairy industry initiatives, and China is now said to have a "thirst for dairy" (Baumes 2004). As noted in a recent article in *China Today*, "It is estimated that only 300 million of the 1.3 billion people in China regularly drink milk, leaving a vast virgin market to be explored by dairy companies" (Lu 2009). The market for milk is focused in urban areas, where intake is more than thirteen times greater than in rural areas (Baumes 2004; Lu 2009) and more common among higher-income groups (Fuller, Huang, Ma, and Rozelle 2006). A survey of dairy purchases in households in three large Chinese cities found that over 90 percent purchased fluid milk, with an average purchase of just over one liter of fluid milk per week (Fuller, Beghin, Hu, and Rozelle 2004). Dairy product sales in China have been growing at the rate of 25 percent per year, and the dairy industry is worth close to one billion U.S. dollars (Dairy Industries International 2006). At present, the dairy industry represents about 10 percent of the Chinese agricultural economy (Fuller et al. 2004), which is comparable to the United States, where it accounts for about 11 percent (United States Department of Commerce 2002).

INDIA

Much like in China, Indian milk promotions reference height and growth and blend these with nationalist goals. For example, a series of ads for the widely distributed "Mother Dairy" brand milk are quite explicit, featuring children in oversized professional clothes, a bottle of milk, and the bold slogan: "The country needs you. Grow Faster."

The association between milk and body size has long had political implications in India, which are best understood in relation to the long history of milking both local zebu cattle (*Bos indicus*) and water buffalo (*Bubalus bubalis*). Cows were central to the subsistence and culture of the Indo-Aryan pastoralists who settled in the north of the South Asian subcontinent, and Vedic literature describes the high esteem in which they were held (Batra 1986). They were symbolically linked to the earth and mothers, both with life-giving properties (Korom 2000). The sacredness of cows, laws protecting them, and religious rituals involving milk or *ghee* (clarified butter) all came to be core tenets of Hinduism. Hindu scriptures identify the cow as the mother of all civilization, its milk nurturing the population; as such, the cow became a potent symbol of "Mother India."

According to William Gould, in the politics of late colonial India "the concept of 'mother cow' could be twinned with the often used depictions of 'Mother India' and the life-giving, pure qualities of cow's milk could be associated in the minds of audiences with the purity and strength of the nation. . ." (Gould 2004: 78). The cow and its protection became important metaphors for the colonized state and the strength of its citizens, especially its men. As Charu Gupta notes, "The cow was now [in the 1920s] more directly linked with building a strong nation, a nation of Hindu men who had grown weak and poor from lack of milk and ghee. For a body of healthy sons, cows became essential . . . Like a mother, she could feed her sons with milk, making them stronger" (Gupta 2001: 4296). The need for protection and improvement of cows to produce milk would correct "the poor physique of many of the population . . ." (Home Poll 1922, quoted in Gupta 2001). Thus links between cow's milk, national strength, and physical growth were articulated as India moved toward nation-statehood, and these remain potent metaphors in the present as India emerges as a major global economic power. Despite the economic importance of water buffalo, its milk never achieved similar recognition (Hoffpauir 1982; Mahias 1988).

A connection between milk and size is explicit in India, but rhetoric about "catching up in size" does not prevail in milk rhetoric, despite average height in India being substantially shorter than either China or the United States (average heights for men and women are ~155 cm and ~152 cm, respectively, in India (Deaton 2008), compared to 166–170 cm for men and 157–159 cm for women in China (Yang et al. 2005), and 177 cm for men and 162 cm for women in the United States (McDowell, Fryar, Ogden, and Flegal 2008). Milk is not a novel food in the Indian diet and has long been valued as a food central to Indian dietary tradition, and thus claims that milk is responsible for greater height in European populations are unlikely to be compelling. That said, greater height is a highly desirable trait for males and females, particularly among the upwardly mobile middle class. A brief survey of recent marriage ads from Pune, India revealed that virtually all—whether it was grooms seeking brides or vice versa—referenced the individual's height, and when the desired height of the partner was indicated, it was always for "tall" regardless of sex. Height is a measure of the success of individuals and their families, and especially reflects on the quality of a mother's care (R. Parameswaran, personal communication).

In addition to growth in height, strength—both physical and mental—is a common theme in Indian milk promotions. Even the ubiquitous "milk biscuits," which contain little milk, are said to be strengthening. For example, Milk Shakti (*shakti* means power) biscuits are advertised by M.S. Dhoni, the famous Indian cricket player: "From boy-next-door to Super Boy—no, that's not the plot for the next Hollywood blockbuster, it's the effect of Milk Shakti" (www.parleproducts.com/brands/biscuits_milkshakti.asp).

On the other hand, lack of access to milk due to price or availability provides a justification for the dairy industry's expansion, and if the growth and strength of its citizens is enhanced as a result, it will be further evidence of India's political and economic ascendancy in the post-colonial period. Increasing milk production has been a fundamental goal for Indian agriculture. In 1970, the National Dairy Development Board (NDDB) initiated Operation Flood, which aimed to generate a "flood" of milk to supply Indian citizens and increase rural incomes by allowing small-scale producers to get a fair price for their milk by joining cooperatives. Import restrictions on dairy products were lifted in the 1990s, and there was increased private and multinational investment in the dairy industry. At present, dairy makes up about 17% of the Indian agricultural economy (C. F. Delgado and Narrod 2002). Milk consumption has been increasing in concert with a rise in incomes and purchasing power particularly among a growing urban middle class populace (Ali 2007). As in China, national data indicate that milk consumption is about 20% greater in urban than in rural areas and positively associated with socioeconomic status (Shetty 2002; Vijayapushpam, Menon, Rao, and Antony 2003).

With regard to the widespread assertion that milk "makes children grow," it is worth noting that the scientific literature does not provide strong support for this view. A review of studies published in the last 30 years indicates no clear effect of milk on growth in height among school children (Wiley 2005), and studies supplementing children with calcium have found that calcium has no effect on height (Dibba et al. 2000). A well-controlled supplementation study in Kenya found that even when children are undernourished to begin with, milk does not seem to have effects on height that are distinguishable from other foods (Grillenberger et al. 2003). In other words, it may simply be the addition of calories to the diet—rather than special components of milk—that enhances growth. On the other hand, there is a body of work that has correlated milk consumption with height in contemporary European and American children (cf. Berkey, Colditz, Rockett, Frazier, and Willett 2009; Hoppe et al. 2004; Wiley 2005, 2009). Thus, while promotions attributing greater height to milk appear to resonate well with, and "make sense" to consumers, the current scientific literature does not provide unambiguous support for these statements.

MARKETING MILK AS MODERNITY

Beyond its linkages with growth, whether real or imagined, milk has other associations with modernity. The tricky aspect of milk promotion is how to maintain its "natural" superiority as a food, which requires at least some recognition of it as a bovine secretion, while marketing it as part and parcel of citizenship in a highly technological twenty-first century. Here is where the three countries diverge somewhat in their views of milk. In China, milk can take on unabashedly positive Western associations, given the relative novelty of milk in the Chinese diet. But in India and the United States, the status of milk as a traditional food with deep local roots requires some ingenuity to imbue it with new positive meanings.

Increased milk consumption has occurred amid economic expansion and urbanization, with urbanites the primary market for milk products, rather than in the bucolic, farm-based subsistence system so often used as a marketing image in all three countries. In fact, despite milk's close affiliation with nature, it requires technological transformations to succeed as a commodity for a mass market and these serve as important means by which milk can serve the diverse desires of the urban middle class. Milk is highly perishable and vulnerable to spoilage by bacteria. The late nineteenth century solution was, and remains pasteurization, which enabled broader circulation. But even pasteurized milk requires refrigeration, and efficient means of transportation and home refrigeration are needed to support wider distribution. Ultra-high temperature (UHT) milk was the ultimate solution to this problem, as it allows milk to be stored almost indefinitely and transported without refrigeration. This type of milk never became popular in the United States, but it is common in India and China, where the "cold chain" is not commonly available. Widespread concerns about its safety remain in both India and China, where milk adulteration scandals gain wide publicity. "Scientific" and technological transformations of milk are welcomed by a public concerned about milk's safety (and the safety of the nation and its economic progress), just as they were in the early twentieth century United States (DuPuis 2002).[1]

Milk's transformations do not end with sterilization. The cream separator, which came into use in 1871, allowed for an efficient separation of the fat from the rest of fluid milk and enabled the production of skim milk and other fat-reduced forms, allowing milk to fit into a "healthful" lowfat diet. But removal of fat results in removal of vitamin A, so fat-reduced forms must be refortified. Dairies begun adding vitamin D to milk in the 1920s, when rickets, a bone disorder caused by a vitamin D deficiency, was widespread. Homogenization causes the fat molecules to break up and become more evenly distributed in fluid milk, creating a more uniform appearance and richer taste, and renders milk more convenient to drink right out of the carton ("without the inconvenient cream layer," as one Indian milk promotion asserts). Milk can be flavored to make it more palatable, especially to children, or fortified with other vitamins or minerals. For those who are lactase-impersistent, lactose-reduced milk became available in the 1980s in the United States, although, somewhat surprisingly, I have seen no Indian or Chinese promotions of such milk. In sum, the milk found in global supermarkets can hardly be considered a "natural" food and is desired precisely for both its intrinsic "natural" qualities and its subjection to the technologies of modern science. Such transformations change over time as well and are used to "fit" milk to whatever health problems or target demographic is seen as most salient or lucrative at a given time (Atkins and Bowler 2001).

In China, milk's associations with modernity, economic progress, wealth, and Western culture are transparent and interpreted in a positive light. In her study of children's diets in the Xi'an Muslim district, Maris Gillette remarks that

> butter and milk in particular were regarded as typical of Western food. Even in snacks produced locally, the presence of dairy ingredients lent them an aura of foreign-ness and luxury. For *Hui* in their thirties and older, dairy products symbolized a high standard of living. Mingxin remembered craving milk as a child, when little was available and his family was too poor to buy it . . . [since] 1978, China's cows have been "science modernized" *(kexue xiandaihua)* and so dairy products were both readily available and affordable. (Gillette 2005: 111)

Indeed, it is the "Western" aspects of milk that are most salient to increasing demand for milk in China. As Gillette notes with regard to Western factory-produced foods, "through these foods parents hoped to introduce their children to things foreign and equip them to live in an industrialized, technologically advanced, cosmopolitan world" (Gillette 2005: 117). That milk might enhance their growth (both physical and intellectual) further consolidates milk's image as a "modern" food and its consumption the means to the modern/Western life.

Milk's equivalence to modernity or Western lifestyles is more ambiguous in India in part due to longstanding cultural valuation of cows and milk. Milk has a variety of traditional symbols that could be used for its promotion, especially the cow. However, most milk in India derives from water buffalo, and, unless otherwise specified, all commercially available milk can be assumed to be a blend from both animals. This is not widely broadcast; instead happy cows predominate in milk advertisements, although it is important to note that they are not the indigenous beloved zebu cattle that serve as potent national symbols, but rather foreign breeds such as the distinctive black-and-white Holstein. This image alone suggests that milk's historical local meanings in India are not being harnessed to sell milk: Western cows with their greater size and productivity are preferred, with perhaps the sense that these qualities are imparted to the consumers of such milk.

Many commercial dairies offer a separate cow's milk, but without any religious references. Mother Dairy notes only that its cow's milk is "easily digestible," which references Ayurvedic understandings of milk. Meera Premium notes that their cow milk is "processed in [sic] a very hygienic conditions in our production unit and contains calcium. It is supposed to be a good supplement for growing children and is considered very essential in the overall development of the health of growing children." Nandini likewise has a separate cow's milk, marketing it as "the good life" with an image of a Holstein cow. Milk is often advertised as "pure," which serves a double purpose of emphasizing its safety and reference milk's religious significance. However, since "pure" is used for all milk products rather than just cow's milk, it is more likely simply a guarantee against contamination or adulteration.

Still, the brand "Mother Dairy" conjures up both the cow-as-mother and the nationalist "Mother India" motifs. Likewise, Nandini is the name of a wish-granting cow and also means "enjoyment" in Sanskrit. Text at the Nandini brand milk Website merges the modern and traditional:

> Milk is nature's ideal food for infants and growing children in our country, except in rare cases of lactose intolerance. The important place milk occupies in our diet has been recognized since Vedic times, and all modern research has only supported and reinforced this view. In fact, milk is now considered not only desirable but essential from the time the

child is born. . . . till he or she is 12 years of age (http://www.kmfnandini.coop/html/knowyourmilk.htm)

While it might seem surprising that the Indian dairy industry does not make greater use of traditional motifs, the fact that water buffalo milk production predominates due to greater productivity is one obstacle. But second, India has a sizeable Muslim population (~140 million; ~14% of the total population) and strong nationalist Hindu political movements. The dairy industry must be careful not to incite communal antipathy by reference to religious symbols in its marketing. One solution is to divorce milk from its traditional roots and highlight nutritional science perspectives that emphasize milk's nutrients, while playing on some familiar—but not divisive—and/or unifying nationalist themes. By and large, the meanings of milk portrayed in milk promotions are squarely "nutritionist," with myriad references to milk as a rich source of protein and calcium and essential to building strong bones (in addition, India uses a U.S.-like food pyramid for its pictorial dietary guidelines). As such, milk is aligned with Western values and a means to achieve the autonomy associated with economic success

U.S. dairy processors continue to struggle to find an image of milk that speaks to twenty-first century consumers. Like their Indian counterparts, they have chosen to blend the traditional with the modern. But what constitutes "modernity" in the United States is decidedly different from its positive valuation in China and India, with their burgeoning economies and rapidly rising standards of living. Milk promotions in the United States offer milk as a salve for the *problems* of modernity—primarily the chronic diseases that threaten to reverse the gains in life expectancy that had typified the twentieth century (rather than the infectious diseases that once threatened child survival) and a sagging economy conditioned to similar expansion. In addition, children, who serve as symbols of the future, are notably absent from the vast majority of milk advertisements (Wiley 2008). As children make up a smaller percentage of the U.S. population, and with ideas about milk and child growth and strong bones well-entrenched, the dairy industry is focusing its efforts on adults. The aging of the U.S. population and its attendant medical problems is reflected in recent milk promotions, which represent a true inversion of milk's evolutionary role as sustenance for the young. The new "Milk is nature's wellness drink!" promotion provides illustration:

> Milk may be nature's wellness drink that has been around for centuries, but the benefits are far from old-fashioned. It turns out that all milk drinkers have a leg up on other folks. For starters, studies suggest that people who regularly drink milk tend to have healthier diets that are richer in nutrients. They're also more likely to be at a healthy weight. Milk drinkers may also have an edge when it comes to cardiovascular health, including blood pressure. Plus, no other beverage offers the

> same array of bone-building nutrients, including calcium, vitamin D, protein and phosphorus, and has hundreds of studies supporting its link to strong bones. And there's also emerging evidence that the nutrients in milk may play a role in reducing the risk of cardiovascular disease, certain cancers, type 2 diabetes and metabolic syndrome (Milk Processors Education Program 2009).

Middle-aged women (all the milk-mustached celebrities used in association with this ad were adult women) are to believe that milk provides a trusted source of goodness in troubling times. As Wendy Bazilian, a dietician writing for MilkPEP, notes: "When you think about all the ways you pursue wellness, drinking milk each day is one small step in the right direction. It's a simple thing you can do for yourself that can provide a powerful payback. With all the new-age beverages on the market, it's hard to know what's best for your family, especially in these tough economic times. One you can feel good about is milk—it offers more nutrition for your dollar than virtually any other beverage you can buy" (Milk Processors Education Program 2009).

Aside from the fact that "wellness" is sufficiently amorphous to preclude scientific evaluation, the promotion attempts a melding of traditional and contemporary themes. Milk has been around for centuries, unlike those "new-age beverages" (it is notable that this statement is found alongside lithe women doing yoga). Milk is also a panacea in "these tough economic times," providing a "powerful payback" of "more nutrition for your dollar." At the same time, milk consumers will be sure to not suffer from the maladies that stem from the "modern" diet. Thus milk, which served as an icon of modernity and technological advance and accompanied U.S. citizens into twentieth-century affluence, unprecedented size, and longevity is now supposed to alleviate the problems attendant to these (chronic disease and the economic downturn) via its age-old value. But Americans appear to be unconvinced by this repackaging and milk consumption continues its downward trajectory. The early twentieth century proponents of milk for children may have unwittingly created an enduring meaning for milk that can spread across the globe but cannot find a new meaning among its local constituency.

LACTOSE INTOLERANCE AND LOCAL TRANSFORMATIONS OF MILK

Anthropological discussions of cross-cultural variation in milk consumption have largely occurred within the discourse about population genetic variation in adult lactase production (i.e., lactase persistence). Yet milk consumption has surged precisely among those traditionally labeled "lactophobic" and lactase-impersistent populations, suggesting that meanings of milk are fluid and not fixed by the biology of milk digestion. How can this biological variation be squared with this rapid upsurge in milk consumption across the globe, including among lactase-impersistent populations?

It is striking how little reference there is to this issue in the discussion of the global ascendance of milk. Lactose intolerance is sometimes referenced in the context of China's new "thirst for dairy," and stomach complaints are common topics for the customer service at the Shanghai Bright dairy (Chen 2003a). The only reference to it in India was the statement in the Nandini milk ad that lactose intolerance is "rare" and hence of little consequence. In a context in which milk is partly a national symbol, discussion of variation in its tolerance is inconvenient. The same is true in the United States, where rates of lactose intolerance are highest in minority populations, and the dairy industry has been forced to recognize this "problem" and provide solutions to "overcome" it (cf. Wiley 2004).

This challenge is met by deploying local culinary traditions, which may ultimately undermine fluid milk consumption while expanding overall dairy product intake. In India, yogurt (*dahi*), which makes use of bacterial fermentation of lactose, is a widely consumed milk product and is often made in a liquid form (*lassi*) that is now commercially available. In China, the rise in drinkable yogurt intake has been double that of the already spectacular increase in milk intake (Fuller et al. 2006). Yogurt's visual and tactile similarity to soymilk and tofu, both created from the fermentation of soybeans, may facilitate its acceptance. It is worth noting that in Japan and South Korea, fluid milk consumption has been declining since the mid-1990s, when per capita intake peaked at around 35 liters per year, well below that of the United States (Dong 2006; Schluep Campo and Beghin 2006). It may be that in Asia there is a lower ceiling for fluid milk consumption, which is, in part, related to high rates of lactose intolerance.

It is worth pointing out, too, that in the United States, while fluid milk has been declining since World War II, with levels now much lower than the early twentieth century, yogurt and cheese consumption have surged. Americans now eat around over 3.6 kg of yogurt and 15 kg of cheese per year, compared to 0.3 and 4 kg in 1970, respectively (USDA/Economic Research Service 2009). While this trend represents a wide range of phenomena (including Americans' taste for pizza and newfound interest in probiotic bacteria, another "salve" for contemporary health problems), it is possible to view it as a reassertion of earlier modes of processing (Wiley 2011). That is, prior to commercial production and widespread consumption of fluid milk in the United States, most milk was processed into cheese or fermented (Mendelson 2008). While the current scale of this processing and the resulting products are notably different, fluid milk intake has given way in favor of older modes of dairy consumption. Thus, ultimately, milk's success as a component of global diets will necessitate the blending of the local and global, much as other icons of modern food have done (e.g., McDonalds or KFC, cf. selections in Watson and Caldwell 2005).

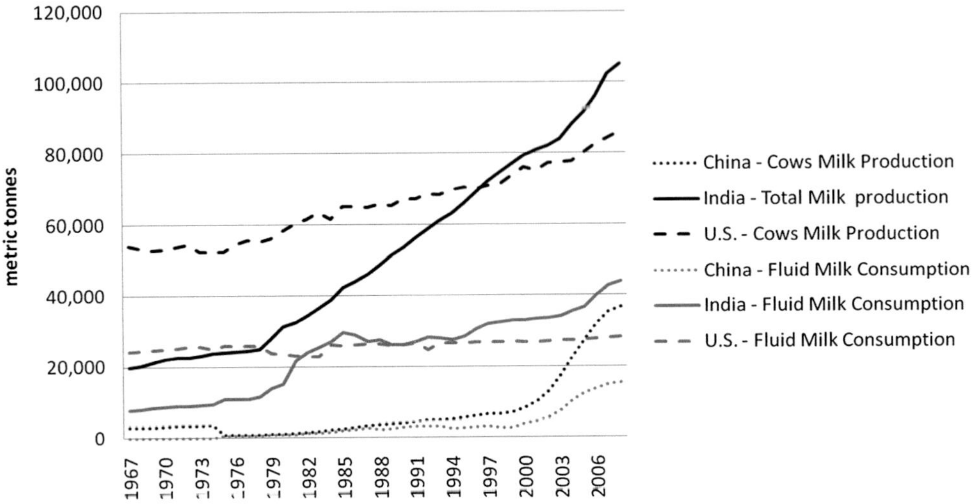

FIGURE 1 China, India, and U.S. trends in milk production and consumption.

CONCLUSION

As milk has become a globalized commodity, produced and consumed in countries that heretofore had not had substantial dairy industries, the "lactophobes" have become the "lactophiles," while consumption among the traditional "lactophiles" continues to slide. In China, milk has become the quintessential modern Western drink, identified with politically and economically strong nations, athletic success, and the means to make up for past "growth deficits." In India, milk has a long history of cultural valuation, yet the current matrix in which milk consumption is rising is not entirely consistent with these ideals. Instead, milk derives from both sacred cows and impure water buffalo, which may preclude the use of local referents in milk promotion. Modern nutritional science overcomes this limitation by positioning the general category of milk as nutrient-rich and hence of benefit to the poor and a science-literate middle class. Meanwhile, in the United States, milk retains the status of a more traditional drink, and beliefs about its contribution to child growth remain but are not sufficient to sell more milk. Current efforts represent attempts to update milk's image as a "wellness" drink suitable for health-conscious and aging adults, especially women, but milk's longstanding association with child growth (as opposed to weight loss or solutions to the health problems of the aged) is proving resistant to change.

Milk's alliance with growth has proven key to the spread of milk consumption around the globe and has overridden historical biases against milk; yet the metaphor of growth has specific local meanings as well and may no longer compel individuals in countries dealing with the consequences of "excess" growth. While India and China are the two largest countries in the world, and growth in relation to population size is resolutely out of fashion in each, enhancement of physical growth (India) or "population quality" (China) provides a viable alternative for the deployment of the growth metaphor by the dairy industry. With larger heights and overall body sizes indicative of individual prosperity and national ascendancy, milk's "natural" connection to growth has provided the mechanism by which milk consumption can meet these goals and provides the rationale for both government promotion of milk and individual dietary choices.

In sum, as it becomes a more globalized commodity, milk is transformed both symbolically to fit local ideologies about both individual and population size and well-being, and physically to fit local biologies, current concerns about them, and existing foodways. Contemporary meanings of milk are locally variable, reflecting unique population subsistence and political histories. While historically positive and negative evaluations of milk mapped onto genetic variation in adult milk digestion, the promise of milk's benefits to one's body and society have proved sufficiently alluring and traditional means of food processing (e.g., fermentation) provide a means to circumvent the gastrointestinal discomfort that may accompany fresh milk consumption.

NOTE

1. Indeed, the 2008 melamine scandal in China, which was but one in a series of scandals involving contaminated milk and milk-based baby formula, caused domestic milk sales to plummet. But the cost of imported milk was prohibitive to many, and consumption of domestic milk is now up to 80% of its previous levels (Huei 2009). Industry analysts have described this as a "speedy recovery is beyond anyone's expectations," but more than anything else it reveals how well-established milk has become as part of the daily diet of many middle-class Chinese citizens.

REFERENCES

Ali, Jabir. 2007. Structural changes in food consumption and nutritional intake from livestock products in India. *South Asia Research*, 27(2), 137–151.

Anderson, E. N. 1987. *The Food of China*. New Haven, CT: Yale University Press.

Arnold, Wayne. 2007. "A Thirst for Milk Bred by New Wealth Sends Prices Soaring." *New York Times*, from http://www.nytimes.com/2007/09/04/business/worldbusiness/04milk.html

Atkins, Peter. 2010. *Liquid Materialities: A History of Milk, Science, and the Law*. Burlington, VT: Ashgate.

Atkins, Peter, & Bowler, Ian. 2001. *Food in Society: Economy, Culture, Geography*. New York: Oxford University Press.

Batra, S. M. 1986. The sacredness of the cow in India. *Social Compass*, 33(2–3), 163–175.

Baumes, Harry. 2004. "China's growing thirst for dairy," from www.globalinsight.com/Perspective/PerspectiveDetail695.htm

Becker, Stanley L. 1983. Will milk make them grow? An episode in the discovery of the vitamins. *American Chemical Society Symposium Series*, 228, 61–83.

Berkey, Catherine S., Colditz, Graham A., Rockett, Helaine R.H., Frazier, A. Lindsay, & Willett, Walter C. 2009. Dairy consumption and female height growth: prospective cohort study. *Cancer Epidemiology, Biomarkers, and Prevention*, 18(6), 1881–1887.

British Broadcasting Corporation. 2007. "China drinks its milk." *BBC News*, August 7, 2007 from http://news.bbc.co.uk/2/hi/uk_news/magazine/6934709.stm

Brownell, Susan. 2005. Food, hunger, and the state. In James L. Watson & Melissa L. Caldwell (Eds.), *The Cultural Politics of Food and Eating* (pp. 251–258). Malden, MA: Blackwell Publishing.

Chen, Kathy. 2003a. "Dairy Firms Churn Out Milk Products in China." Retrieved April 20, 2006 from http://www.tschang.net/articles/20030301.htm

Chen, Kathy. 2003b. "Got Milk? The new craze in China is dairy drinks." Retrieved September 20, 2005 from http://www.mindfully.org/Food/2003/China-Dairy-Drinks28feb03.htm

Cordain, Loren, et al. 2005. Origins and evolution of the Western diet: Health implications for the 21st century. *American Journal of Clinical Nutrition*, 81, 341–354.

Crumbine, Samuel J., & Tobey, James A. 1929. *The Most Nearly Perfect Food: The Story of Milk*. Baltimore: The Williams & Wilkins Company.

Dairy Industries International. 2006. "Chinese dairies made their mark at the IDF World Dairy Summit." Retrieved July 9, 2007 from http://www.dairyindustries.com/story.asp?id=2024211

Deaton, Angus. 2008. Height, health, and inequality: The distribution of adult heights in India. *American Economics Review*, 98(2), 468–474.

Delgado, Christopher F., & Narrod, Clare A. 2002. *Impact of Changing Market Forces and Policies on Structural Change in the Livestock Industries of Selected Fast-Growing Developing Countries Final Research Report of Phase I—Project on Livestock Industrialization, Trade and Social-Health-Environment Impacts in Developing Countries*. Rome: Food and Agricultural Organization.

Delgado, Christopher L. 2003. Rising consumption of meat and milk in developing countries has created a new food revolution. *Journal of Nutrition*, 133, 3907S–3910S.

Dibba, Bakary, Prentice, Ann, Ceesay, Mustapha, Stirling, Dorothy M, Cole, Tim J., & Poskitt, Elizabeth M. E. 2000. Effect of calcium supplementation on bone mineral accretion in Gambian children accustomed to a low-calcium diet. *American Journal of Clinical Nutrition*, 71, 544–549.

Dong, Fengxia. 2006. The outlook for Asian dairy markets: The role of demographics, income, and prices. *Food Policy*, 31, 260–271.

Du, Xueqin, Zhu, Kun, Trube, Angelika, Zhang, Qian, Ma, Guansheng, Hu, Xiaoqi, et al. 2004. School-milk intervention trial enhances growth and bone mineral accretion in Chinese girls aged 10–12 years in Beijing. *British Journal of Nutrition*, 92(1), 159–168.

DuPuis, E. Melanie. 2002. *Nature's Perfect Food: How Milk Became America's Drink*. New York: New York University Press.

Durham, William. 1991. *Coevolution: Genes, Culture and Human Diversity*. Stanford: Stanford University Press.

Enns, Cecilia Wilkinson, Goldman, Joseph D., & Cook, Annetta. 1997. Trends in food and nutrient Intakes by adults: NFCS 1977–1978, CSFII 1989–1991, and CSFII 1994–1995. *Family Economics and Nutrition Review*, 10(4), 16–31.

Enns, Cecilia Wilkinson, Mickle, Sharon J., & Goldman, Joseph D. 2002. Trends in food and nutrient intakes by children in the United States. *Family Economics and Nutrition Review*, 14(2), 56–68.

Enns, Cecilia Wilkinson, Mickle, Sharon J., & Goldman, Joseph D. 2003. Trends in food and nutrient intakes by adolescents in the United States. *Family Economics and Nutrition Review*, 15(2), 15–27.

Fuller, Frank H., Beghin, John C., Hu, Dinghuan, & Rozelle, Scott. 2004. *China's Dairy Market: Consumer Demand Survey and Supply Characteristics*. Ames, IA: Center for Agricultural and Rural Development, Iowa State University.

Fuller, Frank H., Huang, Jikun, Ma, Hengyun, & Rozelle, Scott. 2006. Got milk? The rapid rise of China's dairy sector and its future prospects. *Food Policy*, 31, 201–215.

Ge, K., Jia, J., & Liu, H. 2007. Food-based dietary guidelines in China—Practices and problems. *Annals of Nutrition and Metabolism*, 51(Suppl. 2), 26–31.

Gillette, Maris Boyd. 2005. Children's food and Islamic dietary restrictions in Xi'an. In James L. Watson & Melissa L. Caldwell (Eds.), *The Cultural Politics of Food and Eating* (pp. 106–121). Malden, MA: Blackwell Publishing.

Gould, William. 2004. *Hindu Nationalism and the Language of Politics in Late Colonial India*. New York: Cambridge University Press.

Grillenberger, Monika, Neumann, Charlotte G, Murphy, Suzanne P., Bwibo, Nimrod O., van't Veer, Pieter, Hautvast, Joseph G. A. J., et al. 2003. Food supplements have a positive impact on weight gain and the addition of animal source foods increases lean body mass of Kenyan schoolchildren. *Journal of Nutrition*, 133, 3957S–3964S.

Gupta, Charu. 2001. The icon of mother in late colonial North India: 'Bharat Mata,' 'Matri Bhasha,' and 'Gau Mata.' *Economic and Political Weekly*, 36(45), 4291–4299.

Harris, Marvin. 1985. *Good to Eat: Riddles of Food and Culture*. Prospect Heights, IL: Waveland Press.

Hoffpauir, Robert. 1982. The water buffalo: India's other bovine. *Anthropos*, 77(1–2), 215–238.

Hoppe, Camilla, Udam, Tina Rovenna, Lauritzen, Lotte, Mølgaard, Christian, Juul, Anders, & Michaelsen, Kim Fleischer. 2004. Animal protein intake, serum insulin-like growth factor I, and growth in healthy 2.5-year-old Danish children. *American Journal of Clinical Nutrition*, 80, 447–452.

Huang, H. T. 2002. Hypolactasia and the Chinese diet. *Current Anthropology*, 43(5), 809–819.

Huei, Pei Shing. 2009. "China milk back in favor." *The Straits Times*, January 9, 2009. From http://www.straitstimes.com/Breaking%2BNews/Asia/Story/STIStory_323904.html

Jing, Jun. 2000. Introduction: Food, children, and social change in contemporary China. In Jun Jing (Ed.), *Feeding China's Little Emperors: Food, Children, and Social Change* (pp. 1–26). Stanford, CA: Stanford University Press.

Knips, Vivien. 2005. Developing countries and the global dairy sector Part I: Global overview. Retrieved May 20, 2009 from www.fao.org/ag/AGAInfo/projects/fr/pplpi/docarc/wp30.pdf

Korom, Frank J. 2000. Holy cow! The Apotheosis of Zebu, or Why the cow is sacred in Hinduism. *Asian Folklore Studies*, 59(2), 181–203.

Leighton, Gerald, & Clark, Mabel L. 1929. Milk consumption and the growth of school-children. *Lancet*, 213(5520), 40–43.

Levenstein, Harvey A. 1988. *Revolution at the Table: The Transformation of the American Diet*. New York: Oxford University Press.

Lu, Ethel. 2009. Radical shifts in China's milk market. *China Today*. Retrieved January 14, 2009 from http://www.china.org.cn/business/news/2009–01/14/content_17105973.htm

Mahias, Marie-Claude. 1988. Milk and its transmutations in Indian society. *Food and Foodways*, 2, 265–288.

McCollum, Elmer V. 1957. *A History of Nutrition*. Boston: Houghton Mifflin.

McDowell, Margaret A., Fryar, Cheryl D., Ogden, Cynthia L., & Flegal, Katherine M. 2008. *Anthropometric Reference Data for Children and Adults: United States, 2003–2006*. Hyattsville, MD: National Center for Health Statistics.

Mendelson, Anne. 2008. *Milk: The Surprising Story of Milk through the Ages*. New York: Alfred A. Knopf.

Milk Processor Education Program (n.d.-a). Carson Daly. Retrieved September 20, 2005 from http://whymilk.org/bios/carson_daly.html

Milk Processor Education Program (n.d.-b). "Got Milk? Get Tall!" Retrieved September 20, 2006 from http://www.whymilk.com/facts_gotmilk.htm

Milk Processors Education Program. 2009. "The new face of wellness." Retrieved 1 June 2009, 2009 from http://www.whymilk.com/new_face_of_wellness.php

National Institute of Nutrition. 2006. *Dietary Gudielines for Indians*. Retrieved from http://www.indg.gov.in/health/nutrition/dietary_guidelines_for_indians-en.pdf

Orr, J. B. 1928. Milk consumption and the growth of schoolchildren. *Lancet*, 1, 202–203.

Patton, Stuart. 2004. *Milk: Its Remarkable Contribution to Human Health and Well-Being*. New Brunswick, NJ: Transaction Publishers.

Pollan, Michael. 2008. *In Defense of Food: An Eater's Manifesto*. New York: Penguin.

Popkin, Barry M., Armstrong, Lawrence E, Bray, George M, Caballero, Benjamin, Frei, Balz, & Willett, Walter C. 2006. A new proposed guidance system for beverage consumption in the United States. *American Journal of Clinical Nutrition*, 83(3), 529–542.

Schluep Campo, Isabelle, & Beghin, John C. 2006. Dairy food consumption, supply, and policy in Japan. *Food Policy*, 31, 228–237.

Shetty, Prakash S. 2002. Nutrition transition in India. *Public Health Nutrition*, 5(1A), 175–182.

Takahashi, Eiji. 1966. Growth and environmental factors in Japan. *Human Biology*, 38, 112–130.

Tandon, R. K., Joshi, Y. K., Singh, D. S., Narendranathan, M., Balakrishnan, V., & Lal, K. 1981. Lactose intolerance in North and South Indians. *American Journal of Clinical Nutrition*, 34(5), 943–946.

United States Department of Agriculture. 2008. *Production, Supply, and Distribution Online*. Retrieved May 20, 2009 from http://www.fas.usda.gov/psdonline/psdDownload.aspx

United States Department of Commerce. 2002. *Statistical Abstract of the United States: 2002*. Washington, DC: United States Census.

United States Department of Health and Human Services, & United States Department of Agriculture. 2005. *Dietary Guidelines for Americans*. Retrieved September 10, 2006, from http://www.health.gov/dietaryguidelines/dga2005/document/pdf/DGA2005.pdf

USDA/Economic Research Service. 2009. *ERS Dairy Consumption Trends*. Retrieved February 15, 2010 from http://www.ers.usda.gov/data/foodconsumption/

Vijayapushpam, T., Menon, Krishna Kumari, Rao, D. Raghunatha, & Antony, Grace Maria. 2003. A qualitative assessment of nutrition knowledge levels and dietary intake of schoolchildren in Hyderabad. *Public Health Nutrition*, 6(7), 683–688.

Watson, James L., & Caldwell, Melissa L. (Eds.). 2005. *The Cultural Politics of Food and Eating: A Reader*. Malden, MA: Blackwell Publishing.

Wiley, Andrea S. 2008. *Cow's Milk for "Growth" Across the Lifecycle*. Paper presented at the American Anthropological Association.

Wiley, Andrea S. 2011. *Re-imagining Milk*. New York: Routledge.

Wiley, Andrea S. 2004. "Drink milk for fitness": The cultural politics of human biological variation and milk consumption in the United States. *American Anthropologist*, 106(3), 506–517.

Wiley, Andrea S. 2005. Does milk make children grow? Relationships between milk consumption and height in NHANES 1999–2002. *American Journal of Human Biology*, 17(4), 425–441.

Wiley, Andrea S. 2009. Consumption of milk, but not other dairy products, is associated with height among U.S. preschool children in NHANES 1999–2002. *Annals of Human Biology*, 36(2), 125–138.

Yang, X. G., Li, Y. P., Ma, G. S., Hu, X. Q., Wang, J. Z., Cui, Z. H., et al. 2005. [Study on weight and height of the Chinese people and the differences between 1992 and 2002]. *Zhonghua Liu Xing Bing Xue Za Zhi*, 26(7), 489–493.

Appetites Without Prejudice: U.S. Foreign Restaurants and the Globalization of American Food Between the Wars

AUDREY RUSSEK

Carleton College, American Studies Program, Northfield, Minnesota, USA

The popularity of foreign-themed restaurants grew dramatically in the United States following the Great War. This article analyzes the contradiction between the "Americanization" of food at the same time as native-born Americans enjoyed a growing taste for global cuisines. Distinguishing between foreign and foreign-themed restaurants, this article argues that the latter exposed American palates to a variety of global flavors. In turn, Americans began to conceive of "American food" in more cosmopolitan terms. This article also places material decorations, including the bodies of employees, at the center of its interpretation of the restaurant space and expands the debate over restaurants' use of foreign languages on printed menus to encompass the place of the spoken word. Ultimately, this article argues that the rising popularity of global foodways in the United States not only changed the taste of traditional "American food" but led to a "world citizen" ideal of American national identity.

An American and his Filipino friend walk into a restaurant in the Philippines. The proprietor greets the two men, and then launches into an enthusiastic conversation with the Filipino "in the native dialect" about choices for the meal while the American, "his face wreathed in a huge artificial smile," waits to discover what his friend has ordered. The proprietor disappears to the back, and "within ten seconds there issued from that portion of the house such an odor that the smile literally dropped from the face of the American." In a little time, the chef presents his *pièce de résistance*: an egg that had remained "twelve days under the goose, and six weeks buried in the ground"—"neither an egg nor yet a fowl!" The American, startled and disgusted, roars, "And you expect me to eat that?" Calmly, his Filipino friend replies, "Egg-goose is very sanitary, for the earth has kept it from all the germs which your people fear so much. Funny, Americano, is it not?" After considering the Filipino's point for a while, the American decides, "I guess it all depends on what you are used to, and I suppose there is such a thing as tolerance and narrow-mindedness in the matter of food as in all else. We will put it this way. I am not hungry enough to eat your *balut*, but I grant you that it is a very interesting and, yes, sanitary dish" (Chow 1924: 2–3).

The moral of this tale from 1924, printed in the *Pacific Coast Chef*, one of America's early restaurant trade journals, is that Americans should respect cultural difference, including differences between American and foreign foodstuffs. While the American in the story may not have been "hungry enough to eat" *balut*, throughout the interwar years, Americans' tolerance for foreign flavors blossomed into a preference for the foods, in a large part because of the growth of restaurants representing foreign cultures and cuisines.[1] This essay explains how, from the 1920s through the 1940s, many middle-class, native-born white Americans in urban centers developed a taste for international foods through restaurant dining and took pride in having "appetites that are without prejudice" in contrast to their global counterparts (Brown 1939: 45). Although historians, such as Donna Gabaccia, have argued that "native-born American eaters with little sense of their own ethnic roots. . . . sought out *different* identities by eating new foods [emphasis added]" (Gabaccia 1998: 121), I suggest that these same consumers were simultaneously seeking an affirmation of their *own* American identity through the gastronomic contrast. Dining on foreign foods did not merely expose Americans to global cultures; eating cosmopolitan fare was in essence a nationalist act—it distinguished this population of consumers as *American*.

Advocates of American cosmopolitan dining noted with frequency the reluctance on the part of other foreign nationals and recent immigrants to take part in the crossover culinary experience. "The average American city dweller has a far more cosmopolitan taste when it comes to food than has his counterpart in France and other European nations," argued a journalist for the *New York Times*. "In no other country in the world do people partake of completely foreign meals with the consistency" of Americans in major cities. She continued to explain that while foreign restaurants opened in the United States expecting "to satisfy the demands of their countrymen," by the mid-1930s, native-born Americans constituted the bulk of their clientele (Morgan 1935). The growing popularity of ethnic food occurred, in part, because American restaurant patrons did not conceive of foreign dining establishments in monolithic terms. Instead, they viewed these public dining spaces primarily in one of two ways: *foreign* restaurants and *foreign-themed* restaurants. This difference is not intended merely to split semantic hairs—the two categories help explain how restaurants specializing in reproductions of global cultures and foodways, rather than those serving actual foreign dishes, changed the taste of local American food.

The distinction between foreign and foreign-themed restaurants was not lost on descriptions of public dining places in newspapers, magazines, and industry publications in the years following World War I. Although the terminology might vary, foreign restaurants were usually located in a "foreign colony" of a city and served "native cookery" mostly to a first- or second-generation immigrant clientele from the restaurant's global region (City Eats 1934). The owner of a foreign restaurant almost always claimed a native homeland outside of the United States. White, middle-class Americans tended to regard foreign restaurants as either unappealing, dirty eateries or exotic sites of culinary adventure. On the other hand, foreign-themed restaurants served both foreign dishes and food "commercialized for American consumption" (Houck 1928: K12). They were operated by both foreign-born and native-born Americans; importantly, their goal was to entice a wide variety of customers. One trade journal summarized the criteria for a foreign-themed restaurant in this way: "Foreign-type restaurants feature their national dishes but almost always have a variety of strictly American offerings to meet the demands of those patrons who may like a certain national atmosphere but might not care for the particular type of national cooking" (Study 1944: 29). Foreign-themed restaurants created ambience for effect; they attracted a middle-class American clientele through a dining world of difference.

Paradoxically, in this nativist historical period when a large number of middle-class Anglo Americans advocated "Americanizing" the country, including a reversion back to traditional Early American-style foods, many of these Americans were also priding themselves on their growing preference for foreign foods. While this interest in global cuisine may seem counterintuitive, close examination reveals that by making careful distinctions between foreign and foreign-themed restaurants, native-born and assimilated, naturalized white Americans could measure—qualitatively—first- and second-generation immigrants against cultural standards of citizenship. By rating the extent to which foreign restaurateurs appealed to an American clientele, white customers also rated these recent immigrants as being worthy (or not) of national belonging.

Drawing substantially on restaurant trade journals, as well as lesser-known dining guidebooks, I argue that the global atmosphere and flavors of foreign-themed restaurants helped increase Americans' consumption of foreign foods. Trade journals and dining guides offer a glimpse into the history of small, independent restaurants that constituted over 95 percent of restaurant businesses around 1930 (Marketing Analysis 1930: 12). While historians have more thoroughly documented the stories of chain restaurants, few records or formal archives remain for the vast array of America's historical independent restaurants. Industry publications and regional guides called attention to successful restaurants within a particular moment—albeit from the perspective of operators and customers rather than employees—including small, regional restaurants that have long since disappeared. These sources, which also consider interior decorations and employees' speech and dress, reveal that foreign-themed restaurant owners consciously crafted dining experiences as temporary escapes for white, middle-class customers who sought a highly mediated kind of ethnic encounter. In the process, these proprietors contributed to a more cosmopolitan-tasting American cuisine by introducing foreign flavors into their dishes and broadening white customers' acceptance of foreign foods as part of America's national culinary repertoire.

In his essay "Eating American," Sidney Mintz argues that, historically, immigrants new to the United States have been pressured to give up their cultural traditions—including their way of eating—in the name of "Americanization" (2002: 26). While this sacrifice of tradition is true to an extent, it was not a universal condition for adapting to life in the United States. Instead, the efforts to "Americanize" food in U.S. foreign restaurants between the World Wars mirror the multiple variations of the Americanization movement that took place in the early twentieth century. In his seminal history of American nativism, *Strangers in the Land* (1955), John Higham details how the "Crusade for Americanization" divided into two groups: "100 percent Americanized" and "International Nationalists." The former "opened a frontal assault on foreign influence in American life" by forcing immigrants to "abandon entirely their Old World loyalties, customs, and memories" (247). In contrast, Higham contends, International Nationalists supported the cultural heritage of immigrants, believing that their native traditions enriched the United States and its place in the "world community" (251).

International Nationalists saw the cultural contributions of immigrants—including, I argue, their foodways—as complementary to "the future growth of a still unfinished nationality" (Higham 1955: 251). Similarly, while some in the restaurant industry supported a revival of traditional American cookery, those who operated foreign-themed restaurants embraced the introduction of foreign traditions, including ingredients, into American food (King 1930; Patterson 1933; Ewing 1933). The contained space of the foreign-themed restaurant and its stylized representations of global cultures effectively popularized "foreign-ness" for American restaurant-goers. As a result, foreign-themed restaurants helped infuse Americans' regional palates with global flavors, leading to a more cosmopolitan conception of American cuisine.

THE RISE OF FOREIGN-THEMED RESTAURANTS IN THE 1920S AND 1930S

Prior to the First World War, only a select portion of the native-born American population ventured into foreign restaurants that did not have the culinary stamp of esteemed French or German cuisine. Public eateries serving foreign dishes catered to particular ethnic groups, especially bachelors and recent immigrants. Native-born, middle-class white Americans (usually men) dabbled in these restaurants only when looking for dining excitement; otherwise, foreign restaurants were to be avoided. The growth in number and popularity of foreign-themed restaurants in the United States coincided with a number of political, economic, and cultural changes: the onset of Prohibition, the increase of an urban female workforce, the rising popularity of socializing outside of the home, and the growth of a visual culture produced as part of the burgeoning consumerism associated with movie theaters, department stores, and nightclubs. Many of the high-end *haute cuisine* restaurants that profited from alcohol sales closed their doors as a result of the Eighteenth Amendment. To stay in business, restaurants lowered their prices, changed their designs, and focused on a new clientele: middle-class men and women.

In 1927, the restaurant industry determined that over 20 percent of Americans' meals were eaten outside of the home, a result of increased wealth; a greater desire for travel and leisure facilitated by the automobile; and the "servant problem," which reflected a decline in the availability of domestic help as a result of more restrictive immigration laws (Growth 1927: 19; More Money 1928: 57). However, the industry's first comprehensive marketing survey in 1930 suggested, "Perhaps the most important factor that is causing the growing trend of food consumption away from home is the increasing tendency towards urban dwelling" (Marketing Analysis 1930: 12; Patterson 1928: 25). Men and women who lived in urban areas contributed not only to the general increase in dining out; they also were more likely than their small-town counterparts to experiment with foreign foods as a result of the "cosmopolitan influence" (Smith and Wilson 1938: 27).

Even as early as 1910, food journalists observed that, in New York, "it was quite a common practice for groups to go off to some restaurant serving foreign food and enjoy thoroughly the different manner in which it was served" (Ewing 1935: 68). In 1930, the Childs restaurant chain gathered data on customers around the country and determined that "New York and metropolitan areas are notable for their adventurous spirit at dinner. The New Yorker is eager to try a new dish and seeks variety to keep his appetite whetted" (How American 1930: 68). Visitors and tourists also took advantage of the foreign dining opportunities in big cities. The *Washington Post* reported that 2,000 delegates of the American Home Economics Association, who traveled to New York from places such as Corvallis, Oregon; Burlington, Vermont; and Austin, Texas, chose to dine out in Chinese, Swedish, German, Japanese, and Russian restaurants during their stay (Chinese 1934: 13).

In the 1920s and 1930s, restaurant patrons tended to be white, middle- and upper-class men and women although, as one restaurant study confirmed, "men customers outnumbered women in a large majority of. . .restaurants." This study also showed that "women in secretarial and business work" were the "most important [group] of [female] patrons" (Why 1938: 27). Tourists, including women, also contributed to a large percentage of restaurant sales, especially in urban areas. Marjorie Hillis, in her guide for women vacationists, recommended foreign restaurants, including the East India Curry Shop, Giovanni's Italian restaurant, and the Golden Horn, which served Turkish specialties. All these restaurants qualified as places where "two or more women might go . . . with no qualms or embarrassment" (Hillis 1939: 76–77). The industry was attuned to its clientele. The vice-president of the National Restaurant Association remarked, "The dinner business, at least for most restaurants, doesn't come from the laboring classes. It comes from the families of white-collar workers" (Cooley 1938: 98). Social historian Katherine Leonard Turner points out that in the early to mid-twentieth century, local, small ethnic restaurants that catered to single men and recent immigrants—who did not have the time, means, or ingredients to prepare traditional foods—were some of the only restaurants within reach of the working class (Turner 2006).

Among the overall growth of restaurants, foreign-themed venues, in particular, thrived for several reasons. First, to support U.S. participation in World War I, the federal government, under the leadership of Herbert Hoover, and the U.S. Food Administration (a precursor to the Food and Drug Administration) asked Americans voluntarily to practice food conservation. Several ethnic cuisines were made of economical ingredients that were less in demand than meat and other scarce foodstuffs. Therefore, these diets were budget-friendly and became more acceptable during the war, appearing more frequently on restaurant menus. Also, foreign restaurants that had previously catered to a predominately native clientele witnessed their numbers of customers diminish alongside increasingly tighter immigration restrictions. As the operator of Beliska's Restaurant, which catered to Russian and Hungarian immigrants in New York, described in an interview for the Federal Writers' Project: "Since de immigration is closed, you know, it grows gradjally less people; it is shrinking, yes, business is shrinking liddle by liddle" (Spector 1938). Therefore, restaurant owners became more willing to adapt their restaurant dishes to non-immigrant consumers in order to stay in business (Levenstein 2002).

World's Fairs also played an influential role in introducing Americans to foreign foods. As early as 1876, the simulated displays of world cultures at America's World's Fairs packaged foreign "villages" as part of each fair's "educational" entertainment, and many countries chose to operate restaurants as a way of inviting Americans and other visitors to experience their cultural traditions. The exposure to foreign foods at world's fairs generated curiosity and a taste for these foods long after a fair closed its doors. For instance, at the 1933 Chicago World's Fair, the brother-owner duo of Robert and Max Eitel, who operated several German restaurants in Chicago and Milwaukee, replicated Germany's Old Heidelberg Inn and served traditional German fare by waitresses dressed in "colorful peasant costumes, complete down to the last detail of the leather purse swinging from their belts" (Siekman 1933: 26). Based on the restaurant's popularity at the fair, the brothers reconstructed the restaurant in Chicago the following year so customers could continue to "experience" Germany through its culinary recreation.

Finally, the onset of the Great Depression inspired the creation of novel, escapist dining atmospheres that distracted customers from the grey reality of everyday life. Restaurant trade journals, such as *American Restaurant* and *Catering World*, documented this desire for variety, declaring it an "everlasting call for something new" that took the form of "Chop Suey Week" and nightly "chilly con carne" and "spaghetti a la Caruso" specials, as restaurants sought to "capitalize on this desire for foreign foods" (McKee 1934: 33; Gibbons 1932: 18). Restaurant management books reminded restaurateurs that customers were "yearning for far places," for "strange sights, strange foods, tantalizing odors—without going more than a few miles from their own front doors!" (Gray 1946: 224). As J. O. Dahl, a leading restaurant industry expert, explained in his book *Restaurant Management*: "The mere mention of their names [of foreign countries] inspires dreams. All of us cannot go to these distant places, but in some degree we can bring them to the public" (Dahl 1938: 68). Native-born American customers looking to dabble in world travel over the span of a meal were usually interested in a kind of packaged authenticity, a cultural reproduction that was different enough to feel foreign, but familiar enough to be non-threatening.

VARIATIONS ON A FOREIGN RESTAURANT

The performance of ethnicity within the restaurant space and the cultural reproduction for tourist appeal was not, and had not been, always a part of foreign restaurants. While it was true that many restaurants placed food on the back burner, so to speak, in favor of an exotic, cosmopolitan décor, numerous establishments were owned and operated by immigrants who provided familiar native foods to their community. Guidebook authors were often quick to point out restaurants that fit this description. Konrad Bercovici observed that "the same clients came night after night for their dinner" at a Syrian restaurant in New York, where "the menu was printed in Arabic as if were [sic] in Arabia" (Bercovici 1924: 34). Ruth Thompson described the Tao Yuan Chinese restaurant in San Francisco as "the place where the Chinese and their families, in their native costumes, eat with chopsticks. No American food can be obtained there, but some Americans ... have discovered it and the Orientals will cater to them courteously to the extent of giving a choice of chopsticks or knives and forks" (Thompson 1937: 89). Many Chinese restaurants, motivated by the tourist economy, cultivated exoticism in Chinatown restaurants for non-Chinese tourists seeking "picturesque foreignness" (Takaki 1998: 247). Once the tourists left, these same restaurants served elaborate meals to well-to-do Chinese families, and the restaurants turned into places "where the Chinese felt at ease and the Americans became the foreigners" (Takaki 1998: 253). Similarly, historian Hasia Diner notes in her study of Italian, Irish, and Jewish immigrant foodways, "well through the 1920s, the general public was not the intended consumer" (Diner 2001: 75).

In order to generate more business, especially after immigration restrictions slowed the influx of restaurants' foreign national customers, many foreign-born restaurateurs worked hard to welcome native-born Anglo American guests. At the Red Star Inn, a Bavarian restaurant in Chicago, the proprietor Papa Gallauer attracted customers with "[d]ecorative beer steins. . .and fat waiters with German accents," as well as his own "beaming personality." Guidebook writer John Drury claimed patrons flocked to the restaurant because of the food, "the quiet, old-world atmosphere, and Papa Gallauer" (Drury 1931: 76–77). Morris Ehrlich, who emigrated from the "old country" around 1900, advertised his restaurant to an American-born clientele by emphasizing sanitation, "including an up-to-the-minute water filtering system, for the protection of the patron's health," as part of "a pleasing admixture of Old European-style cookery and modern American restaurant service" (Siekman 1931: 46). The targeted customer, then, was a key distinction between foreign restaurants and foreign-themed restaurants. Revealing the conscientious practice of serving Russian dishes palatable to Americans, Mrs. Valentine A. Varipaeff, the founder and owner of the Russian Tea Room in San Francisco, explained to one guidebook author how it had "taken years of study and experimentation": "I watch my guests and talk to them about what dishes they like, so I have been able to find out the American taste in Russian dishes and cater to it," she explained (Thomson 1937: 138). Although her food remained traditional, it was also selectively foreign to appeal to white, middle-class Americans' tastes.

The interest in appealing to a wide-ranging clientele was critical for a foreign-themed restaurant to be accepted simultaneously as an "American" restaurant, which is best illustrated by George Chappell's 1925 dining guide. In *Restaurants of New York*, Chappell divided New York City's foreign restaurants into two categories; his criteria for differentiation are worth quoting at length. Chappell singled out a "class of restaurant which defies [New York] geographical grouping, namely those of foreign peoples who, *dwelling among us*, still cling to their national cuisine .... French, German, Italian, Spanish, Mexican, Hawaiian, Syrian, Japanese, Chinese, they are found wherever a few of their appetites are gathered together" (8). These "enclave" foreigners were not "foreign citizens"; instead, they were designated outsiders with "queer, unknown tastes" (148). Clinging rigidly to foreign culinary traditions, these restaurants exhibited a loyalty to their homeland that set them apart from American cuisine.

In contrast, Chappell identified foreign restaurants that intentionally invited in "all" Americans. By creating décor and food that appealed to the native-born American palate, they were worthy of the distinction of *not* being designated simply as "Foreign Feeding Grounds."

> In considering the restaurants of *our foreign citizens* it is evident that there are many, particularly among the Germans, French and Italians, which have for many years been favorite meeting and eating places for the general public, *regardless of nationality*. They still retain a national character and their bills of fare are marked by many special dishes which speak eloquently of the Fatherland or La Patrie, but they have also become, to a certain extent, Americanized. *They are the rendezvous of all*. A number of the restaurants of these countries have been mentioned in previous pages of this book. If I recall them under this supplementary heading of "foreign" places, it is because they must be included in the two categories. While patronized largely by the general public, they still remain the gathering places of those who enjoy meeting old friends with whom they can speak their native language and share their native dishes. (149; emphasis added)

In Chappell's view, Americanized foreign restaurants were not really "foreign"; they were representative of cosmopolitan America and therefore foreign-themed. By proving their loyalty to the United States, they earned the title of "foreign citizens."

If the patronage of and enthusiasm for foreign-themed restaurants mirrored the "international nationalist" support of immigrant cultures in the United States, tolerance for foreign languages within the restaurant space also echoed the contradictory demands from proponents of Americanization. Social historians, such as Andrew Haley and Harvey Levenstein, have documented the widespread effort to Anglicize menus in American restaurants in the early to mid-twentieth century (Haley 2003; Levenstein 1988). Middle-class customers tired of the pretension of French terminology and other foreign words begged restaurants to Americanize their menus in the name of national pride and consideration for the tongue-tied patron. The use of foreign terms in restaurants turned Americans into "copycats," claimed dissenters throughout the 1920s. Even into the 1930s and 1940s, restaurant trade journals suggested that American restaurants would finally come into fruition when "terms of French and other foreign origins. . .disappear from the American menu." At that point, "importations of everything will be looked upon with disdain and petulance," claimed Irwin Keeler, editor of the *Pacific Hotel and Restaurant Review*, and "there will be an emphasis on good ole American dishes" (1945: 14). The rising popularity in dining out among Americans occurred, the industry suggested, when menus dropped foreign phrases from the food descriptions—until then, "the American public was too busy to be bothered translating fancy foreign terms into understandable English" (Patterson 1936: 36).

Within the increasingly nativist political climate of the 1920s, much of the debate over menu language tied to the Americanization and English-only movements that were gaining momentum amidst growing nationalist impulses. The *American Restaurant* magazine, one of the industry's leading trade journals, repeatedly printed editorials throughout the early 1920s supporting the idea of a one-language nation. "So we have restaurants on American soil owned and controlled by men from almost every country," the magazine acknowledged in February 1920. However, the article continued, taking a decidedly nativist stance: "We native Americans cannot help but register surprise and even suspicion when we hear foreign tongues spoken. . .in public restaurants." While, for the restaurateur and his foreign-born staff, "it may be hard to twist the tongue around to say it in American," using English was necessary for "restaurant men of foreign birth" to be "one hundred per cent American." According to the restaurant industry, "the taking out of citizen papers does not make an American citizen. The change must take place in the heart"—and, apparently, on the tongue (Americanism 1920: 30). This kind of advocacy for English-only restaurants, however, only tells the part of the story that more closely aligns with the "100 percent Americanization" viewpoint.

Although many Americans pushed to Anglicize the menu, several foreign-themed restaurants still profited from the use of foreign languages and heavy foreign accents as *spoken* by the restaurant workers.[2] The appeal of foreign-language speaking employees was as much—if not more—for the benefit of English-speaking American customers as for foreign nationals. Why would native-born American patrons delight in listening to foreign languages in speech and yet protest menus written in the same languages? Certainly, one reason is likely that hearing another language contributed to the "atmosphere" of the restaurant and the ever-elusive notion of authenticity. Jane Desmond attributes this kind of authorization to the concept of "physical foundationalism," or the belief that the body is an inherently real or authentic indicator of identity because it is "natural." "Live performers," Desmond suggests, "not only authenticate these packaged differences; they also offer the possibility of contact with them," thereby creating an encounter with "people who are 'different' from you." Simultaneously, the production commodifies identity, replacing historical accuracies with an unmediated (and highly subjective) experience (Desmond 1999: xv–xvi). The physical act of speaking a language other than English naturalized the restaurant's recreated foreign environment.

Some restaurants in the late 1920s and early 1930s, such as Childs restaurant in New York, started to hire multilingual waitresses "for the convenience of the foreign patrons who may not be well-versed in English" (Waitresses Are Linguists 1931: 26). Yet, despite the range of languages spoken by the staff—at one restaurant, thirty-two different languages were spoken by the waitresses, collectively—"the expected influx of foreign patrons failed to appear. But plenty of Americans came in" (Beatty 1932: 134). One journalist, describing the appeal of Armenian and Greek restaurants in New York City in 1923 noted:

> The good Anglo Saxons who at first came there out of curiosity, and later brought their friends to show off, have come to like the food. They have learned a little Armenian, a little Greek, have bought curios from the new immigrants who come there and now look like Armenians themselves. Indeed, neither the proprietor nor his waiters have learned English. Last Summer the owner had engaged an English-speaking waitress. He lost many customers because of that. So he became wise. He refuses to speak even the English he knows. (Bercovici 1923)

Many foreign-themed restaurants believed that the use of foreign languages added to the "showmanship" of the establishment and helped increase food sales—foreign languages spoken in restaurants could "season" the atmosphere if used with restraint.

In addition, restaurant staff who spoke a foreign language did not challenge the customer's access to food as long as the staff member *understood* English. Andrew Haley notes that "the struggle over the language of dining was never merely about words, it was about cultural authority" (2003: 33). English-speaking customers rejected foreign language menus if the descriptions hindered their ability to understand what they were ordering. Yet if a foreign language spoken among staff members facilitated the restaurant operation, or provided a kind of musical background for the English-speaking patron, the language could be tolerated as long as it did not prevent the customer from enjoying (and correctly ordering) the meal. "The American linguistic situation produces an almost inescapable paradox," argues Dennis E. Baron in *The English-Only Question*. "Minority-language speakers are encouraged to abandon their native tongues and become monolingual in English to demonstrate their patriotism, their willingness to assimilate, and their desire to enter the economic mainstream. Once they do this, they are encouraged. . .to learn a foreign language in order to strengthen their country's position in the international arena" (1990: 15). Even in the process of "Americanizing" restaurants, foreign languages operated as a tool to create more cosmopolitan American consumers.

American restaurateurs, both native- and foreign-born, recognized the profitable appeal of recreating a global atmosphere for their customers. Childs Company, which operated a chain of nationwide restaurants, noticed its profits declining and responded by opening two new restaurants, recreating the atmosphere of Old France and Old Spain, respectively. In Old France, waitresses "dressed in gay peasant costumes of blue, green, red, and white, with a tiny black hat perched coquettishly on their heads" (Seaburg 1928: 314). At Childs Spanish Gardens, the company even went "to the trouble of picking dark-eyed beauties dressed in suitable multicolored dresses to serve you" (Berliner 1932: 9). The *American Restaurant* magazine praised Colorado restaurateur W. E. Murphy for making "the good Irish name of Murphy synonymous with chile, tamales, and similar Spanish and Mexican delicacies" through his restaurant's Spanish architecture and good food (Lovgren 1937: 44, 108). Similarly, the *Pacific Coast Record* gave credit to Mexican-born Señora Consuelo Castillo de Bonzo, proprietress of the Casa La Golondrina in Los Angeles, who opened the restaurant in 1930 to serve "real South-of-the-Border cuisine" alongside "quaint Mexican atmosphere" (Minster 1961: 38–39). Clearly, performance and representation were integral components of foreign-themed restaurants.[3]

Still, a restaurant could take its culinary modifications too far. One restaurant operator lamented, "the trouble with Chinese [restaurants is that] they try so hard to be Americanized" (Tong 1936: 42). Weighting the scale between exotic foreign interiors and authentic yet palatable food was a difficult balance for Americanized foreign restaurants to strike. At the Aladdin Studio Tiffin Room in San Francisco each customer was encouraged "to imagine he is inside Aladdin's cave" while "Chinese dishes are favored on the menu and Chinese girls in native costume are employed as waitresses" (Dench 1923: 55). Other operators, recognizing the profits and appeal of particular foreign foods, incorporated the production of foreign cuisine and atmosphere into their restaurants, without modifying the original theme. For instance, David L. Stewart, who served American food at his restaurant, The Barn, built a "Chinese Grotto" room and added a Chinese food kitchen, complete with Chinese-born chefs, who prepared Chicken Sub Gum Chow Mein alongside orders for American Turkey dinners (Voegele 1938: 29–31). Philip Gertner, the son of Austrian immigrants, decided "that the Orient had no monopoly on" sukiyaki and added Japanese food, along with French Crepes Suzettes, to his menu. He hired "colorful little Japanese girls" to make the crepes in the window of the storefront using chopsticks, "a fact which the gay *New Yorker* chronicled as an 'international note'" (Marshall 1934: 62, 64).

Harvey Levenstein argues that this "culinary and thematic mishmash" was a direct result of Americans' rejection of strange foreign foods: exotic decorations appealed to the customers' desire for a visually stimulating dining environment, while the food remained familiarly "American" (1993: 49). This explanation, however, does not sufficiently encompass restaurants such as the Aladdin Studio, where the "mishmash" was a collision of two "foreign" themes and foods, neither one decidedly "American." The seemingly random mix of decor and dishes was a response to Americans' longing for "the thrill of having run away for an hour or two from their own too-familiar world," explained one restaurant management guide. "Start with the best decorations you have and the best food you can cook, regardless of period or place" (Gray 1946: 225–228). In other words, a restaurant's success depended on offering customers a change of pace, which could be reflected in the food, the décor, or both. Neither had to be "100 percent American." Rather than clinging to a recognizable "American" dining environment, white middle-class urban Americans delighted in their culinary adventurism—it helped to distinguish their national pride and character.

Restaurant workers played a crucial role in creating the ambience of foreign-themed restaurants, in no small part because of the industry's tendency to view the employees as decorative objects themselves. One design consultant suggested that a "convincing interior" motif could "come from a combination of history and people, or from a race of people" (Harman 1945: 46). "Decoration applies to waiters and dishes too," another restaurant manual reminded readers in the section, "Providing Escape by Decoration," adding as a side note, "You don't even need the same kind of decorations as food" (Gray 1946: 227). Along these lines, Helen Orcutt, "an expert on dress" for waitresses, advised restaurateurs that if a woman "waits in a restaurant of old Spanish flavor, she must dress the part of the señorita, even to the high comb and mantilla" (Proper Costumes for Waitresses 1928: 18). Seeming to follow this advice, "a coffee house has put its girls into the flowered cottons of Spanish peasants," noted the *New York Times* in 1928 (Rice 1928: 136). The view of employee-as-object functioned to naturalize the foreign realism of the restaurant, rather than call attention to its artificiality.

Some restaurants exemplified their reliance on physical foundationalism by advertising the physical features, rather than just the costumes, of their employees. Because the bodies of staff members validated the "foreign-ness" of the restaurant, restaurateurs invested in the "authenticity" of these employees. "Speaking of waiters, they are as imported as the Mouquin delicacies," declared a review of Mouquin's French café in New York City (Mouquin 1923: 45). The Gertner restaurants suggested patrons might enjoy the novelty of Japanese food "concocted by dainty little Japanese girls, complete with kimono, wooden clogs, rice powder, and sloe eyes" (Marshall 1934: 64), while the dining room of the Hotel Californian explained that the "colorful touch" of the "little Chinese maidens . . . had to be sacrificed" and replaced by American girls when three of the Chinese girls married (Stacy 1925: 77). Probably the most extreme example occurred in Portland, Oregon, where a restaurant operator was cited by the state for racial discrimination because he refused to hire waitresses other than those of Asian descent. "I have no prejudice against any race," he declared, "but I am determined to carry out my Chinese theme even to employees. These petite Oriental girls in their brilliant kimonos, which incidentally cost me over $10,000 for the crew are a real attraction" (Chinese 1963: 11). The emphasis on "native" costumes and employees, while pretending to promote a favorable image of foreign cultures, simultaneously objectified the employees, presenting them as caricatures for a dining audience. In the minds of many restaurateurs who operated foreign-themed restaurants that represented a nation or ethnicity different from their own, the characterization of human beings as decoration justified a disregard for cultural sensitivity and respect.

The success of foreign-themed restaurants depended on more than the atmosphere created by the employees. Reproductions—however diluted—of traditional foreign dishes held considerable appeal for Americans bored with the relatively bland standard of typical American fare. Tired of underseasoned food, numerous patrons demanded more from the restaurant industry in the 1920s and 1930s. "Haven't American chefs ever heard of salt, pepper, mustard, paprika, cloves, or the other spices and herbs that European chefs use as a matter of course? Must restaurant food in this country be flat, tasteless, dull, and uninteresting?" one disgruntled patron questioned (Noble 1936: 60). Persons hired to develop recipes for restaurants and other institutions of mass feeding responded accordingly. "Foreign cooking is delicious," recommended one recipe writer for the *American Restaurant* magazine. "The flavorings used abroad are sometimes combinations of our own spices and sometimes herbs and seasonings native to the country. Some of these are anise, cardamom, garlic, ajinomoto, allspice, many kinds of red peppers, citron, dill, rosemary, basil, and many others" (Toevs 1930: 43). The author then advised restaurant cooks in how to prepare dishes using these unfamiliar spices and adapt them to American palates. Anticipating skepticism on the part of American chefs, she cautioned, "Some of the combinations sound outlandish, but if you have never eaten apricots in soup, nor cloves in meat, do not condemn them untried" (43).

On another occasion, the same author remarked that despite Americans' familiarity with foods from India, Mexico, and Spain, too many delicious dishes had been overlooked, potentially because of their "burning spices" flavor profile. Modify the dishes, she recommended, and by "substituting commoner commodities at hand, these [recipes] may be copied with satisfactory results" (Toevs 1931: 35). In the interwar years, numerous popular and industry periodicals offered restaurants and home-cooks alike recipes based on "genuine" foreign restaurants' dishes that could be copied and adapted for everyday American dining (Turner 1939). Through the partnership of recipe developers, experimental chefs, and curious customers, foreign flavorings made their way into restaurants that served a variety of "American" fare.

Among the favorite foreign cuisines of native-born Americans was Italian. Italian restaurants became exceedingly popular between the wars, in part because Americanized Italian-themed restaurants created a space where white, middle-class Americans imagined they could let their hair down, throw their hands up, and play in a more festive, gregarious atmosphere. Hasia Diner's study of Italian immigrant foodways argues that particular foods, including oils, cheeses, and macaroni, reserved for only the wealthy elite in Italy, were available to Italian immigrants in the United States. In part because of this availability of food, and continuing the Italian family-oriented emphasis on food preparation and consumption, "Italian immigrants placed a high premium upon eating certain foods and eating them well," which carried over into the appeal of American Italian restaurants (Diner 2001: 51). Levenstein has also suggested that Italian restaurants were particularly popular because they were frequently run by boarding house operators who specialized in making homemade alcohol. When the Eighteenth Amendment shut down their competition, Italian restaurants thrived among non-Italians because the restaurants continued to serve alcoholic beverages to their customers (Levenstein 2002: 87). Importantly, these restaurants advertised themselves to a native-born American clientele by promising food "such as one gets in Italy," and in the process "enveloped food in the themes of pan-Italian identity, submerging local loyalties" to promote a unified "national" image of Italy to Americans (Diner 2001: 66–67).

The food, however, often was *not* what one could get in Italy. Despite claims that chefs "[prided] themselves on giving Italian home-style cooking in their restaurants," "fine, traditional American specialties called 'spaghetti with meatballs' and 'cotoletta parmigiana'" should be "just for fun called Italian," remarked one Italian-born restaurateur (Barber 1930: 56; Diner 2001: 54). What appealed to native-born American customers was the representation of Italy translated through the restaurant's ambiance and service, preferably a setting that conveyed "cultural rebellion and adventure" within a safely contained environment (Gabaccia 1998: 99). One guidebook suggested customers dine at San Francisco's Riviera restaurant to "[s]ave yourself the price of a trip to Italy . . . if you wish to be transported for the evening . . . to an atmospheric place breathing luxury and Latin feeling which is delightfully stirring and different" (Thompson 1937: 10–11). In a more explicit suggestion of "cultural adventure," a profile on Bigin's Bologna Restaurants in the San Francisco *Bulletin* reprinted one of the restaurant's wall panels, a provocative painting by Guillermo Vercellino titled "Carnival," which helped create an image of the restaurant as risqué (Dodd: 7). These depictions of "ethnic performance," complete with mood music and costume were all part of what some restaurateurs called the "showmanship" of foreign restaurants that "helps the sales and maintains tone for the restaurants that use it" (A La Carte Menus 1939). American restaurant patrons delighted in the escapism associated with Italy, and Italian-themed restaurants worked hard to meet customers' expectations of the perceived exoticism of the country.

At the same time, though, many owners of Italian-themed restaurants tried to move beyond the gimmicks and represent the cultural contributions of their native country while simultaneously asserting their loyalty to the United States. One restaurant review of Enrico & Paglieri's Italian restaurant noted that "though you may not get a chance to see them, Enrico is the owner of a gold spaghetti fork and spoon, presented to him in 1937 when he became the dean of the New York Society of Restaurateurs. This honor, conferred more often in Europe, has been shared by no other American" (News of Food 1946: 34). Here, Enrico is offered a kind of dual citizenship within the "restaurant nation"—his name and his restaurant confer Italian nationality upon him, but he is legally a citizen of the United States. Similarly, Pietro Orcino, a native of Piemonte, Italy, who owned-and-operated the Avignone Freres restaurant in Washington, D.C., was elected president of the Washington Restaurant Association (Restaurateurs 1962: 7). By safely navigating the gastronomic waters between the two countries and providing their customers with an accessible version of Italy, Enrico and Pietro were rewarded with the approval of the American restaurant and dining community.

Certainly, self-identified ethnic restaurant owners had a personal investment in the portrayal of their native country presented to American customers. For example, Hasia Diner shows how Italian Americans, "as a group often stigmatized by the dominant culture for its low aspirations and violent character" used public distribution of their food to "present their cultural distinctiveness as rich and worth preserving" (Diner 2001: 226). As a result, by the middle of the twentieth century, the American restaurant industry credited Italy as "second only to France in the art of fine dining" (Cline 1947: 30). Restaurants provided immigrants the opportunity to become "foreign citizens" who retained ties to their cultural heritage but also carved a legitimized space for their belonging in the United States. In this vein, numerous restaurateurs and foreign-born patrons advocated greater representational accuracy in foreign-themed restaurants. Foreign-themed restaurants could operate as sites of resistance, pushing back against essentialist stereotyped depictions of foreign cultures. In turn, they could work to validate the presence of foreign immigrants in the United States. Italian Americans and other self-identified ethnic groups "had a stake in performing their food identity for others" (Diner 2001: 226). That stake was obtaining "foreign citizenship."

FROM FOREIGN CITIZENS TO AMERICAN CITIZENS TO WORLD CITIZENS: CONCLUSIONS

Americans continued to reveal an affinity for foreign-flavored foods during and after World War II, yet there was an increasing emphasis on how these foods shaped a particularly *American*, rather than decidedly "foreign," cuisine. Even before the war, American food writers were pointing out that "the adaptation . . . of unfamiliar food invading the home and widely adopted, is a phenomenon that exists in the formative years of all countries. It has been strengthened in America by the tremendous number of foreigners who have married John or Mary Smith, or who have entered the restaurant business" (Morgan 1935). The patriotic dimension of wartime eating, however, increasingly emphasized how foreign foods were *becoming* American foods. For example, one New York journalist noted that "immigrants or their offspring still [keep] old country customs going, with American trimmings" (Shippey 1949).

Another noted how "'Americanized' versions of alien comestibles turned a pretty penny for lots of restaurateurs" (Bradfield 1949: G12). The global dimension of American-styled foreign cuisine was more frequently praised as American rather than as cosmopolitan, thereby privileging and taking pride in a *national* way of eating.

The restaurant industry also recognized the war's influence on expanding Americans' preference for foreign foods, and it responded in turn, using cosmopolitan dining as a way of demonstrating patriotism and pride in things American. The suspension of imported foods during World War II "Americanized" foreign dishes simply by the fact that they were prepared using domestic ingredients. "In New York City's 2,000-odd foreign restaurants," reported the *New York Times*, "about the only things left that can rightly be called 'foreign' are the recipes, for since Pearl Harbor halted most imports, the food is now strictly American" (Foreign Dishes 1943). In addition, the restaurant industry's successful efforts to add popular foreign foods to the list of OPA-regulated pricing, as well as their anticipation that returning soldiers' palates would have an increased preference for foreign foods, shows how closely foreign foods were intermingled with a cosmopolitan—and yet distinctly American—national identity. "We are no longer a three-dish people—meat, potatoes, and pie," one industry representative declared.

> We have learned to read a menu, to recognize the difference between shish kebab and Yorkshire pudding. . . .at home we haven't neglected international food appeal. We have come a long way from the chop suey 'palace' with its pseudo-Chinese food, to the splendid restaurants featuring genuine Cantonese cooking; to the German, the Swiss, the French, the Scandinavian smorgasbords; the Italian and Hungarian and Armenian establishments specializing in the tempting dishes of their forbears. At the same time, we are developing our own native dishes. (Wells 1959: 23)

America was finding its national cuisine in the midst of, rather than separate from, foreign food influences.

Between the First and Second World Wars, foreign-themed restaurants not only lent themselves to debates over Americanization and national identity; they also provided the material space in which Americans—native- and foreign-born alike—revised definitions of cultural and culinary citizenship in cosmopolitan terms through performative gestures. As immigrant newcomers became accustomed to living in the United States, native-born Americans adapted the country's cuisine to incorporate global tastes. The exposure to and genuine pleasure found in the addition of spices and other flavors used in foreign foods gradually changed what tasted "American" in American dishes. Through the introduction of foreign flavors to mainstream American dining, facilitated by attractively exotic global décor, foreign-themed restaurants added a cosmopolitan taste to traditionally American foods. This "Americanization" of restaurant food in the United States through the addition of "foreign" ingredients contributed to a broader "world citizen" vision of American identity in the mid-twentieth century.

NOTES

1. Throughout this essay, I assume that it is possible to consider what Americans ate as both food and cuisine. My rationale that such a thing as "American cuisine" exists falls in line with Krishnendu Ray's definition of American cuisine, which treats cuisine as "a particular kind of talk about cooking" imagined into existence by professional food writers and restaurants, where national cuisine is "performed in the public sphere" (Ray 2008: 265, 289).

2. In discussions questioning the existence of an American cuisine, both Sidney Mintz and Krishnendu Ray (despite their different conclusions) support the idea that cuisine is inextricably tied to language and the "talk" about food, not only the tasting of food (Mintz 2002; Ray 2008).

3. The materiality of the restaurant space, and the production of racial and ethnic images within the eating establishments, are part of what Kristin Hoganson calls "performative geography"—the performance of the geographically different through the manipulation of costume, stage settings, and cultural ephemera, thereby producing "representations of difference" (Hoganson 2007: 137). American-born white customers wanted to feel welcomed by the difference, rather than alienated by it. Therefore, successful foreign-themed restaurants tried to invoke foreign places and yet retain some level of familiarity for its patrons. For instance, owners of the Pagoda Inn advertised their restaurant on its menus as "High-Class Chinese and American," stating: "It is the aim of the management to introduce a part of the Chinese civilization to our American friends" (Pagoda). Similarly, businesses such as Green's Chinese American Restaurant in Philadelphia offered "American or Chinese Food—You ask for it, we have it," and San Antonio's Shangri-La Restaurant served "typical Chinese food and also specializes in American steaks and fried chicken dinners" (Green; Shangri-La 1944: 9).

REFERENCES

"A La Carte Menus Found Outmoded." 1939. *New York Times* (November 8): 25.

"Americanism." 1920. *American Restaurant* (February): 30.

Barber, E. 1930. Delicious Italian Food at Its Source. *Better Homes and Gardens* (October): 24, 56.

Baron, D. 1990. *The English-Only Question: An Official Language for Americans?* New Haven, CT: Yale University Press.

Beatty, J. 1932. How People Act in Restaurants. *American Magazine* (December): 134.

Bercovici, K. 1923. "America Europeanized." *New York Times* (September 16): SM 4.

———. 1924. *Around the World in New York.* New York: The Century Co.

Berliner, J. J. 1932. Childs Restaurants Go Over the Top. *Catering World* (April): 9–13.

Bradfield, K. 1949. "Cosmopolitan Cookery." *Los Angeles Times* (August 28): G12.

Brown. 1939. "For Gourmets and Others: Dining Abroad in the City." *New York Times* (January 22): 45.

Chappell, G. 1925. *The Restaurants of New York.* New York: Greenberg Publisher.

"Chinese Food Makes a Hit With Experts." 1934. *Washington Post* (June 28): 13.

"Chinese Restaurant." 1963. *Pacific Coast Record* (July): 11.

"Chow." 1924. *Pacific Coast Chef* (February): 2–3.

"City Eats 800 Tons a Day." 1934. *Washington Post* (October 28): F6.

Cline, J. 1947. Tempting Italian Dishes. *American Restaurant* (February): 30–32, 133–138.

———. 1948. Curries Are Popular and They Save Meat. *American Restaurant* (January): 38–39, 123–125.

Cooley, R. 1938. Streamlining Your Ideas. *American Restaurant* (October): 90, 92, 94, 97–98, 101.

"Culinary Geography While You Eat." 1942. *American Restaruant* (September): 30–31, 75.

"Curry Recipes Offered." 1959. *Pacific Coast Record* (May): 25.

Dahl, J.O. 1938. *Restaurant Management: Principles and Practice*. New York: Harper & Bros.

Dana, R. 1948. *Where to Eat in New York*. New York: Current Books, Inc.

De Gouy, L. 1941. Good Food Hints. *Restaurant Management* (November): 32.

Dench, E. 1923. A Handful of Ideas. *American Restaurant* (April): 55.

Desmond, J. 1999. *Staging Tourism: Bodies on Display From Waikiki to Sea World*. Chicago: University of Chicago Press.

Diner, H. 2001. *Hungering for Americans: Italian, Irish, and Jewish Foodways in the Age of Migration*. Cambridge, MA: Harvard University Press.

"Dining and Wining Around Chicago." 1937. *Restaurant Management* (October): 287.

Dodd, H. B. n.d. Where San Francisco Bohemians Eat: No Monkey Business Here. *The Bulletin Magazine*: 7. San Francisco Public Library clippings.

Dodd, J. L., and H. B. Dodd. 1925. *Bohemian Eats of San Francisco*. San Francisco: [s.n.]

Drury, J. 1931. *Dining in Chicago: An Intimate Guide*. New York: H. Wolff.

"Ellis Island Scenes Pictured." 1927. *New York Times* (June 12): X5.

Ewing, H. 1933. Let's Feature Our American Dishes. *American Restaurant* (May): 28–31, 40.

———. 1935. Desire for Foreign Food. *American Restaurant* (November): 68.

"For Real American Tid-Bits." 1941. *American Restaurant* (March): 62.

"Foreign" Dishes. 1943. *New York Times* (November 14): SM 20.

Freeman, L. 1941. American Foods Hold Spotlight. *American Restaurant* (February): 38, 80, 82, 86.

Gabaccia, D. 1998. *We Are What We Eat: Ethnic Food and the Making of Americans*. Cambridge, MA: Harvard University Press.

Gibbons, T. 1932. What Customers Want Today. *Catering World* (June): 16–19.

Gray, M., and De lo Padua, V. 1946. *How to Be a Success in the Restaurant Business*. New York: Greenberg.

Green's Chinese American Restaurant menu. n.d. Henry Loo Papers, The Historical Society of Pennsylvania.

Growth of the Eating-out Habit. 1927. *Pacific Coast Chef* (October): 19.

Haley, A. 2003. "I Want to Eat in English": The Middle Class, Restaurant Culture, and the Language of Menus, 1880–1930. *Midwestern Folklore* 29: 28–39.

Harman, H. 1945. After You Bring Them *In*. . . . *American Restaurant* (November): 46, 114–116.

Harrison, A. 1917. Chinese Food and Restaurants. *Overland Monthly and Out West Magazine* (June): 527.

Hayden, D. 1981. *The Grand Domestic Revolution: A History of Feminist Designs for American Homes, Neighborhoods, and Cities*. Cambridge, MA: MIT Press.

Hickman, E. 1945. Stretch Red Ration Points With Goat Meat. *Chuck Wagon* (March): 14.

Higham, J. 1955. *Strangers in the Land: Patterns of American Nativism, 1860–1925*. New Brunswick, NJ: Rutgers University Press.

"Higher Mace and Nutmeg Quotas." 1944. *American Restaurant* (March): 54.

Hillis, M. 1939. *New York, Fair or No Fair: A Guide for the Woman Vacationist*. New York: The Bobbs-Merrill Company.

Hoganson, K. 2007. *Consumers' Imperium: The Global Production of American Domesticity*. Chapel Hill, NC: University of North Carolina Press.

Houck, B. 1928. Gastronomic Adventures. *Los Angeles Times* (May 13): K12.

Isbell, M. W. 1944. Foreign Food Tastes Will Be Forgotten. *American Restaurant* (October): 41–42.

Johnson, W. 1921. Dining 'Round the World in Los Angeles. *Los Angeles Times* (January 1): V19.

Keeler, I. 1945. Americanization of the Menu Predicted. *Keeler's Pacific Hotel and Restaurant Review* (July): 14.

King, C. 1930. National Dishes of America. *American Restaurant* (March): 60, 64, 68.

Levenstein, H. 1988. *Revolution at the Table: The Transformation of the American Diet*. New York: Oxford University Press.

———. 1993. *Paradox of Plenty: A Social History of Eating in America*. New York: Oxford University Press.

———. 2002. The American Response to Italian Food, 1880–1930. In C. Counihan (ed.). *Food in the USA. A Reader*. New York: Routledge, pp. 75–90.

Lovgren, K. 1937. Fine Foods and Atmosphere Make Murphy's Famous. *American Restaurant* (April): 44, 108.

Mackenzie, C. 1935. "When the City Dines Out." *New York Times* (March 31): 19.

"Mardikian Sees Opportunities for American Cuisine." 1943. *American Restaurant*. (February): 66.

Marketing Analysis of the Restaurant Industry. 1930. Chicago: American Restaurant Magazine.

Marshall, R. 1934. A Profitable Business Built on Other People's Ideas. *American Restaurant* (May): 35, 62, 64.

McKee, P. 1934. The Everlasting Call for Something New. *American Restaurant* (November): 33, 62.

"Menus Will Be Changed More When War Is Over." 1943. *Chuck Wagon* (May): 9.

Minster, J. 1961. Los Angeles Landmark. *Pacific Coast Record* (October): 38–39.

Mintz, S. 2002. Eating America. In C. Counihan (ed.). *Food in the USA. A Reader*. New York: Routledge, pp. 23–34.

More Money Means More "Eating Out." 1928. *Mixer and Server* (January 15): 57.

Morgan, H. 1935. "Our Wide Taste in Food." *New York Times* (October 13): SM 17.

"Mouquin's Famous for Its French Cuisine." 1923. *The Restaurateur* (April 7): 45.

"News of Food." 1946. *New York Times* (June 24): 34.

Noble, S. 1936. And Season to Taste. *American Restaurant* (October): 60–61, 100–102.

Pagoda Inn menu. n.d. Henry Loo Papers, The Historical Society of Pennsylvania.

Patterson, C. 1920. 1928. The Outlook for 1928 in the Restaurant Business. *American Restaurant* (January): 25.

———. 1933. Popularizing the American Cuisine. *American Restaurant* (May): 23.

———. 1936. Pat's Page. *American Restaurant* (June): 36.

———. 1949. 30th Anniversary Convention. *American Restaurant* (May): 37, 76.

Pennell, E. R. 1918. A Stranger in My Native Land. *The North American Review* (June): 880.

Pillsbury, R. 1998. *No Foreign Food: The American Diet in Time and Place*. Boulder, CO: Westview Press.

Podd, G. 1943. Have Your Menus Gone to War? *American Restaurant* (February): 32–33, 71.

"Postwar Nutrition." 1944. *American Restaurant* (July): 50.

"Proper Costumes for Waitresses." 1928. *New York Times* (May 30): 18.

Ray, K. 2008. Nation and Cuisine: The Evidence from American Newspapers ca. 1830–2003. *Food and Foodways* 16: 259–297.

"Recipes of All Nations." 1938. *American Restaurant* (June): 107.

"The Restaurant Library." 1940. *American Restaurant* (March): 18, 21.

"Restaurants Show Record Gain in Survey." 1930. *American Restaurant* (February): 33.

"Restaurants Serving Exotic Foods to Get OPA Prices." 1944. *New York Times* (July 20): 21.

"Restaurateurs Elect Pietro Orcino." 1962. *The Restaurateur* (February): 7.

Rice, D. 1928. "The Waitress of Today Is Trained for Her Job." *New York Times* (May 20): 136.

Ripperger, H. 1934. "Appetite's Pride and Prejudice." *New York Times* (November 11): SM 14.

"Round the World Menus." 1932. *American Restaurant* (August): 38.

Seaburg, N. 1928. In Old France: The Latest Childs. *Restaurant Management* (June): 312–314.

"Shangri-La Offers Chinese Food." 1944. *Chuck Wagon* (August): 9.

Shippey, L. 1949. Lee Side. *Los Angeles Times* (February 24): A5.

Siekman, H.C. 1931. Old-Time Dishes in a Modern Way. *American Restaurant* (September): 46–48.

———. 1933. "A Century of Progress Restaurants." *American Restaurant* (June): 25–27, 50, 53.

Smith, B. and C. M. Wilson. 1938. *Through the Kitchen Door: A Cook's Tour to the Best Kitchens of America*. New York: Stackpole Sons.

Spector, H. C. 1938. *Nobody Boddas You (Beliska's Restaurant)*. Library of Congress, Manuscript Division, WPA Federal Writers' Project Collection. http://memory.loc.gov/ammem/wpaintro/wpahome.html (1 August 2009).

Stacy, A. 1925. Shears Salad. *Hotel Monthly* (October): 77.

"A Study of an Italian-Type Restaurant." 1944. *American Restaurant* (February): 29.

Takaki, R. 1989, 1998. *Strangers From a Different Shore: A History of Asian Americans*. Boston: Little, Brown and Co.

Thompson, R. 1937. *Eating Around San Francisco*. San Francisco: Suttonhouse, Ltd.

Toevs, E. 1930. Foreign Foods in America. *American Restaurant* (June): 43–44, 82.

———. 1931. Winter Dishes From Abroad. *American Restaurant* (January): 35–36.

Tong Y. Chin and the Golden Dragon. 1936. *American Restaurant* (December): 42–42, 84–88.

Towe, E. 1944. Servicemen's Tastes and Knowledge Broadened by Quartermaster Corps. *Washington Post* (January 2): B2.

Turner, G. 1939. Give Your Meals a South-Sea Tang. *Los Angeles Times* (September 24): I11.

Turner, K. L. 2006. Buying, Not Cooking: Ready-to-Eat Food in American Urban Working-Class Neighborhoods, 1880–1930. *Food, Culture, & Society* (Spring): 13–40.

Voegele, W. O. 1938. He Doesn't Know the Restaurant Business But. *Restaurant Management* (September): 27–31, 50, 52, 54.

"Waitresses Are Linguists." 1931. *New York Times* (March 5): 26.

Wells, A. 1959. It's a Two Way Street. *Pacific Coast Record* (August): 23.

Why the Survey. 1938. *American Restaurant* (September): 26–33, 79–80, 82.

Wyman, A. D. 1921. "Foreign Quarter Chefs Tell Many Secrets." *Los Angeles Times* (February 23): II3.

Virginia Ham: The Local and Global of Colonial Foodways

MEGAN E. EDWARDS

Department of Anthropology, University of Chicago, Chicago, IL, USA

The Virginia ham, a regional delicacy, provides a unique opportunity to explore the local and global dynamics at play in the colonial foodways of the British North Atlantic. Moving beyond the simple question of origins, I ask why people ate this food with such gusto in this period and place and seek to explain the ham's development and rise to fame. Whereas earlier scholarly fixation on the food as object provides important insights, the interests of this article lie with the broader universe of people and practices within which production and consumption were embedded. Evidence demonstrates the transfer of Old World techniques to the Chesapeake Bay, and the fusing of these traditions with native practices in the creolizing social and physical environment of colonial Virginia. My contextualization provides for a deeper understanding of the historical and social processes that influenced the development of this food and the culinary heritage of Tidewater Virginia.

> "No self-respecting Southern pig can imagine a higher distinction than becoming, in due course, a Virginia ham—spicy as a woman's tongue, sweet as her kiss, as tender as her love." (Fishwick 1964, 131)

With this lusty imagery the *American Heritage Cookbook* introduces the near-mythical history of Virginia's famed ham. The ubiquity of this food item in the marketed cultural landscape of the Commonwealth's Tidewater region astounds first-time visitors. A trip up the Delmarva Peninsula, where every souvenir shop sells country-cured hams, affords countless examples of a regional fixation extending from Virginia's Eastern Shore to the southern banks of the James River. Isle of Wight County, where the acclaimed

Smithfield ham is still salted and smoked for a global market, represents itself as the birthplace of this modern American *terroir* food.

In a refrigerated age, Virginia ham has become a food trapped in time; a throwback that seems natural in an American South where the past is never further than one's local plantation house museum. A tourist or food connoisseur—raised in and possibly acting against the homogenizing culinary landscape of modern industrial foodways—encounters such location-specific *terroir* foods as islands of time, embodying in pungent flavors the traditional approaches to food that stand in defiance of the crush of global modernity. And yet it was the *grande dame* of globalizing forces herself—trans-Atlantic colonialism—that descended on the Chesapeake Bay in the seventeenth and eighteenth centuries to act as midwife in the birth of this *terroir* food. This article explores the confluence of global and local factors in the colonial emergence and early development of Virginia's much-touted ham. The analysis begins in the early seventeenth century and culminates with the American War of Independence, although much more could be written about the subsequent history of this ham in the global marketplace of *terroir* foods.

PERSPECTIVES ON VIRGINIA HAM: TOWARD A METHOD AND THEORY OF COLONIAL FOODWAYS STUDIES

The methodology pursued here is a foodways approach focused on one particular foodstuff—the Virginia ham. Foodways analysis entails parsing the material and social factors effecting the production, distribution, and consumption of foods. Virginia ham is here interpreted as representative of a colonial locale's foodway and thus as an intersection of the global and local. On a local scale, food presents us with a powerful opportunity to think of people in both their social and natural settings, as foodways tie humans to their environments as well as to one another. Here I explore the historical anthropology of how people and groups survived and adapted, through their foodways, to a new world in seventeenth and eighteenth-century Virginia. The two-hundred-year span of this study was an era when global cultures, through Britain's colonial project, were tossed together in particular places—locales where individuals and groups had to negotiate unconventional social orders and what for immigrants were alien environments. And yet these locales and their colonial inhabitants were not isolated. They lived at one point on the increasingly global map, engaged imaginatively and materially with peoples both near and far.

Undertaking a study of the historical development of colonial Virginia foodways, through a focus on one iconic preserved meat, requires a tacking back and forth between the local and the global. After a brief introduction to the food in question, addressing the nature of this ham as productive process, the stage will be set for exploring the historical development of this foodway. The first global aspect of this preserved meat foodway to be scrutinized will be those distinct food cultures that converged in the Chesapeake over the course of the colonial period—English (with broader European influences), Algonquian, and African (initially by way of the Caribbean). From this trans-Atlantic inquiry into those cultural approaches to meat preservation that were present in the colony, our attention shifts to the supremely local factors of climate, the environment, and colonial demographic and settlement patterning that impacted the development of particular foodways in this historic locale. Stepping back to the global, the international flows of key ingredients in meat preservation will be examined to understand why the particular preservation method embodied in Virginia ham persevered through the Revolutionary era. This wider perspective then focuses on another locale, that of the colonial metropole London, to understand the growth of an international demand for ham that not only fueled an emerging export market in this colonial food, but ensured its place on elite tables in Virginia, bringing us back to a conclusion in the local.

A mix of primary and secondary sources helps us understand Virginia ham as a colonial foodway. A reconstruction of the internalized subsistence and culinary toolkit of early English settlers, specifically pertaining to meat preservation, is based on the prescriptive literature on housewifery and husbandry potentially present in settlers' minds and on their shelves. Insight into how these practices and ideas transferred to the colony comes from primary colonial sources with pertinent food references. The line between primary and secondary sources is not always clear, as many primary narrative accounts, used here to understand the local conditions of colonial Virginia, are culled from later transcriptions. Indigenous meat preservation practices are teased from primary accounts, as seen through the lens of Englishmen using cognitive analogies to understand alien foodways in this newly settled land. The research of scholars of the African diaspora is employed to draw African-descended foodways into this globally constituted local picture.

True of all these cultures at the time of colonization, the treatment of food has generally been an oral tradition passed from one generation of cooks to another over the hearth and butcher block. Prescriptive texts, from receipt books to housewifery manuals, offered fashionable variations on familiar techniques and served as cultural ideals that may or may not have been subscribed to, whatever their popularity in print. The problems with using these English sources are only exacerbated when one considers the unique social and material landscapes and climate that confronted the English coming to live in seventeenth-century Virginia. The beauty of this space between distantly produced prescriptive ideal and local colonial reality is the opportunity it affords for observing a colonial process known as "creolization."

"Creolization," a process of trans-cultural practical improvisation, provides the analytical teeth for a more anthropologically informed approach to the historical development of foodways in a locale such as the colonial Chesapeake. The term "creole" has floated through colonial and post-colonial discourse for 500 years. Beginning with Iberian New World colonialism, and spreading to French and British contexts in the seventeenth century, this term came to designate those of Old World descent born in the New. It invoked a perceived modification of life forms necessarily changed by foreign soils and climates. Over time, the usage of "creole" began to slip closer to that of "mestizo," taking on a sense of the genetic and cultural mixing of peoples in the Americas (Stewart 2007, 7–8; Dawdy 2000).

Creolization, as the process implicit in "creole" divergence from parent stock, was first applied academically to the study of New World languages. From here, anthropologists of the Caribbean, focusing largely on African American cultures, took up the concept. The popularity of designating colonial items as "creole" has, however, risked grinding this concept's analytical teeth to nubs. The term, thus applied, can become mere definition, reducing history to stasis and concealing past social processes and ambiguities (Palmié 2006). Such has been the case with those under-theorized foods dubbed "creole" within the context of New Orleans and popular Louisiana cuisines (Gaudet 2003).

The application of creolization models to the study of colonial British North America is hardly a novelty. James Deetz and Leland Ferguson pioneered such work with their historical archaeologies of African American sites (Dawdy 2000). Moving from marginalized racial groups to socially dominant Anglo-Virginians, Carole Shammas explored the uses of pejorative "creole" designations on the part of a metropole judging its colonial subjects (1979). The inspiration for the present research comes, however, from L. Daniel Mouer's essay on the archaeology of colonial Virginia. Mouer boldly asserts a variety of proofs for the creolization of dominant white Virginian culture through exposure to native and African-descended traditions in the colonial Chesapeake. The material remains of Mouer's "Chesapeake Creoles" thus reveal to us those interactions between Europeans, Africans, and Native Americans that subsequent racial ideology and historiography strove to obliterate from local and national memory (Mouer 1993; Dawdy 2000; Joseph and Zierden 2002).

Moving beyond proofs of creolization in Virginia, my research argues for a model of creolization as local process. The key to such a study is to historicize and contextualize the creole phenomenon in question. I incorporate regional scholarship on local colonial demographics, ethnic compositions, and social structures—as well as antecedent food traditions—to thus deepen my analysis (Trouillot 2002; Chaudenson 2001). And so, while actual acts of creolization may evade our gaze, we are able to imagine the moments of creativity where redundancies and similarities cut across cultural boundaries as individuals negotiated new physical and social worlds—worlds nonetheless structured by harsh hierarchies of exclusion and domination (Price 2001; Gundaker 2000: 124–133; Brown 1996). The use of a creole analytic allows us to move beyond food as object to understand food as a manifestation of the social and cultural processes in play at the intersection of the local and global that was the colonial world.

VIRGINIA HAM AS COLONIAL FOODWAY

Norman G. Marriott and Herbert W. Ockerman, authors of a connoisseur's guide to America's country hams, cast Virginia's varietal as the progenitor of an American country ham-curing tradition seen throughout the South (2004). Ham-curing, as a form of meat preservation, represents man's effort to overcome the decay that sets in as soon as an animal is slaughtered. A brief entrée into the general logistics of meat preservation, including salting and smoking, provides insight into preserved meat as a foodway linking people and the environment. This emphasis highlights the impact of locality on the emergence of this culinary tradition. Some familiarity with those ingredients that enter into the curing process proves equally instrumental in understanding how the commerce and politics of empire have shaped the development of local colonial foodways.

In contrast to what passes for hams in most supermarkets and delis across America, country hams are rubbed with dry salt and allowed to sit for weeks in salt tubs as moisture is drawn out of muscle fiber. Both salting and smoking draw water out of freshly butchered meat, depriving microorganisms of the moist environment through which they render dead muscle tissue inedible. The cure mixture in which the hams sit can vary from salt alone to a mixture of salt, sugar, and saltpeter. Variations in cure content and ratio subtly affect the flavor and texture of the resulting meat.

In southeastern Virginia, hams are smoked to speed up drying and add flavor. Hardwoods such as hickory stoke low-burning smokehouse fires over which hang hams spaced far enough apart to allow smoke to engulf all exposed flesh. The specie of wood is critical, as softwoods deposit a resin during smoking that imparts a bitter flavor to the meat (Everett and Barham 1993: 4–5). While resin is undesirable, the formaldehyde deposited on a ham's surface in the smokehouse further retards the oxidation of fat that turns salted meat rancid (Lawrie 1985: 155–156). The end product of this process is a ham with a deep red color and extreme saltiness, especially to modern palates (Everett and Barham 1993: 5–6; Graham et al. 1998).

CUISINES COLLIDING: DISTINCT FOOD CULTURES IN COLONIAL VIRGINIA

Given that spoiling meat has always troubled omnivorous humans, the practices and ideas that different peoples have brought to the problem of meat preservation are many and diverse. In the colonial Chesapeake, society eventually settled on a foodway that produced an identifiable Virginia ham. Primary sources, including prescriptive food manuals and narrative accounts, attest to the knowledge bases from which English and native Algonquin men and women drew in preserving animal flesh in early colonial Tidewater Virginia. By contrast, those of African descent appear to have had less influence on the earliest preservation practices, as white landowners did not completely shift from indentured English servants to African slaves until the middle of the seventeenth century (Brown 1996: 114). By this time salted and smoked meat was already making its mark in local foodways.

By 1670, landowners were already erecting custom-made smokehouses specifically for ham production (Hodges 1993: 203). Similarly, preserved pork's potential as a trade good was already employed to entice members of England's lower social orders to the colony. Bacon's sale, it was advertised, could enable humbler men to earn a little pocket change to "woo a good man's daughter" and establish a family of their own in Virginia (Bullock 1649: 53). Preserved pork's local culinary significance was, nonetheless, reinforced by West African tastes and cooking practices (Shiflett 2004). Slaves coming from the Caribbean may also have brought the practice of *boucanage*—smoke-curing meat over wooden hurdles—with them to Virginia, adding yet more cultural force to the durability of this culinary practice in the multiethnic locale of the colonial Chesapeake (Chaudenson 2000: 229–230; Wilk 2006: 30).

Two preservation traditions appear in the Tudor and Stewart period English prescriptive literature held in the collections of Colonial Williamsburg's Rockefeller Library and the British Library. The earlier strain focuses on brining or potting, with air-drying an accepted additional step (Tusser [1573] 1593; Heresbach [1577] 1658; Dawson [1585] 1596; Partridge [1585] 1639; Anon. [1588] 1660; Platt 1594). Alongside these preservation techniques a tradition of chimney-smoked meats emerges, initially linked with Dutch or Westphalian methods (Platt [1602] 1615; Digby 1699; Wolley 1672; Price [1681] 1974). Hams, as a pork product distinct from bacon, appear in tandem with this imported smoking technique, bearing the French-derived designation gammon, anglicized into 'ham' only in the eighteenth century (W. M. 1658: 75; Wolley 1672: 172–174). There appears to be little evidence to support the contention that any particular smoking technique was inherently English at the time of initial colonization in Virginia. Furthermore, there is no evidence from this period for the erection of detached smokehouses on estates in England for the sole purpose of processing pork (Hodges 1993: 203).

If we turn to evidence of Algonquian meat preservation in the Chesapeake, we do see something of an indigenous meat smoking tradition. John Smith, in his 1612 *A Map of Virginia,* described Virginia Indians broiling fish and flesh on hurdles over the fire. Virginia Indians are also described as turning flesh on a spit, after the Spanish fashion, till it is "drie as jerkin beefe in the West Indies," keeping over a month without putrefying (Spencer 1982: 340). William Strachey, in 1612, provided the only early colonial description of a separate structure built by the Virginia Indians to preserve meat. The "scene or high stage" he noted was raised near the house—a scaffold covered in mats to form a shelter. Men sat and talked in such huts, where corn and fish was laid on hurdles to dry. Otherwise, meat was dressed in the single chambers that constituted native houses, where a continual fire was kept burning night and day (Haile 1998: 636–637, 684). So a tradition of smoked foods appeared on the ground in the Chesapeake from the very onset of English settlement there, although it was uniquely non-English in its initial manifestation.

Evidence for actual meat preservation practices among early English settlers in the colonial Chesapeake is scant. In his *General History* of 1624, John Smith recalled the 1608 case of a man purportedly powdering (salting) his wife to eat during the "Starving Time" (Haile 1998: 340). The contemporary employment of this preservation technique is further supported, though in less appalling circumstances, by Silvester Jourdain's account of the shipwreck of Virginia Company men on Bermuda in 1610. Here the ship's crew powdered (salted) hogs on the spot to victual the ship for its passage on to Jamestown (Spencer 1982: 329–330). All of these techniques conform to the earlier strain of English meat preservation practice.

Yet, by the late eighteenth century, a major shift is evident in settlers' preservation of meat, whereby Algonquian and Afro-Caribbean smoking techniques have been incorporated in step with continental European food traditions. Nicholas Cresswell noted, from 1774–1777, that hams in the region were rubbed with salt, sugar, and either saltpeter or hickory ash before being hung in a smokehouse over a slow, smoky fire of hickory. Later, in his *Journal of the War in America*, the Frenchman de Robertnier highlighted the separate smokehouses of Virginia, where salted pork was hung over a small fire for six weeks to attain its singular quality (Brandau 1984).

THE LOCAL CREOLE IMPERATIVE: NEW SOCIAL AND PHYSICAL CONTEXTS FOR COLONIAL FOODWAYS

As members of these global cultures converged on the Chesapeake, they were confronted with the reality of new social configurations set against a climate and environment that would pose a number of challenges to old practices, necessitating the mutual cultural improvisations that constitute a creolization of foodways (Oliver 2005).

Regional scholars have discussed at length the lack of social and demographic stability at Jamestown, immediately after the English arrival in 1607, as tied to colonists' inability to provision themselves adequately (Bowen and Andrews 2000; Brown 1996; Gleach 1997). Beyond quick material exchanges of provisions, extended interactions also took place between the Jamestown community and their Algonquian neighbors. One such relationship, critical to the colonists' survival, involved the Indians Kemps and Tassore being held in bondage to teach the English the proper ordering of fields for New World crops ([Strachey 1612] Haile 1998: 673). When conditions in the Jamestown fort became especially dire in 1608, men were dispersed among neighboring Indian villages to be "billeted amongst the savages, thus knowing all their passages, fields, habitations, how to gather and use their fruits as well as themselves" ([Smith 1624] Haile 1998: 322). Having eaten, on numerous occasions, the preserved meats of the Powhatan chiefdom, the colonists were now given a chance to observe and possibly practice native foodways in close quarters. This process of cultural exchange was still underway in the 1650s, when Colonel Norwood received instruction from an Indian "king" on how to dress venison over an open fire in the same fashion outlined by Smith earlier (Spencer 1982: 95).

A massive influx of European settlers over the course of the seventeenth century brought with it a measure of social and demographic stability to the English colony, though on a very different order than that of the Old World. High mortality rates remained a marked feature among Europeans in the seventeenth-century Chesapeake. A population of only 64,000 ushered in the eighteenth century from some 120,000 immigrants who made the journey to Virginia over the course of the preceding century. The sex ratio was also disproportionately male, and the postponement of marriage among female servants prevented the formation of nuclear households and further hindered the reproductive success of a population already "seasoned" by disease and climate (Horn 1994; Brown 1996).

The average immigrant during this first century of settlement was a middling yeoman, between the ages of 15 and 24. All-male households, with a notable lack of generational continuity or family life, were common (Spencer 1982: 55–61). While living conditions may have been strikingly similar to London or Bristol, whence many of the immigrants departed, colonial social units were scattered across the rural, riverine landscape of the Tidewater. Settlement and trade patterns in the early colonial Chesapeake remained non-conducive to the emergence of market towns, where ready-made provisions would otherwise have been on hand for males living without female domestic producers (Horn 1994; Tames 2003).

With men performing the duties of housewives and female servants in the Chesapeake, precisely how English foodways were transferred in the absence of traditional gender roles is an important consideration. While gender roles were not adhered to at all times in the Old World, English females were more likely to acquire male roles than vice versa (Brown 1996: 84). The gender hierarchy of the time, which placed women subordinate to men, meant that male servants were generally disinclined to perform work perceived as women's work (Brown 1996: 24–26, 84; Tames 2003: 50–51).

Another aspect distinguishing life and society in the Chesapeake from that of England was its multiethnic nature. While a differential racial hierarchy was ever-present in the minds of those resident in Virginia, such a barrier did not prevent intercultural exchange between the English, Algonquians, and enslaved Africans comprising the colonial population (Opie 2008; King 2002). The sex ratio imbalance among English settlers in the seventeenth century left early colonists dependent on trade and contact with Algonquians for food. Englishmen simply lacked sufficient females of their own stock to engage in gendered domestic production, including the dressing and preservation of meat (Gleach 1997; Brown 1996). Over the course of the eighteenth century, as the female settler population rose, the role of housewife in elite households was increasingly allocated to enslaved African women working in tandem with English servants. In such colonial contexts, intimacy and shared foodways went hand-in-hand with the elaborate dance of social and racial hierarchy that kept the master class at a safe cognitive distance from social inferiors (Sobel 1987; Brown 1996).

The advantage of this multiethnic local society lay in the diversity of cultural approaches to meat preservation that helped English colonists overcome local Chesapeake heat and humidity to ensure the prolonged edibility of their precious meats. English writers of the late-sixteenth century understood that the "contagion of weather" could spoil even the most thoroughly salted and barreled meat. The need for alternatives to standard English preservation techniques became an especially marked issue as England's mariners increasingly victualed themselves in tropical climates, where flesh was purported not to last 24 hours when traditionally preserved. Sir Hugh Platt's 1594 call for the prompt publishing of innovations and experiments in meat preservation alludes to this necessity. The problem in tropical latitudes was that flesh could not be made to take up salt in the traditional manner, owing to a putrefying heat and humidity that was only ever encountered during particularly unseasonable summers in England (Platt 1594: 8–9). The same problems pertained to the permanent settling of Virginia.

The heat and humidity of the Tidewater posed serious problems to early settlers. By 1610, when William Strachey arrived and made note of the conditions of Jamestown, settlers had already begun adapting their architecture along Algonquian lines to accommodate Virginia summers (Strachey [1610] 1998: 430). The higher temperatures and unpredictable fluctuations that typify Virginia's fall weather made dry-curing, as opposed to pickling, more favorable—as a government curing pamphlet advised farmers as late as 1917. The same holds for smoking, which would have further ensured the preservation of meat from fall slaughter through to summer consumption. The choice of pig flesh for preservation, in a climate so antithetical to meat's durability, stacked the odds in favor of colonists, as pork is high in saturated fat and, therefore, is somewhat slower to oxidize and spoil than the meat of other domesticated animals (Bowen 1990: 136).

The woodlands that covered colonial Virginia not only provided an ample source of hardwoods for smoking meats, they also provided the natural feed of those pigs whose hindquarters were destined to become the region's famed hams. As early as the 1620s, English husbandmen had made the connection between a pig's diet and the quality of its flesh. Gervase Markham noted that raising animals in woodlands or champion country produced the whitest, fattest, and best flesh (1625). John Lawson noted in 1709 that local pork in the Carolinas was better than any in Europe because of the variety and excellence of mast, or nuts, in the woods where Carolina pigs fed (Spencer 1982: 396). Bringing this issue home, a colonial tract from the mid-seventeenth century noted the favorable qualities of Virginia bacon, produced from the numerous pigs running free in the colony's woodland ([Wodenoth 1649] Spencer 1982: 347). Traditional English pannage, whereby hogs foraged freely in the woods for mast (Markham 1623/1625), became the dominant practice in the colonial Chesapeake. The woodlands produced ample acorns and tubers for pigs, while the marshes adjoining many rivers and creeks proved an equally rich source of food for livestock (Bowen 1996, 1999: 358–359; Bowen and Archer 2005).

A GLOBALLY REINFORCED LOCAL TRADITION

The locale in which the Virginia ham foodway was developing, at the intersection of a culturally diverse society and obdurate environment, was not isolated from the influence of global commercial politics and international fashion. The first of these broader-scale factors sheds light on the histories of the commodities that came together in the curing process, including salt, sugar, and saltpeter. These commodities influenced how meat was preserved, as fluctuations in supply pressured colonists to favor local creole practices.

The British colony in Virginia, like so many up and down the Atlantic coast of North America, was constantly in need of flesh-preserving salt. John Rolfe may have noted the establishment of a salt-works in the colony by 1616, but a 1621 Virginia Company dictum cites continued complaints of a local salt shortage in ordering the immediate establishment of this industry in the colony (Spencer 1982: 344–345). Virginia relied heavily on Liverpool salt to feed its small-scale fisheries and cottage salt-pork operations. And American salt production was routinely undercut by English imports, actions that eventually drove local salt-works out of business (Kurlansky 2002: 218–222).

With the Revolution, the salt crisis came to a head following shipping blockades by the British. The Continental Congress went so far as to subsidize salt-works, a vital force in provisioning the army with a steady supply of meat protein (Kurlansky 2002: 218–222). Even the *Virginia Gazette* lent its communicative might to rallying production of this critical commodity (Brandau 1984: 34–38). With such a tight supply of salt in Virginia, the employment of more frugal preservation techniques that incorporated smoking, as opposed to long-term storage in salt consuming pickles or powdering barrels, held considerable appeal.

Saltpeter made its debut in curing processes in the mid-seventeenth century (M.W. 1658). Saltpeter, the vernacular of potassium nitrate, extends the life of cured meats by retarding salt-tolerant microbial activity, as well as preserving original coloration (Lawrie 1985, 102–103). Saltpeter is also a main ingredient in gunpowder, a fact that contributed to its relative availability as a food preservative. While early modern England continued to rely on continental producers and traders for the bulk of its saltpeter, measures were taken by Tudor and Stuart monarchs to secure an independent source for this key munitions ingredient, contributing to the establishment of the East India Company in the mid-seventeenth century (Crocker 1999: 5–6). As with salt itself, saltpeter was in short supply during the American Revolution, being diverted to meet more pressing armament needs (Brandau 1984: 42–43).

Sugar followed saltpeter in the evolution of English curing practices. The reason for sugar's absence prior to the appearance of saltpeter is that its main function in the cure is to counter the harsh effects of the latter, which has a tendency to toughen meat (Ashbrook and Anthony 1917: 14–15). Matching the timing of sugar's appearance in English cures, the mid-seventeenth century was the period when Barbadian sugar plantations finally saw enough output to effect home markets in England (Mintz 1986: 37). Virginia invariably stood on the edge of this trade, however, being neither a sugar producer nor refiner.

The vagaries of global trade networks, subject as they were to political struggles, provided yet another inducement for the creolization of colonial Virginia's local meat preservation foodway. Colonial inhabitants had to make full use of the variety of food cultures and preservation traditions present in the colony to overcome supply-side uncertainties. And yet the popularity of Virginia ham as the choice of local and farther-flung Anglo elites was equally tied to international intellectual trends and changing culinary fashions emerging within Europe. During the seventeenth and eighteenth centuries the full spectrum of European culinary tastes were undergoing a transformation from the aromatic creations of the medieval to those more simplified flavors familiar to modern gastronomes (Schivelbusch 1992). This was, in effect, a culinary extension of the Renaissance penchant for seeking the European roots of culture in classical antiquity—an alimentary quest for antique antecedents. Among other writings, Renaissance men published compendia detailing the dietary habits of the ancients, affecting how European elites conceived of proper nutrition and the ordering of their own dining habits (Peterson 1994; Pinkard 2009; Albala 2009).

The meat of the humble pig garnered considerable culinary acclaim on the resurrected word of these ancients. Jean Bruyerin-Champier, sixteenth-century physician to the kings of France, praised the versatility of pork, whose fifty flavors the Roman historian Pliny was said to have touted. Conrad Gesner, a Swiss botanist and zoologist resident in sixteenth-century France, went so far as to chart antique cuts of meat, comparing these to what he saw in contemporary Swiss shops and homes (Peterson 1994: 90, 98). Such a fixation on Roman dietary habits helps contextualize the otherwise dubious lineage asserted by Conrad Heresbach for Westphalian hams as the "Celtick Gammons" praised by Strabo and Atheneus (1658: 283). Heresbach's statement mirrors that of Bruyerin-Champier, who traced the ancestry of the contemporary hams of Gaul to a favored delicacy in ancient Rome. The secret of these hams' production, the court physician claimed, had passed through the ages from Mainz into the environs of Bayonne in France (Peterson 1994: 139). Salted pork products, especially hams, thus became the province of a European gentry seeking to display its knowledge of current gastronomic fashion and theory as respected the wisdom of the ancients.

Although France might have witnessed the birth of a more modern palate, such tastes soon spread throughout Western Europe. The political turmoil of England in the seventeenth century provided a fertile ground for culinary borrowing. English courtiers and intellectuals followed the future Charles II to France during Cromwell's rule in the 1640s and 1650s, there gaining an intimate knowledge of new continental tastes. Robert May, Hannah Wolley, and Sir Kenelm Digby were just a few of the Restoration cooks, returning to England with the "restored" Stewart monarchy, to bring what they had learned in exile back to English readers through their published cookery books (Spencer 2002: 141–143, 159). The resulting culinary carry-overs were accentuated by the prestige attached to employing foreign cooks in English gentry households from the late seventeenth century onward (Wheaton 1983: 162–163).

By the turn of the eighteenth century the notoriety of hams from Mainz and Bayonne was well established in England. Ham shops, grocers, and cheesemongers populated the streets of London during the first half of the eighteenth century, purveying hams imported from these prized European regions (Peterson 1994: 139, 145). The timing of this specialized retail boom paralleled the proliferation in contemporaneous cookery books of attempts to imitate these imported luxury meats, some directed specifically to producing items for retail in metropolitan centers. And yet, as of 1750, the best flesh for curing hams for British luxury consumption was seen to come from the "wild" black hogs of Continental Europe and Virginia (Ellis [1750] 2000: 168). The superior-quality pork coming out of these regions was tied to these hogs' traditional woodland diets, whereas pigs were increasingly fed on industrial urban waste in England at this time (Thirsk 1990: 46–47).

Smoked hams were as highly valued an item in Virginia as they were in England and on the continent in the later eighteenth century. A 1770 inventory of the Governor's Palace in Williamsburg records a detached smokehouse, powdering tubs, and four purchased hams within the household of the governor. The high value of smoked meat products can even be seen in the anti theft devices built into period smokehouses. One technique was to turn one of a pair of hinges upside-down, ensuring that the smokehouse door could not simply be lifted from its hinges to access the precious commodities held therein (Brandau 1984: 54–55).

These hams were, as one might suspect from their lofty value, destined for local elite tables. Robert Beverly, in 1705, observed an emulative desire among Virginia's home-grown creole gentry to have their hospitable victuals dressed and served as nicely as those gracing the best tables in London (Spencer 1982: 387; Brown 1996: 271). The ubiquity of hams in elite recipe collections and on formal tables in Virginia attests to this food's role in a transnational culinary repertoire attuned to a taste for salt-acid flavors and preserved meats (Harbury 2004). A palate common to Europeans and Anglo-American colonials explains the praise lauded on Virginia hams by the Frenchmen de Robertnier and Rochambeau during the American Revolution (Brandau 1984: 54; Kurlansky 2002: 218). Virginia culture and foodways did not develop in a backwater cut off from European social trends. Virginia ham was simultaneously a local and global food—rooted in a particular landscape, but holding to allusions of international grandeur.

The road to an international trade in Virginia hams is hinted at in the provisioning of Continental Army troops with locally produced hams at the time of the American Revolution (Hörandner 1986: 56; Hatfield 2004; Kurlansky 2002: 218). The presence of those same cottage operations that provisioned the army, incorporating the labor of slaves and poorer white families (Spencer 1982: 379; Shiflett 2004: 72), no doubt contributed to the 1779 appearance of Capt. Mallory Todd in Smithfield, Virginia. In the midst of international conflict, Todd set up shop and was soon shipping hams to the Caribbean island of St. Eustatius. An in-depth study of this emerging industry, while laying beyond the scope of the present article, would be a rich and worthwhile vein to pursue in future research on Virginia ham.

CONCLUSION

While Virginia ham serves today to mark a particular food locality, its past reveals an intrinsically global, multicultural colonial and creole foodway. The production and consumption of Virginia ham was a knot that bound one end of the expansive social and political net of global colonialism that ever-increasingly drew together the peoples and cultures of the world for the sake of European profit and prestige. Migrating settlers, slaves, and native groups, encountering strange environments and new social orders, improvised through the sharing of foods and preparation techniques across seemingly impermeable barriers of race and identity. In the end it was this trans-cultural, trans-national, and trans-regional mobility of people, foodstuffs, and culinary knowledge that lay behind the perseverance of Europe's overseas colonial ventures.

The story of Virginia ham is so much more than a dry telling of the origins of a dry-cured meat. The tale of Virginia's ham serves as a most excellent lens through which to understand the intersection of the creolizing local and homogenizing global in global foodways. This begins with the intensely local and "creole" (i.e., "born in the colonies") nature of colonial food products—tied, as they must be, to the people and land that have given them form. And yet the forces that combined to produce the locality of Virginia's Tidewater were global from the region's very inception as colonial venture. To complicate the picture even more, the creole (as in culturally mixed) origins of Virginia's ham were effaced as local Virginia elite strove to regain a sense of ethnic identification with their distant British homeland through acts of emulative consumption, whether at private feasts or in the more public Williamsburg coffeehouse (Brown 1996; Stewart 2007: 19; Bowen, personal communication). Elite tastes across the Atlantic thus held sway over the growing renown of a food whose origins lay in the improvised creolization of local colonial foodways.

ACKNOWLEDGMENTS

Many thanks to Dr. Joanne Bowen, of the Colonial Williamsburg Foundation, and Dr. Audrey Horning, then of the College of William and Mary, for their enthusiasm and guidance in approaching this research. The collections and librarians at the CWF Rockefeller Library and British Library were indispensable. I must also thank Mr. Frank Batten, whose grant enabled my research in London. Thank you, again, to Carolyn de la Peña and Benjamin Lawrance for coordinating the *Tasting Histories* conference and providing such fruitful comments in their effort to hone the interpretive edges of this paper. And thank you to the Lichtstern Student Travel Fund at the University of Chicago for enabling travel to this wonderful meeting. Finally, I wish to dedicate this article to the memory of my dearly departed grandmother, Alethea Cheney Serpell Patrick Edwards—a Virginian to the end, who always held a place in her heart for country ham and a highball.

REFERENCES

Primary Sources

Anon. 1597. *A new book of cookery. The good huswiues handmaid for cookerie in her kitchen in dressing all manner of meat, with ither wholsom diet for her and her houshold, etc.* London: E. Allde.

Anon. 1576. *A Proper New Booke of Cookery. Declaring What Maner of Meates Be Best in Season for Al Times of the Yeere, and How They Ought to Be Dressed.* London: Antony Kytson.

Anon. 1588. *The Good Hous-wiues Treasurie.* London: Edward Allde.

Ashbrook, F. G., and G. A. Anthony. 1917. *U. S. Farmers' Bulletin 913: Killing Hogs and Curing Pork. Department of Agriculture.* Washington, DC: Government Printing Office.

Boss, Andrew. 1903. *Farmers' Bulletin No. 183: Meat on the Farm: Butchering, Curing, and Keeping.* U.S. Department of Agriculture. Washington, DC: Government Printing Office.

Bullock, William, Gent. 1649. *Virginia Impartially Examined, and left to publick view, to be considered by all judicious and honest men ...* London: John Hammond.

Dawson, Thomas. 1596. *The good huswifes Iewell.* London: Edward White.

Digby, Sir Kenelm. 1699. *The Closet of the Eminently Learned Sir Kenelm Digby Kt opened ... Published by his son's consent.* London: EC for H Brome.

Dodoens, Rembert. 1606. *Rams Little Dodeon. A Briefe Epitome of the New Herball.* London: W. Ram.

Ellis, William. 2000. *The Country Housewife's Family Companion.* Facsimile of 1750 ed. Totnes, Devon: Prospect Books.

Fitzherbert, John. 1562. *The Boke of Husbandrye Verye Profitable and Necessarye for Al Manner of Persons.* London: John Awdely.

Glasse, Hannah. 1995. *The Art of Cookery, Made Plain and Easy.* Totnes, Devon: Prospect Books.

Haile, Edward Wright. 1998. *Jamestown Narratives.* Champlain, VA: RoundHouse.

Hartlib, Samuel. 1658. *The Compleat Husband-man; or, a Discourse on the whole art of husbandry; both forraign and domestick, etc.* London: Edward Brewster.

Heresbach, Conrad. 1658. *The Perfect Husbandman or the Art of Husbandry in four Books by CH, BC, and CM.* London.

Hess, Karen. 1981. *Martha Washington's Booke of Cookery ... copied by and unknown hand sometime in the Seventeenth-century.* New York: Columbia University Press.

M., W. 1658. *The Compleat Cook. Expertly prescribing the most ready wayes, whether Italian, Spanish, or French, for dressing of flesh and fish etc.* London: for Nathaniel Brooks.

Markham, Gervase. 1625. *A Way to Get Wealth, by the Approved Rules of Practice in Good Husbandry and Huswiferie.* London: for Roger Iackson.

Partridge, J. 1639. *The Widowes treasure.*

Partridge, John. 1584. *The treasurie of commodius conceits and hidden secrets. Commonly called, The Good Huswives Closet of provision for the health of her houshold.* London: Richard Jhones.

Platt, H. 1615. *Delights for Ladies, to adorne Their Persons, and Tables, Closets, and Distillatories: With Beauties, Banquets, Perfumes, and Waters.* London: by HL for A Johnson.

Platt, Sir Hugh. 1594. *The Jewell House of Art and Nature.* London: Peter Short.

Price, Rebecca. 1974 [1681]. *The Compleat Cook: or Secrets of a Seventeenth-Century Houaewife.* 1681 manuscript compiled by Madeleine Masson. Researched by Anthony Vaughan. London: Routledge and Kegan Paul.

Randolph, Mary. 1984 [1824]. *The Virginia Housewife*. Facsimile of 1824 ed., with addition of text from 1825 and 1828 eds. Compiled by Karen Hess. Columbia, SC: University of South Carolina Press.

Spencer, Maryellen. 1982. "Food in Seventeenth-Century Tidewater Virginia: A Method for Studying Historical Cuisines." Ph.D. diss., Virginia Tech.

Tusser, Thomas. 1593. *Fiue Hundreth Pointes of Good Husbandrie, as well for the champion or Open Countrie, as also for the woodland or severall*. London: R. Yardley & P. Short.

U. S. Department of Agriculture. 1949. *Farmers' Bulletin No. 1186: Pork on the Farm: Killing, Curing, and Canning*. Washington, DC: U.S. Government Printing Office.

Wolley, Hannah. 1672. *The Ladies Delight: Or a rich closet if choice experiments and curiosities*. London: T. Milbourn for N. Crouch.

Worlidge, John. 1669. *Systema Agriculturae; the mystery of husbandry discovered. To which is added, Kalendarium rusticum; or the Husbandman's monethly directions*. London: J.W. Gent.

Secondary Sources

Albala, Ken. 2009. History on the Plate: The Current State of Food History. *Historically Speaking* 10, 6–8.

Bowen, Joanne. 1991. "The Zooarchaeologist's View of the Importance of Pork in the Southern Diet." Unpublished paper presented at SHA Conference in Richmond, Virginia. Colonial Williamsburg Foundation.

———. 1996. Foodways in the 18th-century Chesapeake. In *The Archaeology of 18th-century Virginia*. Theodore R. Reinhart, ed. Richmond: Archaeological Society of Virginia.

———. 1999. The Chesapeake Landscape and the Ecology of Animal Husbandry. In *Old and New Worlds*. Geoff Egan and R. L. Michael, eds. London: Oxbow Books.

———. 1990. "A Study of Seasonality and Subsistence: Eighteenth Century Suffield, Connecticut." Ph.D. diss., Brown University.

Bowen, Joanne, and Susan T. Andrews. 2000. "The starving time at Jamestown: Faunal analysis of pit 1, pit 3, the bulwark ditch, ditch 6, ditch 7, and midden 1, James City County, Virginia." Report submitted to: William M. Kelso, Jamestown Rediscovery, Association for the Preservation of Virginia Antiquities, October.

Bowen, Joanne and Steve Archer. 2005. "Towards an Archaeological Understanding of the Changing Landscape Ecology of Tidewater Virginia's Plantation System," unpublished paper presented at SHA Conference in York, England.

Brandau, Rosemary. 1984. "The Butchering and Processing of Pork in Eighteenth Century Williamsburg." Paper for Colonial Williamsburg Foundation, August.

Brown, Kathleen M. 1996. *Good Wives, Nasty Wenches, and Anxious Patriarchs: Gender, Race, and Power in Colonial Virginia*. Chapel Hill, NC: University of North Carolina Press.

Chaudenson, Robert. 2001. *Creolization of Language and Culture*. New York: Routledge.

Crocker, Glenys. 1999. *The Gunpowder Industry*. Princes Risborough, Buckinghamshire: Shire Publications.

Dawdy, Shannon L. 2000. "Preface" and "Understanding Cultural Change Through the Vernacular: Creolization in Louisiana" *Historical Archaeology* 34(3), 1–4, 107–123.

Everett, Marion G., and Patsy D. Barham. 1993. *A History of the Smithfield Ham Industry*. Smithfield, VA: Isle of Wight County Museum.

Fishwick, Marshall. 1964. Southern Cooking. In *American Heritage Cookbook & Illustrated History of American Eating and Drinking*. New York: Simon and Schuster.

Gaudet, Marcia. 2003. "Mardi Gras, Gumbo, and Zydeco: An Introduction to Louisiana Culture" and "Is It Cajun, or Is It Creole?" In M. Gaudet and J.C. McDonald (eds.) *Mardi Gras, Gumbo, and Zydeco. Readings in Louisiana Culture*. Jackson, MS: University Press of Mississippi, vii–xvi, 150–153.

Gleach, Frederic W. 1997. *Powhatan's World and Colonial Virginia: A Conflict of Cultures*. Lincoln, NE: The University of Nebraska Press.

Graham, Paul P, N. G. Marriott, and R. F. Kelly. 1998. "Dry-Curing Virginia Style Ham." Virginia Cooperative Extension. Blacksburg, VA: Virginia Tech.

Gundaker, Grey. 2000. "Discussion: Creolization, Complexity, and Time," in *Historical Archaeology* 34(3): 124–133.

Hatfield, April L. 2004. *Atlantic Virginia: Intercolonial Relations in the Seventeenth Century*. Philadelphia: University of Pennsylvania Press.

Hodges, Charles T. 1993. Private Fortifications in 17th-century Virginia: A Study of Six Representative Works. In T. R. Reinhart and D. J. Pogue (eds.) *The Archaeology of 17th-century Virginia*. Richmond, VA: The Dietz Press.

Hörandner, Edith. 1986. Storing and Preserving Meat in Europe: A Historical Survey. In *Food in Change: Eating Habits From the Middle Ages to the Present Day*. Alexander Fenton and Eszter Kisbán, eds. Edinburgh: National Museums of Scotland.

Horn, James. 1994. *Adapting to a New World: English Culture in the Seventeenth-Century Chesapeake*. Chapel Hill, NC: University of North Carolina Press.

Joseph, J. W., and Martha Zierden. 2002. Cultural Diversity in the Southern Colonies. In J.W. Joseph and M. Zierden (eds.) *Another's Country: Archaeological and Historical Perspectives on Cultural Interactions in the Southern Colonies*. Tuscaloosa: University of Alabama Press, 1–12.

King, Julia A. 2002. "Foreword" to J. W. Joseph and M. Zierden (eds.) *Another's Country: Archaeological and Historical Perspectives on Cultural Interactions in the Southern Colonies*. Tuscaloosa: University of Alabama Press, xiii–xvii.

Kurlansky, Mark. 2002. *Salt: A World History*. New York: Walker and Co.

Lawrie, R. A. 1985. *Meat Science*. 4th ed. New York: Pergamon Press.

Marriott, Norman G., and Herbert W. Ockerman. 2004. *The Ultimate Guide to Country Ham: An American Delicacy*. Deborah G. Lowery, ed. Radford, VA: Brightside Press.

Mintz, Sidney W. 1986. *Sweetness and Power: The Place of Sugar in Modern History*. New York: Penguin Books.

Mouer, L. Daniel. 1993. "Chesapeake Creoles: The Creation of Folk Culture in Colonial Virginia." In *The Archaeology of 17th-century Virginia*. Theodore R. Reinhart, ed. Richmond: Archaeological Society of Virginia.

Oliver, Sandra L. 2005. *Food in Colonial and Federal America*. Westport, CT: Greenwood Press.

Opie, Frederick Douglass. 2008. *Hog and Hominy: Soul Food From Africa to America*. New York: Columbia University Press.

Palmié, Stephan. 2006. Creolization and its discontents. *Annual Review of Anthropology* 35, 433–456.

———. 2007. "The 'C-word' Again: From Colonial to Post Colonial Semantics" in C. Stewart (ed.) *Creolization: history, ethnography, theory*. Walnut Creek, CA: Left Coast Press, 66–83.

Peterson, T. Sarah. 1994. *Acquired Taste: The French Origins of Modern Cooking*. Ithaca, NY: Cornell University Press.

Pinkard, Susan. 2009. *A Revolution in Taste: The Rise of French Cuisine, 1650–1800*. New York: Cambridge University Press.

Price, Richard. 2001. The miracle of Creolization: A retrospective. *New West Indian Guide* 75(1–2), 35–64.

Shammas, Carole. 1979. "English-Born and Creole Elites in Turn-of-the-Century Virginia" in T. W. Tate and D. L. Ammerman (eds.) *The Chesapeake in the Seventeenth Century*. Chapel Hill, NC: University of North Carolina Press, 274–296.

Shiflett, Lisa R. 2004. "West African Food Traditions in Virginia Foodways: A Historical Analysis of Origins and Survivals." MA thesis, East Tennessee State University.

Sobel, Mechal. 1987. *The World They Made Together: Black and White Values in Eighteenth-Century Virginia*. Princeton, NJ: Princeton University Press.

Spencer, Colin. 2002. *British Food: An Extraordinary Thousand Years of History*. London: Grub Street.

Stewart, Charles. 2007. "Creolization: History, Ethnography, Theory" in C. Stewart (ed.) *Creolization: History, Ethnography, Theory*. Walnut Creek, CA: Left Coast Press, 1–25.

Tames, Richard. 2003. *Feeding London: A Taste of History*. London: Historical Publications.

Thirsk, Joan, ed. 1990. *Agricultural Change: Policy and Practice, 1500–1750*. New York: Cambridge University Press.

———. 2000. *The English Rural Landscape*. New York: Oxford University Press.

Trouillot, Michel-Rolph. 2002. "Culture on the Edges: Caribbean Creolization in Historical Context" in B.K. Axel (ed.) *From the Margins: Historical Anthropology and Its Futures*. Durham, NC: Duke University Press, 189–210.

Wheaton, Barbara K. 1983. *Savoring the Past: The French Kitchen and Table From 1300 to 1789*. Philadelphia: University of Pennsylvania Press.

———. 1991. *"Waste Not, Want Not": Food Preservation from Early Times to the Present Day*. Edinburgh: Edinburgh University Press.

Wilk, Richard. 2006. *Home Cooking in the Global Village: Caribbean Food From Buccaneers to Ecotourists*. New York: Berg.

Making White Bread by the Bomb's Early Light: Anxiety, Abundance, and Industrial Food Power in the Early Cold War

AARON BOBROW-STRAIN

Associate Professor of Politics, Whitman College, Walla Walla, Washington, USA

This article explores U.S. policymakers and consumers' engagements with global bread politics in the early Cold War. This provides a glimpse into the making of a particular form of postwar "American alimentary exceptionalism" premised on the universal choiceworthiness of industrial foodways. This alimentary exceptionalism did not assume that the U.S. industrial diet was gastronomically superior to other countries' diets, but rather that it offered a unique foundation of strength, stability, choice, and abundance on which world peace could rest in the uncertain postwar world. Thus, the article contends that Americans' confidence in industrial foodways and industrial food production systems—something whose legacies we still grapple with today—was forged, in part, on the imperial landscape of Cold War competition. In that sense, the article traces the largely unexamined flipside of postwar food imperialism: how the exercise of food power abroad shaped Americans' understandings of their own diet and its place in the world.

"The U.S. is not loved or hated because it is a citadel of political liberty ... [it is] measured by its ability and willingness to contribute from its own comfortable fat to strengthen Europe's shivering frame.... At the moment the tendency [in Europe] is to judge the United States rather severely and to make allowances for Soviet Russia ... *[but] bread comes from America and it does not come from Russia.*"

—Hamilton Fish, 1947

"Bread: It Is the First Concern of a Hungry World. Trouble Looms for the Nations Which Cannot Provide it."

—*Los Angeles Times* headline, August 10, 1947

"WHERE IS THE WHITE BREAD?"

After six weeks of fierce fighting for Sicily in the summer of 1943, Allied forces established their first occupation government in former Axis territory. Quick victory in Sicily would help turn the tide of the European war, but the question on the minds of many of the island's half-starved residents was far more quotidian: "In many a liberated town," *Time* magazine reported, "the first question asked was: 'Where is the white bread?'"[1] The war's end was still years away, but *Time's* focus on hungry Sicilians' demands offered a glimpse into how the United States would see itself in the postwar world—a world that seemed to clamor desperately for bread that only America could provide.

This article explores U.S. policymakers and consumers' engagements with global bread politics during the early Cold War. It does that with an eye toward understanding the making of a particular form of "American alimentary exceptionalism" premised on the universal choiceworthiness of industrial foodways.[2] This alimentary exceptionalism did not assume that the U.S. industrial diet was gastronomically superior to other countries' diets, but rather that it offered a unique foundation of strength, stability, choice, and abundance on which world peace could rest in the uncertain postwar world.

During World War II, homefront food production and everyday dietary choices had been explicitly enlisted in U.S. national defense efforts. Diet, patriotism, and military readiness had become inextricably linked, as Amy Bentley masterfully shows in *Eating for Victory: Food Rationing and the Politics of Domesticity*.[3] With victories in Europe and Asia, however, American kitchens appeared to demobilize. In Amy Drake McFeely's words, "Relieved of their pseudo-military roles, women embraced new assignments as consumers ... With sugared words and pictures, the ads reminded the public once again that abundance is at the core of the American dream. The war in the kitchen was over."[4]

Or had it simply taken on new forms? A growing number of scholars have begun to note how Cold War propaganda explicitly mobilized "the American kitchen"—with its shining new appliances, sleek lines, and dazzling surfaces—"as an icon of the Western way of life."[5] But what about American food itself? To what extent was America's burgeoning taste for abundant industrial food linked to what Daniel Yergin, in his classic history of the early Cold War, called the country's newfound commitment to "permanent military readiness"?[6]

That question place this article in conversation with debates about the United States' exercise of "food power" during the Cold War. For decades, a well-developed line of scholarship has shown how the United States's postwar projection of food power abroad through food aid and technology transfer constituted a form of cultural, economic, and dietary imperialism.[7] Not surprisingly, debates about these alimentary projections have largely centered on the nature of their impact abroad; how they affected the culture, diets, and livelihoods of people outside the United States. This is an important subject, but *not* this article's focus.

Instead, this article explores the largely unexamined flipside of postwar food imperialism: how the exercise of food power abroad during the early Cold War shaped Americans' understandings of their diet and its place in the world. It argues that Americans' strong confidence in the choiceworthiness of its industrial foodways and industrial food production system—something whose legacies we still grapple with today—were forged, in part, on the imperial landscape of Cold War competition.

The United States's alimentary imperialism and its faith in industrial food both pre-date the Cold War,[8] but this article contends that they took on a new form in era of superpower competition.[9] In the end, Cold War practices of food aid, reconstruction, and propaganda reinforced a particular kind of American alimentary exceptionalism—one less explicitly racialized than previous versions, and more grounded in ideologies connecting consumer abundance to global stability.

This fusing of industrial foodways with the imperatives of national security instilled a particular, narrow vision of "good food" with geopolitical urgency (and marginalized alternative visions). More than a half-century later, even as critiques of industrial foodways mount from all directions, this urgency has not disappeared. Indeed, it energizes key attempts to defend industrial food production against proponents of slow, local, and organic eating.[10] By placing American industrial foodways in a Cold War context, this article reminds us that, even when couched in the language of humanitarianism and world peace, the present-day eliding of industrial food production and global security by authors such as James McWilliams or Nina Federoff normalizes a state of emergency in which the enormous social, economic, environmental, and health costs of industrial must be accepted without question or critique.[11]

ANXIETY AND ABUNDANCE: COLD WAR CULTURAL POLITICS AND U.S. FOODWAYS

The argument introduced above owes a debt to feminist food historians who first framed postwar foodways as *political*—a site of struggle over household gender relations, constructions of masculinity and femininity, and the meanings of domesticity in a nation of industrial power.[12] This article builds on those insights by placing household- and national-level food politics in global relief. It suggests that our understanding of the role domestic discourses of "healthiness," "abundance," "choice," "newness," and even "convenience," played in shaping postwar foodways will benefit by being brought into conversation with global Cold War history.

This, in turn, inserts the article into a larger engagement with Cold War cultural history—particularly debates over whether and how anxieties about global conflict affected ordinary Americans immersed in postwar celebrations of consumer abundance. Cold War historians have long traced the ways that concerns about global superpower conflict reinjected values of military readiness and competitive toughness into many arenas of everyday life, including constructions of masculinity, child rearing practices, popular fiction, Hollywood films, and Broadway musicals.[13] Although it has received less attention than other areas of Cold War popular culture, it seems likely that American foodways were shaped by those same anxieties. At the same time, however, historians have also begun to warn against ascribing too much agency to Cold War anxieties. During the late 1940s and early 1950s, the argument runs, Americans may have worried about their country's ability to compete with Communists, but they also had a lot of other things on their minds. As Leo Ribuffo suggests, "Documentary filmmakers who retrospectively cherish images of suburban school children ducking under their desks during air raid drills should also show them rushing Good Humor trucks to buy ice-cream cones."[14]

This article takes a different tack in its approach to the question of anxiety and consumption. By placing U.S. foodways—specifically, the taste for industrially processed bread—in their larger geopolitical context, it blurs implicit divides between anxious thoughts of military readiness and joyful celebrations of consumer abundance. While McFeely and Ribuffo's points are well taken, this article suggests that duck and cover drills and Good Humor bars were not as different as we might think. Fueled by the successes of postwar food relief, an explosion of new convenience foods, and the messages of Cold War propaganda, celebrations of American alimentary abundance at home and abroad provided a reassurance at a time when the country seemed to be falling behind the Soviets in many other arenas. Wonder Bread might not have tasted as good as French baguettes or contained the natural nutrients of Soviet "black bread," as many consumers readily acknowledged, but, unlike those other breads, they were fortified, plentiful, and cheap—and world peace seemed to depend on them.

Located at the nexus of cultural and geopolitical history, this article deploys a diverse set of sources ranging from women's magazines, domestic advice columns, advertising, and popular food writing to the records of the Foreign Agriculture Service (FAS), U.S. Information Agency (USIA), and Supreme Commander of the Allies in the Pacific Japanese Occupation Authorities (SCAP). The article proceeds as follows: First, it places postwar breadways in the historical context of ongoing struggles over industrially produced loaves. The next two sections examine the European food crisis of 1946–1948 and early 1950s anti-Soviet propaganda, respectively, showing how American bread, industrially farmed wheat, and other modern convenience foods came to be seen as critical elements in the fight against Communism. Finally, two more case studies—efforts to convert Japanese diets from rice to wheat and the mid-1950s craze for French bread—illustrate sites of uncertainty and struggle over the universal choiceworthiness of U.S. foodways. In both cases, policy makers, tastemakers, and ordinary consumers found their confidence in the universal choiceworthiness of American industrial foodways challenged by alien diets. In many ways these global encounters ultimately reinforced assumptions about the superiority of U.S industrial bread, but they also exposed cracks in the architecture of alimentary exceptionalism, creating space for the resurfacing of long-held doubts about the meaning of industrial bread. Not coincidentally, by the late 1960s, "natural" Asian diets and "authentic" French food would emerge as important icons of resistance to American industrial food (and the imperial politics it seemed to represent). And industrial white bread would emerge as a leading icon of all that was wrong with *Amerika*.[15]

INDUSTRIAL BREAD AND ITS DISCONTENTS

In 1890, ninety percent of American bread was baked in homes by women, and the country's few commercial bread bakeries were nearly all tiny one-oven shops with a few employees serving urban neighborhoods. Less than forty years later, this had changed dramatically: in 1930, ninety percent of the country's bread was baked outside the home by men in increasingly distant factories, neighborhood bakeries were in decline, and bread had begun to take on the form in which we know it today—a standardized, homogenous product of food science and assembly line manufacture. From the beginning, however, this revolutionary process of industrialization came accompanied by virulent protests from diverse quarters.[16]

From the 1910s to the 1930s, anyone reading women's magazines, health newsletters, domestic advice columns, or listening to popular radio programs could not have escaped an overwhelming sense that the country's new staff of life was broken. "The whiter your bread, the quicker you're dead," Dr. Clark jingled on his Home Health Hour radio show, while other prominent food gurus accused industrial bread of contributing to, among other ills, anemia, cancer, diabetes, blood poisoning, criminal tendencies, tuberculosis, polyneuritis, neurasthenia, gout, bursal rheumatism, tooth decay, liver disease, kidney failure, overstimulated nervous systems, physical disfigurement, and acidosis.[17]

During World War II, highly successful campaigns to synthetically enrich industrial bread and train consumers about the value of vitamin-charged loaves silenced most of this criticism. Industrial bread was, once again, seen as vital and strong—a weapon of national defense. While, many of industrial bread's most prominent critics disliked synthetic enrichment, they reluctantly rallied to the cause in the name of wartime expediency.[18] By the late 1940s, however, they once again felt free to vent.

In fact, even during the industrially infatuated 1950s, it would have been difficult to find anything positive written about industrial bread's flavor or texture in venues ranging from women's magazines to newspaper food columns. It was "cottony fluff," "cotton batting," "fake," "purposeless perfection," "inedible," "limp," and "hot air." Consumers, for their part, echoed many of these concerns. In the largest multiyear study of American bread habits ever, a third of respondents described supermarket bread as "doughy; gummy; soggy; not well baked," about 15 percent thought the taste was terrible, and as much as eighteen percent thought it too airy. Only about a third to a quarter (depending on the year of the study) could find nothing in their bread flavor or texture to complain about. Importantly, however, the one thing consumers *could* agree on was that their bread was good for them. With the memory of wartime enrichment campaigns still fresh in their minds, 96–100 percent of respondents believed industrial bread had the nutritional strength to build strong bodies.[19]

Whether they liked it or not, in the late 1940s and early 1950s, Americans ate a lot of industrial bread—even though, with rising prosperity, the end of wartime shortages, and the dawning of a new age of techno-food marvels, they had many other options; perhaps more options than any group of eaters in history up to that point. But the vast majority of households in the United States ate store-bought white bread at all three meals—totaling some 8.6 billion loaves a year in 1954 (not including home-baked bread, and store-bought whole wheat, raisin bread, and "ethnic" breads). According to another study 98.8 percent of the country ate bread daily. Most people consumed 3–7 slices a day, but an astounding 33 percent of the population finished off more than 8 slices a day. And this level of bread consumption cut across class: while the wealthiest 10 percent of the country consumed bread in slightly smaller quantities, the remaining nine income deciles varied little in their daily intake. Age seem to matter either: adults and children ate bread at exactly the same rate. Only gender seemed to differentiate bread eaters: women, forbidden the staff of life by many popular diets of the time ate the least, while men and boys, associating bread with body-building strength, ate the most.[20]

During World War II, bread consumption, driven by the rationing of other staples, accounted for as much as 40 percent of all calories consumed in the country daily. After the war, Americans could have abandoned bread, just as they traded Victory Gardens for backyard barbecues. Instead, the proportion of calories derived from bread settled in at 25–30 percent and then, despite the absolute certainty with which food economists and baking industry specialists predicted rapid declines in consumption, hovered around the same point for the 1950s. Studies remarked at the high percentage of daily vitamins, iron, and protein consumers derived from the much-derided staff of life.[21]

Why did postwar consumers continued to eat so much industrial bread, despite widespread popular condemnation of its flavor and texture? The answer wasn't that consumers lacked options. Americans could have abandoned bread as a staple, or purchased breads other than industrial white. They didn't. When, from time to time, big baking companies attempted to launch lines of whole wheat bread, they invariably fell flat. And, despite the continued survival of small specialty bakeries, especially in cities, rye, whole wheat, and other "ethnic" loaves offered little competition, accounting for only 8–12 percent of bread consumption during the postwar period. Likewise, convenience and habit can't entirely explain bread's salience. As marketing experts discovered convenience and habit ranked low in consumers' reasons for buying bread, while quality, value, and nutrition topped the list.[22]

So why *did* postwar America uniformly stick to gummy bread, at least across class and age lines? A complete answer to that question is beyond the scope of this article. Instead it focuses on one unexamined element: the way that American industrial bread's place in Cold War politics created a metric with which consumers could compare their limp, fluffy, and much-derided bread positively to the world's dense, hearty loaves.

IF BREAD DOESN'T COME, BOMBS WILL

During the winter of 1945–1946, while the United States celebrated peace by consuming 3,000 calories a day per person and singing "Let it snow! Let it snow! Let it snow!" with Vaughn Monroe, severe weather nearly destroyed Europe's entire bread grains crop. Historic drought that summer followed by another bad winter finished the job. In a region where most people got 40–55 percent of their daily calories from bread, nearly 125 million European faced starvation.[23] Bread riots rocked France, which had seen its worst wheat harvest in 132 years. Italy's flour stocks dwindled and Britain reported that its bread situation was worse than the darkest days of the war. Wheat stocks were so low in the UK that government officials were forced to extend and deepen wartime bread rationing, despite fierce popular opposition. Winston Churchill called the decision, "One of the gravest announcements [he] had ever heard in the House in a time of peace."[24] Things looked even less promising in Asia. China faced a massive rice crisis, famine gripped Korea, and millions of conquered Japanese survived on 520 calories per day. In total, the United States estimated, 500 million people—1 in 5 people on the planet—faced famine conditions between 1946–1948.

Some relief supplies shipped to Asia, but for racial and geopolitical reasons, Truman and the country's attention was riveted on Europe. Mobilizing his bully pulpit, grain exporters' eagerness to exploit new markets, and almost every Liberty ship in the U.S. Navy, Truman mobilized the largest movement of wheat and flour in world history—almost 900 million bushels between 1946 and 1947; enough to bake, conservatively, 70 billion loaves of white bread.

The United States's role as the postwar world's most important source of bread did not take policymakers by surprise. Even before Pearl Harbor, military strategists commonly argued that food "would win the war and write the peace," and agriculture officials planned for that peace even as they mobilized to fight. Most importantly, they wanted to make sure that the country avoided a devastating rural recession like the one triggered after World War I, when war stimulated grain production collided with a large postwar drop in demand for U.S. wheat. This time around, the country would use its agricultural advantage strategically, killing two birds with one stone: supporting farmers at home while projecting food power into the uncertain political terrain of the future. What surprised the Truman administration was not the fact that the United States survived the war as the only power in the world with its agricultural system not only unscathed, but in peak form—the most important player in the world food system. What shook Washington was just how quickly and forcefully this role thrust itself on the country.

To free up wheat for the world, Truman called on the country to voluntarily conserve bread, prohibited the use of wheat in alcohol production, and mandated a higher extraction rate for white flour.[25] When Americans complained about the new, supposedly "gray" high-extraction loaves,[26] Truman scolded them, saying that not getting "exactly the kind of bread that [you] prefer" was a tiny price to pay for saving lives and establishing lasting peace.[27] Publications such as *Life, Look, Parents' Magazine, Time,* and *American Home* backed the president, running heart-wrenching stories of hunger in Europe and offering readers advice on how to conserve wheat. Thousands of women signed pledges to conserve bread in their households, and food magazines went back on war footing, publishing tips and recipes for saving bread.

While Americans felt generally sympathetic toward humanitarian efforts to help allies and even former enemies in Europe, public support for wheat conservation, high-extraction loaves, and possible bread rations was short-lived.[28] Letters to newspaper editors reveal widespread skepticism about Americans' willingness to suffer bread restrictions for altruistic reasons. Instead, humanitarian concern for "starving European children" segued into self-interested thinking about wheat exports and national security. As *Consumers' Guide* assured readers, American bread "cast upon the waters" would return, "in the form of preventing a generation of rickety European children from growing into a sickly, embittered, and grasping people bent on war. It will, in other words, return to us in the form of the better chances of peace and security in our own homes which only a healthy and peaceful Europe can assure."[29]

An August 10, 1947 article in the *Los Angeles Times* summed up the new attitude in the headline, "Bread: it is the first concern of a hungry world. Trouble looms for the nations that can't provide it." If bread doesn't come, the article continued, "bombs—in one form or another—will." The *Farm Journal*, which, granted, had its own interest in food exports, put the matter bluntly, "better to win friends now with flour, than have to face their guns later." "Baukhage," a nationally syndicated D.C. pundit and popular radio personality, made the case even more explicit in his Associated Press column: "The history of Europe since the war is that every government fall when the bread ration is reduced ... The free world is at stake." The only thing that can "save Europe for democracy," he continued, is "the American farmer."[30]

The news from France appeared particularly grave. The country's 1947–1948 wheat harvest was as disastrous as the previous year's, and even with emergency shipments from France's North African colonies the government could not maintain its basic bread ration at 300 grams per person. Foreign Agricultural Service field officers in France wrote urgent telegrams to the State Department in Washington warning officials to expect a general breakdown of the French food distribution system by the end of May 1948 if even larger U.S. wheat shipments weren't forthcoming. This would likely trigger widespread protests and strikes, as it had in 1946 and 1947, but it might even get worse. Opposition groups were already using the country's puny bread ration as a central wedge issue. French Communists, in particular, had made impressive political hay out of a single 5,000-ton wheat shipment from Russia, and U.S. officials complained that the country didn't seem to appreciate the United States' far greater contributions. If bad harvests forced the government to lower the bread ration to 250 grams, they predicted, it might tip France's delicate political balance toward Communist forces. At the very least, the pro-government wing of organized labor might seek rapprochement with the Communists.[31]

In Paris, the May Day parade that year featured a contingent of workers carrying placards reading, "Give us a slice of bread," while back in the United States, syndicated columnists Joseph and Stewart Alsop warned readers that smaller bread rations "would geometrically increase the chances of very unfortunate results in the polls ... If France starved, it would go Communist ... If France goes to the Communists in the spring elections, the great struggle for Europe between the Soviet and western political systems will almost certainly be ended in Russia's favor." The fate of Europe seemed to hang on French bread rations.[32]

Whether these fears were reasonable or not, the U.S. responded with stepped up wheat shipments. On May 10, 1948, after two years and 900 shiploads of stop-gap aid to France, the Liberty Ship John H. Quick docked at the Port of Bordeaux bearing the first official Marshall Plan wheat. Lavishly praising the United States for its help, government officials announced that the bread ration could be maintained. This averted full-fledged crisis in France, although bread-related protests and political instability would continue into the 1950s.

For long-term stability, pundits agreed that France needed industrial baking and American-style competition. The French baking industry had too many inefficient subsidies, lax sanitation regulations, archaic distribution networks, and monopolistic guilds. When ergotism, a rare form of hallucination-inducing poisoning caused by fungus-infected rye, sickened two hundred residents in the small village of Pont Saint-Espirit during the summer of 1951, U.S. media reveled in the sensational story. The gory details of a *pain maudit* (damned bread)—a "medieval disease [illegible] never seen in the United States"—splashed across newspapers and magazines for days.[33] Tales of villagers convinced they were jet planes, hordes of peasants fleeing imaginary tigers, and rumors that "the village idiot had hexed the baker" seemed to confirm the larger sense of French baking: it was irrational and archaic. Campbell's Soup Company president William B. Murphy captured this attitude at a U.S. Information Agency symposium on food and the Cold War: French foodways, he declared, were "charming" and something to "keep . . . happily in mind while we survey most of the other half of mankind," but certainly no model for global security.[34]

In Iran, another quickly emerging Cold War battleground, U.S. and Soviet strategists mobilized bread grains in the fight for control over oil. Through the late 1940s, with bad wheat harvests in Iran's Azerbaijan breadbasket triggering bread riots throughout the country, Soviet propaganda spread rumors that Tehran was sending the nation's wheat to the United States to pay for arms. A 1942 episode where Axis agitators allegedly stirred up anti-Ally bread riots in Tehran was still fresh in U.S. officials' minds, and they worried Soviet propaganda would turn Iran against them. What worried them even more than propaganda, however, was the Soviet's concrete commitment to provide the country with 100,000 tons of wheat in 1949. Luckily for U.S. strategists, the Soviet wheat traveling overland trickled into the country slowly, while American Liberty ships filled with wheat arrived with great fanfare in 1949.[35]

Bread and flour shipments were also credited with undermining Communist forces in Greece, where, in 1948, 96 percent of the nation's staple was made from U.S. flour or wheat.[36] Turkey followed a similar pattern. And the Berlin blockade, for its part, confirmed policymakers' sense of the strategic importance of fresh bread, giving civil defense experts a first-hand glimpse of the effects of bread deprivation on civilian populations. Although it would have made more sense to airlift light, nutrient dense foods instead of flour and baking fuel, officials observing the situation in Berlin quickly concluded that, in times of crisis, "ample freshly baked bread . . . was essential to civilian morale." Later, they would apply this lesson to U.S. civil defense planning, which stressed the importance of bread supplies.[37]

Things did not go as well in Czechoslovakia. In 1948, Truman's failure to extend bread grain shipments to East-leaning Czechoslovakia was credited with pushing the country definitively into the Soviet camp, and the president publically vowed never to allow something like that to happen again. In a soon-to-be-famous St. Patrick's Day speech, the president declared, "There are times in world history when it is far wiser to act than to hesitate," demanding quick passage of the Marshall Plan, which, at first, consisted largely of stepped-up bread grain shipments. In the same speech, the president called for universal peacetime military training and the reestablishment of the Selective Service system. With bread grains leading the way, the country was going to (cold) war.[38]

By the early fifties, Main Street would no longer be asked to "save a slice a day" for humanitarian reasons. From that point on, food power would be the sole concern of an emerging national security wielding a golden arsenal of grain. Whether average consumers thought explicitly about their bread's place in the world, the postwar European experience had strongly cemented a deep association between U.S. bread and security.

This association was not new. It built on strong currents of pre-war thinking that linked industrial white bread with national vitality and eugenic fitness as well as highly successful wartime efforts to convince consumers of enriched white bread's pivotal role in national defense.[39] But, in the postwar context of polarized global competition, it took on more global significance. American industrial bread's association with national security—forged in the crucible of European relief efforts—helped reinforce the idea that American industrial foodways were universally choiceworthy and necessary elements of the fight against Communism.

BREAD COMES FROM AMERICA

In a June 1952 commencement address, President Eisenhower, despairing at the country's decline into red-baiting and book banning, implored Dartmouth College graduates, "to fight Communism with something better." But, as Secretary of State John Foster Dulles noted, increasingly visible poverty and racial tensions were "ruining" the United States's image abroad. The country's Cold War propaganda machine was struggling to speak convincingly of America's lofty ideals. It was getting harder and harder to point, concretely, to what that "something better" was that America offered the world.[40]

To make matters worse, by the end of the decade, the United States appeared to be losing ground to the Soviets in almost every arena that mattered—education, science, technology, weapons. Every arena except consumer goods and food production, that is. In this context, visions of domestic consumer affluence displaced Freedom and Equality as the most important weapon in U.S. propaganda efforts. As Eugenia Kaledin notes, "When Vice President Richard Nixon challenged Soviet Premier Nikita Khrushchev . . . he did not argue that Americans had little poverty, nor did he champion the civic freedoms that define American democracy. Instead he made a big issue of American consumer production for easier living."[41] U.S. efforts to combat the appeal of Communist "workers' paradise" with glamorous images of life in a "consumers' paradise" filled with sleek Chevrolets, color TVs, and Populuxe living room sets have been well-documented.[42] The important role that industrial food played in creating the image of an American consumer paradise is less well known.

Over-the-top portrayals of luxurious gadget-filled American homes did not even convince Americans all the time, and Soviet propaganda frequently countered images of affluence with stories of race, class, and gender inequality.[43] But it was much harder to convince anyone that the Eastern Bloc ate better. Even as confidence in the superiority of U.S. military readiness, technology and education wavered at home and abroad, Americans sensed that, as the influential pundit Hamilton Fish put it during the height of the European food crisis, "bread comes from America and it does not come from Russia."[44] This sentiment was widely echoed in many realms: from popular media to the floor of the U.S. Senate, where Hubert Humphrey declared, "Russia cannot supply food. The United States can."[45]

During the 1959 American National Exhibition in Moscow, where Richard Nixon famously accused Nikita Khrushchev of making lousy dishwashers, U.S. newspaper headlines across the country positively crowed over the way American food "Dazzle[d] Ivan." Modern food processing was "Our Secret Weapon"—"The Newest Weapon in America's fight against communism."[46] "Johnny" might not be able to read as well as "Ivan," as Rudolf Fleisch warned in his best-selling attack on the U.S. educational system, but few Americans doubted that Johnny could eat better than the Soviets (even as the U.S. fretted about its own bout with soaring bread prices in the early 1950s). Campbell's Soup Company president William B. Murphy again captured this attitude speaking at the USIA in Washington: "Communism is utterly incompatible with the production of food" while "The best example of the American dream of plenty is in food."[47]

To be sure, U.S. food propaganda typically focused on more glamorous modern food concoctions—TV dinners and ready-mix cakes—but industrial bread was basic and U.S. industrial foodways were often juxtaposed with the Communist world's scarce, "dark bread." A 1946 *Woman's Home Companion* feature on "life behind the iron curtain," for example, held white bread up as a key example of the "*produkti*" Russian people craved, but only America could provide. While some critics of fluffy American bread praised hearty Soviet loaves, they generally conceded that the U.S. baking system was still better at providing affordable abundance. The *Los Angeles Times* proudly declared that, "a Soviet worker must work half a day or longer to earn enough money to buy a kilogram of rye bread, while an American needs to work only 12 minutes," while the U.S. Bureau of Labor trumpeted statistics indicating that American workers had to work six minutes to buy a loaf of bread compared to 25 for the Russian worker.[48]

Similarly, the U.S. press reveled triumphantly in stories of bread hoarding and shortages caused by crop failures and poor distribution under Khrushchev—from Gaston, North Carolina ("Reds Stand in Breadlines") to Lima, Ohio ("Bread Scarce in Soviet Cupboards").[49] Accounts of daring escapes from the Soviet bloc run frequently by popular magazines during the early 1950s invariably mentioned bread prices and bread lines as a motivating factor in the flight from Communism. And even when American reporters in Russia observed abundant high-quality and nutritious dark bread, the staff of life was still a symbol of U.S. superiority: the Russian food system was so inefficient, they argued, consumers had few other options and could afford little else beyond dark bread.[50]

Finally, with Soviet military technology advancing at frightening speeds, some comfort could be taken from the fact that bread shortages occasionally crippled its army. "A loaf of bread induced many Russian troops in Hungry to lay down their arms," the *Chicago Daily Tribune* reported, citing witnesses who "saw them hand over their tanks for a couple kilograms of bread because they were so badly supplied."[51]

Thus, abundant modern food, including industrial white bread, helped constitute one of the Cold War's most reassuring dreams: the idea of alimentary affluence in the West and dark Soviet bread lines in the East. In industrial bread, U.S. policymakers, manufacturers, and consumers had definitively fused the assumed universality of their foodways with the imperatives of national security.

Armed with this confidence—and sense of geopolitical urgency—America set out to transform the world's bread; sometimes literally, sometimes figuratively. U.S. corporations, with government support, built American-style industrial bakeries in Iran and struggled for similar footholds in Western Europe. But what happened when the iron triangle of wheat, industrial baking, and global security set down in countries with other staple foods? The results were far more complicated than both proponents and critics of American industrial foodways acknowledge, as the cases of Japan and Mexico reveal.

RATIONALIZING RICE EATERS

In the early 1950s, U.S.-trained public health officers, and agribusiness representatives combined forces to spread the gospel of white bread to the conquered rice-eaters of Japan. Their efforts—particularly the targeting of Japanese school children's palates through school lunch programs—are frequently held up as the ultimate example of U.S-backed agribusiness forcing its industrial foods on defenseless populations; of the premeditated destruction of healthy, "holistic" eating.[52] But the story is quite a bit more complicated than that, not least because the Japanese taste for white bread long predates the end of WWII. Indeed, American occupation officials faced an imperial conundrum: Japan welcomed white bread and industrial baking technology transfers with open arms, but fiercely resisted cultural assumptions about the nutritional and political superiority of a white bread diet.[53] This two-sided response divided occupation official, creating room for debate about white bread's role in securing the Asian front against Communism. While some officials argued for rebuilding Japan on a foundation of rice and fish protein, others insisted on bread and milk

Japan had been home to a small, but flourishing baking industry since the late 19th century, with white bread serving as a popular novelty food and sometimes status symbol.[54] Indeed, as occupation officials quickly discovered, the most forceful complaint levied by the Japanese against U.S.-supplied bread was that it was *not white enough*. As one fifty-year-old housewife polled by SCAP sociologists in 1950 recalled, "We have always liked bread before the war, and always ate it on Sundays. So we can get used to it [as a new staple], but if it is not white bread we will be very unhappy about it."[55]

After the devastation of war, however, bread of any color was nothing to scoff at. The final years of the war had been a nutritional disaster for the islands' population, as Japan lost control over food producing territories abroad. The average weight of Japanese children plummeted and even affluent children suffered marked deficiencies of vitamin B, C, and D. After the war, the United States had far greater sympathy for starving white Europeans than it did for the Japanese, and the great food aid machinery doled out stingy rations to the East until the crisis in Europe was resolved. Thus, early school lunch programs consisted of less than an ounce of dry milk per child, thin miso broth, scavenged military surplus rations, and whatever vegetables parents could provide. Schools struggled to meet the 500 calorie per child goal.[56]

When, in 1949, officials could finally announce that, "Owing to the goodwill of SCAP, the complete lunch program will be carried out by providing each child with pure white bread and butter," 100 g of bread per child 20 days a month at a heavily subsidized price looked extremely good. Children protested at the "odious flavor" of many SCAP-imported foods—especially dry milk, which students flat-out refused to drink—but white bread was popular. Students and parents overwhelmingly praised the school lunch program and lobbied for its continuation.[57]

At the same time, Japanese consumers balked at the idea that bread could sustain a nation, despite the fact that, even before the war, Japanese leaders had tried to connect wheat diets with modernization and military might.[58] Sounding not unlike a European-American complaining about sushi, one housewife spelled out the problem: "With a bread diet, one becomes hungry immediately; with a rice diet it lasts longer." "With bread alone," another housewife bemoaned, "people like my husband, who does carpentry work, get tired." Although, thanks to subsidized ration coupons, 93 percent of the islands' population ate bread once a day and the majority told pollsters that they enjoyed it, few would choose bread over rice if given a choice.[59]

This attitude generated debate among occupation officials, public health officers, and agribusiness representatives. From early on in the occupation, public health officials—whose cultural understandings of what constituted a "real meal" had a tendency to mix freely with their understanding of scientific nutrition—saw the occupation as a watershed chance to "rationalize" and "improve" the Japanese by liberating them from their polished rice staple. Officials' frustration and disappointment are palpable in documents complaining of the inability to provide a "complete" or "real" lunch for Japanese school children—by which they meant that they could not provide bread and butter along with what they recognized as more culturally appropriate table of miso stew, fish protein, and vegetables. Even as their capacity to provide calories and protein expanded dramatically through the late 1940s and early 1950s, the lack of bread constituted a gaping hole in planners' visions of a full meal.[60]

Only when school districts finally had the flour, baking facilities, and cooking fuel to produce bread would they deem their program a true success—the school lunch program had much loftier goals than mere calorie distribution. Its larger mission was to "rationalize" or "correct" the Japanese diet, while fostering, "the scientification of the Japanese kitchen; [and the] permeating of democratic thought." "Democratic spirit," SCAP headquarters insisted could be nurtured in school cafeterias through the "substitution of reason and scientific practices in place of local customs and superstitions regarding cooking practices."[61] Propagating American meals was part of a strategy of forging civilized citizens, and without bread—the perceived core of a civilized diet—a local school official complained, how can we teach these lessons to our children?[62]

In 1950, J. L. Locke, a U.S. milling industry representative summed up these cultural assumptions in an appeal to "improv[e] the health and attitude of the Japanese people by supplementing their diet with enriched white bread": "There is some reason to believe that a change in diet might so change the health and attitude of that warlike people that we could live with them in improved peace and harmony." Locke's self-interested motives were transparent and occupation officials, hoping to develop a domestic milling industry in Japan, roundly rejected the U.S. milling industry's appeals. But in many ways they accepted the basic premise of Locke's argument.[63] The occupation offered a historic opportunity to transition Japan toward wheat, and this, in turn, had important political ramifications. As SCAP Commander General Douglas MacArthur wrote in 1950, finding a reliable substitute (i.e., wheat) for rice was a key to "block[ing] the rapacious encroachment of Communism" in the region.[64] When Secretary of Agriculture Ezra Taft Benson talked with *U.S. News and World Report* about his 1958 trip to Japan, the sight of "kiddies at their desks—each kiddie . . . with a big wheat roll made of American-grown wheat products and a bowl of reconstituted milk," wasn't just a gift for U.S. farmers it was a good sign for world peace.[65]

This perceived relation between rice-eating and weakness built on a longstanding popular discourse in the United States. During the 1910s, for example, an advertising campaign for Veribest Bread in the Midwest declared, "Bread-eating nations lead the world," with a drawing of a U.S. soldier towering over a caricatured Japanese man. "An interesting fact," it continued: "Rice eating nations are not so strong or progressive as bread eating nations."[66]

The conservative columnist George Sokolsky worried that rice would not fortify Asia against Communist incursions and urged the government to deploy America's genius for advertising in the service of shifting Japan toward more vital foods.[67] To support this idea, Sokolsky pointed to the popular radio adventure character Jack Armstrong, "the All American Boy," who so effectively cemented connections between fortitude and Wheaties in the 1930s. This, in turn, might have reminded readers of the central plotline of many Jack Armstrong shows: the handsome wheat-fueled All-American Boy travels to an exotic, non-Western land, where he accomplishes heroic feats unimaginable to the natives.

Reporting on an eleven-fold increase in Japanese wheat consumption during the occupation, a widely reprinted 1957 news story gave this plot a new twist: thanks to the presence of bread in Japanese school lunches, "Japan's youth is literally outgrowing and outweighing its parents." This effect could also be observed in Japanese beauty pageants where bread was producing "long-limbed beauties."[68]

Ultimately, however, U.S. bread subsidies, school lunch programs, bread festivals, baking classes, advertising campaigns, and sandwich recipe contests had only marginal impact. Bread production increased dramatically during the fifties, but the association of bread with vigor, and civilization—did not stick. Even the founder of one of the country's largest postwar bakeries—a pioneering force behind the Americanization of Japanese baking—complained in 1967,

> I find myself the only one in my family who stubbornly sticks to eating bread. I eat bread with beer, bread with anything, and I have done my best over the years to get the other members of my household to understand that it is in our interests to eat bread. My children, who went off to study overseas, have come home and now won't touch anything but rice. What's a father to do?[69]

This left policymakers pondering the best route to a secure Asia. Officials connected with the USDA and farm lobby continued to present wheat exports and bread habits as central to peace, but others wavered. By the 1960s, talk of transitioning Japan to a wheat diet had faded, and rice supplies topped the list of food security concerns. Wheat exports and American bakery technology transfer continued, but with fewer of the trappings of a civilizing mission. The association between American bread habits and military strength was durable, but not unshakeable.[70] When it came to creating a secure foundation for peace, local tastes and traditions did matter—perhaps rice could be a source of strength.

Of course, industrially refined white rice shared certain affinities with American white bread that allowed for this culturally flexible embrace of rice as a security food. When it came to artisanal French bread, however, this was not the case. With French bread—relatively similar to U.S. bread in its basic contents, but the product of a very different approach to food provisioning—taste and tradition carried the taint of frailty.

GOOD BAGUETTE, BAD BAGUETTE

By the mid 1950s, Americans could increasingly compare their supermarket bread to the golden products of western European bakeries. Subsidized by Marshall Plan money, U.S. tourists had begun traveling to France in record numbers.[71] And they returned from those tours with stories of ungodly good bread. At the same time, in New York and other big cities, affluent consumers could purchase what would today be called "artisanal" European breads from "real" French, Italian, and English bakeries—bakeries that stood a class above "ethnic" bread shops that had served immigrant neighborhoods for decades. By 1962, New Yorkers could even duck into Bloomingdales and come out with baguettes that had been baked in Paris the night before.[72]

Not everyone had this type of access or would want to pay the hefty premium for authentic European bread, of course, but anyone who read the newspaper could form an opinion about the difference between American white bread and its European counterparts. The message was clear: European bread might taste divine, but it lacked system and fortitude. And, for better or worse, in a dangerous world system fortitude had to trump taste.

What is striking is that this attitude didn't just emanate from jingoistic Francophobes. Francophiles also replicated the divide between taste and security. A 1955 article by *New York Times* food editor Janet Nickerson exemplified this trend. Pitting American white bread against its European counterparts, Nickerson argued that opposition to American white bread divided into two camps, one based on health and the other on flavor. The epicurean critics held a special place in her heart; indeed they were incontrovertibly correct. Fluffy, limp-crusted, and bland industrial white bread couldn't hold a candle to crisp, nutty-flavored French and Italian breads. Alas—and one can almost hear her sigh echoing across the decades—"health values deal with fact while flavor considerations deal with opinion." Thus, in the end, she advised readers were better off buying industrial white bread. A baguette or *pan de como* might brighten the table on a special occasion, but "the fact that they are made with water rather than milk impairs their nutritional value."[73] Growing fascination with "charming" French foodways in the 1950s and early 1960s had the ironic effect of reinforcing U.S. nationalism: "Superiority in food and wine [made] France itself seem suspect."[74]

Although Francophobia and Francophilia hold a special place in U.S. nationalism, this logic easily applied to other "exotic" lands and their breads. For example, New York gourmets such as Silas Spitzer might wax poetic about Middle Eastern breads, made in ways "unchanged from the earliest days" by "tribesman" with "native skill," but without an influx of modern baking techniques and "rationalized" distribution networks, U.S. observers concluded many countries faced bread riots and ugly political situations. "We are the only people in the world who subsist largely on commercial bread, manufactured by impersonal machinery on an assembly line, limp white bread that is pre-sliced, prepackaged, and all but predigested," Spitzer lamented, "Yet there is an articulate and growing minority, only partially made up of people of foreign blood, that rejects white bread."[75]

The *Holiday* article continued on to praise "exotic" breads—"fascinating loaves of strange size and contour"—but, of course in the end, returned to France, "whose sanitary regulations are notoriously few, but whose bread is truly wonderful." The author hoped to tempt skeptical readers into New York's ethnic bakeries, but, in singing the praises of strange loaves of uncertain hygiene, enjoyed by a small "minority, only partially made up of people of foreign blood," he reaffirmed the overarching sentiment presented in this paper: at some level—as intangible yet as real as newfangled television waves—*not* having white bread on hand, whether in the kitchen cupboard or on the international stage, was somehow risky.

CONCLUSION

During the 1950s, American food writers, diet advisers, and consumers lambasted the country's industrial loaves. They were "gummy," "underbaked," and "cottony." Yet only a small minority doubted enriched white bread's nutritional strength and vigor—fortitude clearly needed in an age of looming global threats. As this article has shown, however, industrial bread's strength and vigor was also seen as something needed *from* America. Early Cold War practices of food aid and alimentary propaganda gave America's much-derided loaves a central role in the ongoing drama of global superpower competition. The "successes" of these efforts, in turn, confirmed the country's sense that its industrial bread and processed foodways were universally choiceworthy elements of a stable world order. Thus, through the bread politics of the early Cold War, U.S. industrial foodways and the imperative of national security became fused in policy makers and the general public's minds.

Forged in the crucible of European relief efforts and postwar reconstruction, the elision of industrial food and geopolitical stability helped construct one of the key binaries through which Americans perceived Cold War geopolitics: the contrast between an efficient American system of alimentary abundance made possible by the industrialization of eating on one hand, and the rest of the world's inefficient, backwards food systems, on the other. Visions of America's unique ability to feed the world and expand consumption through abundant industrial food—American alimentary exceptionalism—helped underpin the larger formations of Cold War American exceptionalism.

The binary between America's efficient food system and the world's more questionable, systems could be reversed or blurred, as seen in the cases of French food and Japanese school lunches, but it still placed American industrial bread in an architecture of dietary hierarchy. This, in itself, was nothing new. U.S. food writers, consumers, and public health experts had long compared America's sliced white industrial bread to "foreign" loaves—but this had almost always been done in the context of figuring out the internal boundaries that made up "America." It had largely taken the form of comparison between modern bread, eaten by "real Americans," and the stuff devoured by dark, swarthy European immigrants and poor Southerners.

During the early Cold War, as this article has shown, that changed. The country, more willing to include various European immigrant populations under the heading of "white" (if unchanged in its attitude toward blacks and non-European immigrants), used white bread to confirm the *national* boundaries of America in a context of international competition. As U.S. foodways grew increasingly homogenous in postwar period, food fights that had, in the past, raged within the United States (e.g., between modern white bread and backwards Southern cornbread) were transplanted to the international stage. In this way, past contrasts between industrial white bread eaten by eugenically fit white populations and the "dark, dusky" loaves of immigrant populations gave way to more *global* hierarchies of dietary progress. In many ways, it was through imperial encounters around bread, flour, and wheat described in this article that modern industrial bread truly became "American bread."

Over the next two decades, many Americans come to reject that imperial boundary making project altogether. Sixties and seventies counterculture held up factory-made bread an icon of all that was wrong with industrial, imperialist America. The technocratic system of order and efficiency that simultaneously churned out reassuring loaves, sustained Cold Warriors, and held social chaos at bay, gave way. When, amidst the upheavals of 1968, John G. Fuller published *The Day of St. Antony's Fire*, a best-selling account of the Pont Saint-Espirit ergotism outbreak, hallucinatory French bread symbolized freedom and resistance, not dangerous disorder.

NOTES

1. "Where Is the White Bread?," *Time*, August 2, 1943. The article's title evokes Paul Boyer's classic Cold War cultural history, Paul S. Boyer, *By the Bomb's Early Light: American Thought and Culture at the Dawn of the Atomic Age* (Chapel Hill, NC: University of North Carolina Press, 1994). Versions of this article were presented at the UC Davis Robert Mondavi Institute "Tasting History" conference and the University of Arizona School of Geography and Development colloquium series, where I received important feedback. Comments from Carolyn de la Peña, Melanie DuPuis, and three anonymous reviewers proved invaluable in helping me rework and clarify my argument.

2. By "industrial food," I refer to sustenance produced through capital-intensive agriculture and processed into homogenous, standardized products to maximize efficiencies and returns to scale. By "industrial foodways," I refer to the collective *habitus* of consuming industrial foods. The phrase "American alimentary exceptionalism," is, of course, intended to evoke the larger concept of American exceptionalism. That term has many meanings with different emphases, but all highlight the perception that the United States has a unique and privileged place among the nations of the world and in the march of human history. Seymour Martin Lipset, *American Exceptionalism: A Double-Edged Sword* (New York: W.W. Norton, 1996).

3. Amy Bentley, *Eating for Victory: Food Rationing and the Politics of Domesticity* (Urbana, IL: University of Illinois Press, 1998).

4. Mary Drake McFeely, *Can She Bake a Cherry Pie?: American Women and the Kitchen in the Twentieth Century* (Amherst, MA: University of Massachusetts Press, 2000).

5. Victoria De Grazia, *Irresistible Empire: America's Advance through Twentieth-Century Europe* (Cambridge, MA: Belknap Press of Harvard University Press, 2005). See also Laura A. Belmonte, *Selling the American Way: U.S. Propaganda and the Cold War* (Philadelphia: University of Pennsylvania Press, 2008); Walter L. Hixson, *Parting the Curtain: Propaganda, Culture, and the Cold War, 1945–1961* (New York: St. Martin's Press, 1997).

6. Daniel Yergin, *Shattered Peace: The Origins of the Cold War* (New York: Penguin Books, 1990).

7. Although it served as a central pillar in U.S. geopolitical strategies dating back to at least WWI, the basic premise of "food power" was most bluntly stated by Secretary of Agriculture Earl Butz in the 1970s: "Hungry men listen only to those who have a piece of bread. Food ... is a weapon in the U.S. negotiating kit." Under the doctrine of food power, the U.S. would use its undisputed agricultural might and advancing food processing technologies as both a carrot and a stick in geopolitical struggles. See Robert L. Paarlberg, *Food Trade and Foreign Policy: India, the Soviet Union, and the United States* (Ithaca, NY: Cornell University Press, 1985). Writing on "food imperialism" has generally cleaved between political economy (with its focus on the ways U.S. food power impacted agrarian systems and livelihoods, particularly in the Third World) and cultural politics (with its focus on struggles over the "Americanization" of diets around the world). Examples of the former include: H. Friedmann, "Feeding the Empire: The Pathologies of Globalized Agriculture Source," *The Socialist Register* (2005); John H. Perkins, *Geopolitics and the Green Revolution: Wheat, Genes, and the Cold War* (New York: Oxford University Press, 1997); Peter Rosset, *Food Is Different: Why We Must Get the WTO out of Agriculture* (New York: Zed Books, 2006); Vandana Shiva, "The Geopolitics of Food: America's Use of Food as a Weapon," *Economics and Politics Weekly* 23, no. 18 (1988). Examples of the latter include: Hixson, *Parting the Curtain: Propaganda, Culture, and the Cold War, 1945–1961*; Richard F. Kuisel, *Seducing the*

French: The Dilemma of Americanization (Berkeley, CA: University of California Press, 1993); Reinhold Wagnleitner, *Coca-Colonization and the Cold War : The Cultural Mission of the United States in Austria after the Second World War* (Chapel Hill, NC: University of North Carolina Press, 1994).

8. See, for example, Nick Cullather, "The Foreign Policy of the Calorie," *American Historical Review* 112, no. 2 (2007); Mona Domosh, "Purity and Pickles: Discourse of Food, Empire, and Work in Turn-of-the-Century USA," *Social and Cultural Geography* 4, no. 1 (2003); Dan Morgan, *Merchants of Grain* (New York: Viking Press, 1979).

9. A few historians have referenced the reciprocal effects of postwar food power on how people in the United States thought about their food. This article builds on their insights. Warren Belasco, *Meals to Come: A History of the Future of Food* (Berkeley, CA: University of California Press, 2006); Bentley, *Eating for Victory: Food Rationing and the Politics of Domesticity*.

10. Nina V. Fedoroff and Nancy Marie Brown, *Mendel in the Kitchen: A Scientist's View of Genetically Modified Foods* (Washington, DC: Joseph Henry Press, 2004); James E. McWilliams, *Just Food: Where Locavores Get It Wrong and How We Can Truly Eat Responsibly* (New York: Little, Brown and Co., 2009).

11. *Ibid.* For a history of this kind of crisis narrative and its effects, see: Belasco, *Meals to Come: A History of the Future of Food*. This might also give us pause at the way in which proponents of local food production have begun to invoke national security, e.g., Michael Pollan, "An Open Letter to the Next Farmer in Chief," *New York Times*, October 9, 2008.

12. Steven Gdula, *The Warmest Room in the House: How the Kitchen Became the Heart of the Twentieth-Century American Home* (New York: Bloomsbury, 2008); Sherrie A. Inness, *Dinner Roles American Women and Culinary Culture* (Iowa City, IA: University of Iowa City, 2001); McFeely, *Can She Bake a Cherry Pie?: American Women and the Kitchen in the Twentieth Century*; Jessamyn Neuhaus, *Manly Meals and Mom's Home Cooking: Cookbooks and Gender in Modern America* (Baltimore: Johns Hopkins University Press, 2003); Laura Shapiro, *Something from the Oven: Reinventing Dinner in 1950s America* (New York: Viking, 2004).

13. See for example: Boyer, *By the Bomb's Early Light American Thought and Culture at the Dawn of the Atomic Age*; K. A. Cuordileone, *Manhood and American Political Culture in the Cold War* (New York: Routledge, 2005); Cynthia Hendershot, *Anti-Communism and Popular Culture in Mid-Century America* (Jefferson: McFarland, 2003); Guy Oakes, *The Imaginary War: Civil Defense and American Cold War Culture* (New York: Oxford University Press, 1994); Lisle Abbott Rose, *The Cold War Comes to Main Street: America in 1950* (Lawrence, KS: University Press of Kansas, 1999); Stephen J. Whitfield, *The Culture of the Cold War*, 2nd ed., The American Moment (Baltimore: Johns Hopkins University Press, 1996); Peter J. Kuznick and James Burkhart Gilbert, *Rethinking Cold War Culture* (Washington, DC: Smithsonian Institution Press, 2001).

14. Peter Filene, "'Cold War Culture' Doesn't Say It All," in *Rethinking Cold War Culture*, ed. Peter J. Kuznick and James Burkhart Gilbert (Washington, DC: Smithsonian Institution Press, 2001); Leo P. Ribuffo, "Will the Sixties Never End? Or Perhaps at Least the Thirties? Or Maybe Even the Progressive Era? Contrarian Thoughts on Change and Continuity in American Political Culture at the Turn of the Millennium," in *Rethinking Cold War Culture*, ed. Peter J. Kuznick and James Burkhart Gilbert (Washington, DC: Smithsonian Institution Press, 2001).

15. See Warren James Belasco, *Appetite for Change: How the Counterculture Took on the Food Industry*, 2nd ed. (Ithaca, NY: Cornell University Press, 2007).

16. For a more detailed history of the industrialization of bread see: Aaron Bobrow-Strain, "White Bread Bio-Politics: Purity, Health, and the Triumph of Industrial Baking," *Cultural Geographies* 15, no. 1 (2008). Data on bread production drawn from: "Flavor of Today's Bread Is Much Better Than Many Critics Are Willing to Admit," *Western Baker*, January 1937; "The Story of American Efficiency," *The U.S. News*, October 31, 1938; W.J. Panschar, *Baking in America*, vol. 1 (Evanston, IL: Northwestern University Press, 1965); Donald R. Stabile, "Bakery Products," in *Manufacturing: A Historiographical and Bibliographical Guide*, ed. David O. Whitten and Bessie Emeric Whitten (Wesport, CT: Greenwood Press, 1990).

17. Aaron Bobrow-Strain, "Kills a Body Twelve Ways: Bread Fear and the Politics of "What to Eat?," *Gastronomica* 7, no. 3 (2007); Bobrow-Strain, "White Bread Bio-Politics: Purity, Health, and the Triumph of Industrial Baking"; Aaron Bobrow-Strain, *White Bread: The History of a Dream* (Boston: Beacon Press, 2012).

18. Aaron Bobrow-Strain, "White Bread Bootcamp: 'Good Food' as National Defense in the Campaign for Vitamin Enrichment" (manuscript under review, available on request from the author).

19. USDA Agricultural Marketing Service, "Consumers' Preferences among Bakers' White Breads of Different Formulas: A Survey in Rockford, Illinois, Marketing Research Report No. 118" (Washington, DC: USDA, 1956).

20. *Ibid*. and National Millers' Federation, "What People Think About Bread: A Summary of Research Studies Among Consumers and Nutrition Authorities" (1948), found at: Records of the Food and Drug Administration, Division of General Services, General Subject Files, 1938–1974, Box 1435, National Archives II at College Park, College Park, MD (hereafter, NARA-CP).

21. Data on consumption patterns in the preceding paragraphs drawn from Marguerite C. Burke, "Pounds and Percentages," in *Food: The Yearbook of Agriculture, 1959*, ed. United States Department of Agriculture (Washington, DC: U.S. Government Printing Office, 1959); Panschar, *Baking in America*; Esther F. Phipard, "Changes in the Bread You Buy," in *Crops in Peace and War: The Yearbook of Agriculture, 1950–1951*, ed. United States Department of Agriculture (Washington, DC: U.S. Government Printing Office, 1951); "Boost for Bread," *Business Week*, February 28, 1948; Thomas C. Desmond, "Bread-Your New Perfect Food," in *Food in War and in Peace, Consolidated Report of the New York State Joint Legislative Committee on Nutrition*, ed. New York State Joint Legislative Committee on Nutrition (Albany, NY: New York State Legislature, 1944); Richard G. Walsh and Bert M. Evans, *Economics of Change in Market Structure, Conduct, and Performance: The Baking Industry, 1947–1958* (Lincoln, NE: University of Nebraska Studies, 1963); Ronald L. Wirtz, "Grain, Baking, and Sourdough Bread: A Brief Historical Panorama," in *Handbook of Dough Fermentation*, ed. Karel Kulp and Klaus Lorenz (New York: CRC, 2003); M. L. Way and H. B. McCoy, *Establishing a Retail Bakery, Industrial (Small Business) Series, No. 29* (Washington, DC: United States Department of Commerce, 1946).

22. National Millers Federation, "What People Think About Bread."

23. European bread consumption statistics from, "Rural Dietaries in Europe. Annex: Report on Bread League of Nations," August 26, 1939, Foreign Agricultural Service Correspondence (hereafter FAS) RG 166, France 1950–1954, Box 152, NARA-CP. Background on the 1946–1948 crisis in this section drawn from: Bentley, *Eating for Victory: Food Rationing and the Politics of Domesticity*; Harry Fornari, *Bread Upon the Waters; a History of United States Grain Exports* (Nashville, TN: Aurora Publishers, 1973); Thomas J. Knock, "Feeding the World and Thwarting Communists," in *Architects of the American Century*, ed. David Schmitz and T. Christopher Jesperson (Chicago: Imprint Publications, 2000); Morgan, *Merchants of Grain*; Paarlberg, *Food Trade and Foreign Policy: India, the Soviet Union, and the United States*.

24. FAS Field Office in London to U.S. Secretary of State, July 19, 1946, FAS RG 166, United Kingdom, Breadstuffs, 1946–1949, Box 966, NARA-CP, MD.

25. Extraction rate refers to the percentage of the whole wheatberry retained in flour after the milling process. Thus, true whole wheat has an extraction rate of 100 percent. In the United States, white flour has an extraction rate of around 72 percent. Increasing extraction rates to 80 or 90 percent conserves flour by utilizing more of the bran and germ of the wheatberry, while yielding a flour somewhere between white and whole wheat.

26. Extraction rate refers to the percentage of the whole wheat kernel retained in flour after milling. Thus, true whole wheat has an extraction rate of 100 percent. Standard white flour contains 70–75 percent of the whole wheat kernel, while high extraction white flours utilize 80–85 percent.

27. Quoted by Bentley, *Eating for Victory: Food Rationing and the Politics of Domesticity*. See also: "Truman's Remarks to Citizen Food Committee," *New York Times*, October 2, 1947.

28. Bentley, *Eating for Victory: Food Rationing and the Politics of Domesticity*.

29. "Bread on the Waters," *Consumers' Guide*, May 6, 1946. See also "How to Do With Less Bread," *Life*, May 6 1946; "New Dark Bread Is Part of U.S. Contribution to the Grave World Food Crisis," *Life*, March 4, 1946; "Greatest in History," *Time*, June 10, 1946; "Conserve Bread," *Parent's Magazine*, May 1946; "Save Wheat," *American Home*, May 1946.

30. "Bread: It Is the First Concern of a Hungry World. Trouble Looms for the Nations Which Cannot Provide It," *Los Angeles Times*, August 10, 1947; "Guns, Bread, and Butter," *Farm Journal*, September 1953; Baukhage, "U.S. Farmer Will Beat Communism," *Associated Press Syndication*, October 2, 1947. Examples of American skepticism about bread conservation cited in Paul Mallon, "Overhauling of UNRA by Hoover Expected," *Western Newspaper Union Syndication*, April 28, 1947.

31. FAS Field Office in Paris to U.S. Secretary of State, "French Import Requirements, Food Items," May 12, 1947; FAS Field Office in Paris to U.S. Secretary of State "Food Situation and Related Political Developments in France," February 20, 1947; FAS Field Office in Paris to U.S. Secretary of State, "The Breadgrain Situation in France," April 9, 1947; FAS Field Office in Paris to U.S. Secretary of State, June 11, 1946. All found in FAS RG 166, France, Breadstuffs, 1946–1949, Box 9, NARA-CP, MD.

32. "Marshall-Aid Ship Cheered in France," *New York Times*, May 11, 1948; Joseph Alsop and Steward Alsop, "Food Is Politics," *Los Angeles Times*, May 4, 1946.

33. See for examples, stories in *Life, Time,* and *The New York Times*. Ergotism had less of a presence in the United States because Americans consumed relatively little rye flour, but this explanation did not factor heavily in media coverage.

34. Murphy, "The Challenge of the Future: An Overview."

35. U.S. Ambassador in Tehran, "Irano-Soviet Wheat Agreement," December 3, 1949, FAS RG 166, Iran, Breadstuffs 1946–1949, Box 780, NARA-CP.

36. FAS Field Office in Athens to U.S. Secretary of State, August 31, 1948, FAS RG 166, Greece, Breadstuffs, 1946–1949, Box 724, NARA-CP, MD. A similar story played out in Turkey. See also Yergin, *Shattered Peace: The Origins of the Cold War*.

37. "Food in Civil Defense," *The Technology Review* 55, no. 4 (1953). On the effect of the Berlin airlift on civil defense planners' understand of bread's role in the Cold War see also: "Food in Civil Defense"; Majorie M. Heseltine, "Feeding of Mothers and Children under Emergency Conditions," *Public Health Reports* 67, no. 9 (1952).

38. Yergin, *Shattered Peace: The Origins of the Cold War*.

39. See Bobrow-Strain, "White Bread Bootcamp: 'Good Food' as National Defense in the Campaign for Vitamin Enrichment"; "White Bread Bio-Politics: Purity, Health, and the Triumph of Industrial Baking."

40. Eugenia Kaledin, *Daily Life in the United States, 1940–1959 Shifting Worlds*, Greenwood Press "Daily Life Through History" Series (Westport, CT: Greenwood Press, 2000); Belmonte, *Selling the American Way: U.S. Propaganda and the Cold War*.

41. Kaledin, *Daily Life in the United States, 1940–1959 Shifting Worlds*. See also Ruth Oldenziel and Karin Zachmann, *Cold War Kitchen: Americanization, Technology, and European Users*, Inside Technology (Cambridge, MA: MIT Press, 2009). For a classic rationalization of the shift in understanding of what made America exceptional and choiceworthy, see David Morris Potter, *People of Plenty Economic Abundance and the American Character*, Charles R. Walgreen Foundation Lectures (Chicago: University of Chicago Press, 1954).

42. Belmonte, *Selling the American Way: U.S. Propaganda and the Cold War*.

43. U.S. press coverage of the Moscow exhibition sparked considerable debate over whether its vision of American life was realistic or representative; see also Oldenziel and Zachmann, *Cold War Kitchen: Americanization, Technology, and European Users*. Soviet critiques were even more cutting. For example, during the Moscow exhibition, one Soviet journalist issued a damning, and still relevant, critique of U.S. consumer domesticity: "The numerous daily appliances used by Americans seem to bind the woman forever to the mission of housewife, wife, and cook. They lighten her role as such, but at the same time for eternity place her daily life in the profession of housewife." "Reflections about the American National Exhibit (from *Izvestiya*) Marietta Shaginyan, " August 23, 1959, Records of the U.S. Information Agency (hereafter USIA), American National Exhibition, Moscow, 1957–1959, Box 2, NARA-CP, MD.

44. Quoted in "With Both Bread and Freedom," *Time*, June 30, 1947.

45. Quoted in Knock, "Feeding the World and Thwarting Communists."

46. USIA, Moscow 1957–1959, Press Clipping File, Box 3, NARA-CP, MD.

47. William B. Murphy, "The Challenge of the Future: An Overview," in *Food and Civilization, a Symposium* (Washington, DC: USIA Voice of America Lecture Series, 1966).

48. "Russian Works Longer for His Food ECA Says," *Los Angeles Times*, August 22, 1949; Oriana Atkinson, "Mt Life Behind the Iron Curtain," *Woman's Home Companion*, October 1946; De Grazia, *Irresistible Empire: America's Advance Through Twentieth-Century Europe*; J. A. Livingston, "U.S. And Soviet Price Systems Far Apart," *Big Spring Daily Herald*, June 10, 1956.

49. "Bread Scarce in Soviet Cupboards," *The Lima News*, September 24, 1963; Jay Axelbank, "Russians Forced to Stand in Line to Buy Most Goods," *Eau Claire Daily Telegram*, October 16, 1963.

50. Livingston, "U.S. and Soviet Price Systems Far Apart"; Lauren Soth, "Consumer Goods Scarce," *Corpus Christi Times*, August 30, 1955. Interestingly, these articles subtly (and not so subtly) introduce criticisms of U.S. industrial bread. They reverse the binary of good American bread versus bad Soviet bread, while reinforcing the larger architecture of alimentary exceptionalism.

51. Willard Edwards, "Soviet Troops Confused," *Chicago Daily Tribune*, December 19, 1956.

52. See, for example, Mark Hammond and Jacqueline Ruyok, "The Decline of the Japanese Diet: From Macarthur to Mcdonalds," *East West* October (2008).

53. On Japan's long struggles over the place of foreign foods in its diet, see Emiko Ohnuki-Tierney, "We Eat Each Other's Food to Nourish Our Body: The Global and the Local and Mutually Constituent

Forces," in *Food in Global History*, ed. Raymond Grew (Boulder, CO: Westview Press, 1999); Katarzyna J. Cwiertka, "Popularizing a Military Diet in Wartime and Postwar Japan," *Asian Anthropology* 1(2002).

54. {Company, 1996 #412}

55. "Survey of Bread and Flour Utilization by the Japanese People," 1950, Records of the Supreme Commander of the Allies in the Pacific (hereafter SCAP), Public Opinion and Sociological Research Division, NARA-CP, MD.

56. Public Health and Welfare Bulletin, "Supplementary School Lunch Program, " June 1948, SCAP, Civil Affairs Section, Tohoku Civil Affairs Region, Public Health and Welfare Activities, 1946–1951, Box 258, NARA-CP, MD; "Report on Public Health and Welfare in Japan," n.d. c. 1949–1950, SCAP, Economic and Scientific Section, Price and Distribution Division, Food Branch, 1946–1951, Box 6428, NARA-CP, MD.

57. "Supplementary School Lunch Program; "Tabulation of Public Opinion of School Lunch," July 25, 1951, SCAP, Economic and Scientific Section, Price and Distribution Division, Food Branch, 1946–1951, NARA-CP, MD.

58. On Japanese attempts to connect wheat diets and military strength, which predate the postwar period: Cwiertka, "Popularizing a Military Diet in Wartime and Postwar Japan."

59. "Survey of Bread and Flour Utilization by the Japanese People."

60. "The Complete School Lunch—Providing Bread and Butter," August 9, 1949, SCAP, Civil Affairs Section, Hokkaido civil Affairs Region, Civil Affairs Files, 1945–1951, Box 2534; "Instruction from Ministry of Education Concerning School Lunch, " n.d., SCAP, Civil Affairs Section, Hokkaido Civil Affairs Region, Civil Affairs Files, 1945–1951, Box 2534; Vice Education Minister to Prefectural Governors, "Concerning the Encouragement and Popularization of the School Lunch Program," December 11, 1946, SCAP, Headquarters Division, Public Welfare Files, 1945–1951, Box 2278; "Recent Tendencies of School Lunch Program and Counter Measures," August 22, 1949, SCAP, Civil Information and Education Section, Education Division, Physical Education and Youth Affairs Branch, Topical Files, 1946–1951, Box 5721; Chief Manager of School Lunch, Hokkaido Board of Education to SCAP General Headquarters, "Nowadays Condition of School Lunch in Hokkaido," handwritten letter, n.d., SCAP, Civil Affairs Section, Hokkaido Civil Affairs Region, Civil Affairs Files, 1945–1951, Box 2534. All in NARA-CP.

61. "Instruction from Ministry of Education Concerning School Lunch, #419.

62. Chief Manager of School Lunch to SCAP General Headquarters.

63. J. L. Locke to SCAP General Headquarters, "Suggestions for Improvement of the Health and Attitude of the Japanese People by Supplementing Their Diet With Enriched White Bread," August 3, 1949, SCAP, Price and Distribution Division, Food Branch, 1946–1951; SCAP General Headquarters to J. L. Locke, September 26, 1949, SCAP, Price and Distribution Division, Food Branch, 1946–1951. Both in NARA-CP, MD.

64. General MacArthur to Ambassador Gasciogne, UK Political Representative in Japan, October 6, 1950, SCAP, Price and Distribution Division, Food Branch, 1946–1951, NARA-CP, MD.

65. Reprinted in "Feeding the World's Hungry: Cure for Farm Troubles? An Interview with Ezra Taft Benson," *The Altoona Mirror*, March 22, 1958.

66. "Bakeries in Ogden Are Praised by Expert," *Ogden Standard*, July 2, 1915.

67. George E. Sokolsky, "China's Rice," *Hearst Newspaper Syndication*, January 17, 1953.

68. "Japanese Eat Various Types of Bread, Grow Taller," *Associated Press Syndication*, December 24, 1957.

69. Company, *From a Corn of Wheat: Yamakazi*.

70. Recall that even occupation officials debated whether rice might be a more culturally appropriate bastion of strength. Strains of U.S. popular opinion had also made this argument. For example, a widely reprinted 1951 news piece argued, "The most important thing for to the majority of the people of Asia is not democracy, nor Communism, nor any political ideology—but food, which means life itself. And in most of Asia food is rice." "Who Controls Rice Supply Controls Asiatic Destiny," found in *The Richwood (OH)* Gazette, June 22, 1951, among other newspapers.

71. Christopher Endy, *Cold War Holidays American Tourism in France* (Chapel Hill, NC: University of North Carolina Press, 2004).

72. "Bread from France," *New York Times*, May 16, 1962.

73. Janet Nickerson, "Bread Gets an Airing," *New York Times*, March 13, 1955.

74. Kennan Ferguson, "Mastering the Art of the Sensible: Julia Child, Nationalist," *Theory and Event* 12, no. 2 (2009).

75. Silas Spitzer, "Break Bread With the World," *Holiday* 1955.

"To Avoid This Mixture": Rethinking *Pulque* in Colonial Mexico City

DANIEL NEMSER
University of California, Berkeley, California, USA

On June 8, 1692, a popular uprising left Mexico City in ruins. The colonial government blamed the violence on pulque, *an indigenous alcohol made from the fermented juice of the maguey. Not all* pulque, *however, was considered equal. While ostensibly pure* pulque blanco *(white* pulque*) was seen as medicinal,* pulque mezclado *(mixed* pulque*), which contained certain additives, was condemned as a threat to political stability. This essay takes this often-overlooked distinction as a point of departure for examining the political and social significance of* pulque *by way of the grid of intelligibility that gave it meaning. For colonial elites, the mixing of* pulque *had a magnetizing effect on the social world, drawing the urban poor together in the space of the* pulquería *(*pulque *tavern) and making possible multiple forms of contact—from solidarity to sex. But it also had epistemological implications: the study of mixed* pulque *offered elites a language for talking about race mixing (*mestizaje*), while simultaneously constituting* pulque *consumers as a seditious collective subject—a* plebe *(plebeian masses) defined, like* pulque, *by mixing.*

Food and drink occupy a central place in the colonial contact zone. Four decades ago, J. H. Elliott described the long and difficult process of "assimilation" by which Europeans incorporated the newly discovered Americas into their mental horizons. "[I]n many respects," he wrote, this process "was still far from completed by the middle of the seventeenth century."[1] Elliott was most interested in the big picture, the history of ideas and macroeconomics, but recently food scholars and colonial historians have used his framework to trace the integration of New World foods into Old World diets (and systems of knowledge), complicating earlier notions of acculturation or one-way cultural flow from colonizer to colonized.[2] Transatlantic commerce, and the global foodways it fosters, have thus revealed not only economic activities but also intricate circuits of cultural change.[3] Often overlooked, however, are the ways in which colonial space itself constitutes a global stage upon which local knowledges, practices, and materials—including the elements of everyday life *not* exported to the metropolis—are "assimilated." Colonialism complicates easy distinctions between local and global, mapping them over or embedding them in each other; in the colonial context, global foodways may have less to do with the geopolitics of mercantilism and the circulation of commodities than with particular formations of colonial governance.[4]

This essay examines the attempts of the Spanish colonial apparatus in New Spain to understand and regulate *pulque*, a traditional indigenous alcohol made from the fermented juice of the maguey plant, at a moment of political crisis in the late seventeenth century. Through close readings of a set of official reports about this drink, I trace an elite obsession with *mixing*, real or imagined, that shapes the contours of colonial politics while revealing both the grid of intelligibility through which these politics are perceived and the authoritative language through which they are articulated. The epistemological work of the contact zone is not just interpretive, in the sense of passively apprehending and organizing raw data, but productive as well: it generates categories of meaning and sites for state intervention. Although the Spanish obsession with blood purity—and its corollary mixing—is well known, the extent to which this genealogical obsession infused the world of material culture is less apparent. In the eyes of colonial elites, the mixing of pulque had material effects on the social world through its magnetizing function, drawing the urban poor together in the space of the *pulquería* (pulque tavern) and making possible multiple forms of contact—from solidarity to sex. But it also had epistemological implications: the study of mixed pulque production would provide a language for talking about race mixing (*mestizaje*) and racial categorization, while at the same time constituting pulque consumers as a (seditious) collective subject—the *plebe* (plebeian masses). Both objects of knowledge, pulque and plebe, are defined precisely by their indefinability, a state in which internal differentiations are necessarily elided and glossed, simply, as *mixed*.

MEXICO CITY, 1692

On the afternoon of June 8, 1692, in the context of widespread food shortages, an uprising broke out in the central plaza of Mexico City that would leave the royal palace and other government buildings in smoldering ruins by nightfall.[5] The scale of the destruction at the very center of colonial authority in New Spain took many elites by surprise, as they tended to see the populace as incapable of effective organization.[6] According to what would become the "official history" of the uprising, best seen in a descriptive letter written by well-known intellectual (and close friend to the Viceroy Conde de Galve) Carlos de Sigüenza y Góngora, the blame fell squarely on the city's indigenous population.[7] Instead of admitting the government's failure to provision the city with grains, which would have provided a reasonable cause for the indigenous poor to rise up, Sigüenza attacked the inebriating and seditious effects of indigenous *pulque*. "From the very moment that the riot began," he wrote, "everyone raised the cry, inspired by Heaven perhaps, that 'This is the result of pulque!'"[8]

Sigüenza's history stands as both the best-known account of the uprising today and the hegemonic explanation of its causes and trajectory for his contemporaries. But his letter, dated August 30, 1692, merely gave the conventional wisdom a more official form, providing an *ex post facto* logic for the viceroy's principal policy response to the uprising: the regulation of pulque. Already on June 9, with the palace still burning in the background, the viceroy announced an edict prohibiting pulque "absolutely" within Mexico City because of its role in provoking the violence.[9] Ten days later the prohibition was extended throughout the whole of New Spain.[10] The government also acted immediately to demonstrate its will to enforce the new law. The very same day it came into effect, according to the contemporary diarist Antonio de Robles, a mulatto was publicly whipped "for a jug of pulque."[11] But Robles also recorded an incongruous detail. On July 31, less than two weeks after the consolidation of the ban, the government legalized the sale of "pulque without roots, which is medicinal" in the plaza.[12]

Many scholars—often following Sigüenza's lead—have glossed over this distinction, anachronistically flattening pulque's multiple forms and reducing to a single voice or overlooking entirely the debates that shaped its prohibition.[13] By highlighting the density of these debates, I am interested in teasing out the political and social significance of this drink, as well as the authoritative discourses that surrounded and infused it with meaning, in the context of the 1692 insurrection. For this reason, my sources are a set of 45 *informes* (official reports) written about a month after the uprising by individual or institutional members of New Spain's colonial elite, both ecclesiastical and secular. These reports, now housed at the Archivo General de Indias (AGI) in Seville, Spain, were sent to the viceroy in response to his request for advice about whether the pulque prohibition should be lifted or maintained. Across the board, the *informes* perhaps unsurprisingly supported extending the blanket prohibition. But many writers went beyond what had been asked of them, offering analyses of not only what they saw as the problematic effects of pulque consumption but also impressions of the pulque economy, the procedures of its production, the social milieu in which it was consumed, and, of course, its material qualities and composition.

My point of departure is this materiality, the foundation for elaborating the distinctions that give name to the subtraction gestured at above: if "pulque" is to be prohibited, then "pulque without roots" belongs to, and constitutes, a different type. The *informes* expand on and develop these regimes of classification. While the ostensibly pure *pulque blanco* or *puro* (white or pure pulque) was generally taken as medicinal, *pulque mezclado* (mixed pulque), which contained certain difficult to pin down additives, was seen as, in the words of the Franciscan friar Juan de Luzuriaga, "the universal cause of sin."[14] Attacks on mixed pulque, furthermore, blurred together with attacks on its consumers, also—and not coincidentally—designated as mixed. When the Royal University advised the viceroy in its *informe* "to avoid this mixture" (*evitar esta mezcla*) above all other considerations, I argue, it was in fact articulating a more generalized politics in reference not only to pulque as an (al)chemical body but by extension to the racialized individual and social collective bodies of its consumers, as well as the urban cityscape in which that consumption took place.[15] Throughout the *informes*, the production of mixed pulque—the transformation or corruption of natural purity through nefarious mixing—resembles, and at times is analogous to, the production of mixed racial subjectivities through social, cultural, and biological mixing. If Foucault's interest in sexuality has made scholars attentive to this "pivot" that connects individual and population bodies and serves as the target of state intervention, my reading decenters the human body by tracing mixing back to the materiality of foodstuffs and foodways.[16] In this case, pulque, and not sex, was identified as the primary force that united bodies on and between multiple levels of scale, drawing them into the city's pulquerías to drink, dance, sing, make love—and presumably plot against the colonial state.

But the *informes* go beyond straightforward associations of mixed pulque's role in the material production of a mixed plebe. The grid of intelligibility that led colonial elites to conceive of the category of mixed pulque at the same time constituted as its mirror image a plebeian imaginary as a newly defined object of governance and political horizon to be regulated by the colonial state.[17] In spite of the best attempts of Spanish elites to probe, decipher, and document its many unknowns (ingredients, production processes, even etymology), this indigenous foodway remained stubbornly opaque and was, therefore, lumped together under the umbrella category of "mixed"; likewise, the racially fluid and indefinable plebeian bodies of Mexico City were channeled into a single collective mass whose principal characteristic was mixing.[18] *Pulque mezclado* and the *mixturada plebe*, I argue, are structurally identical.[19]

THE MAKING, AND MIXING, OF PULQUE

Central in precolonial ceremonial and food cultures, pulque (*octli* in Nahuatl) has been produced for thousands of years.[20] The maguey generally takes six to eight years to mature, at which point an artisan known as a *tlachiquero* makes a deft cut in the heart, releasing a sweet juice called *aguamiel*. Once the juice becomes sufficiently dense, the *tlachiquero* uses a long tube to collect and deposit it in a barrel or vat, along with a small amount of pulque from a previous batch to facilitate fermentation. The frothy and mildly alcoholic result is known as *pulque blanco*.[21] To this "pure" form, a variety of ingredients were added for flavor and as preservatives. In his *informe* to the viceroy, Doctor Francisco Antonio Ximénez listed as additives "orange and melon peels, peppers or chili, mineral lime, the root of *ocpatli* (which because of its strength they call wine medicine), Peru tree, the seeds of the *Pipilzizintli*, and other things that make it stronger and more alcoholic."[22] Other *informes* named stranger ingredients that pulque makers were thought to add as well, including herbs, meat, animal excrement, "a burning rock that the Indians call *tezontle*," and even "a jet-black, live lizard in a sealed tube" that an astonished inquisitor claimed to find in a vat of fermenting pulque ("It was horrifying to see," he confessed in his *informe*).[23]

The exaggerated and inconsistent laundry list that can be compiled from the *informes* suggests a profound interest in mixing in general on the part of elites, but at the same time an imperfect grasp of what exactly was being mixed. The otherwise confident vicar general of the Mercedarian Order, Francisco Martínez Falcón, who advanced a sophisticated scientific argument distinguishing mixed pulque from *aguamiel*, was certain that some root or other was implicated but added parenthetically that "in all of Mexico [City] I have not been able to discover, nor has anybody been able to tell me, what root it is."[24] Along with its precise composition, the minutiae of pulque production also remained obscure. The Franciscan friar Agustín de Vetancurt argued that pulque was impossible to regulate because it was produced "in the *pueblos*," out of the reach of Spanish administrators.[25] To be inserted into the vast urban pulque economy, of course, the drink had to be brought into Mexico City, which theoretically opened it up to supervision (not to mention taxation). But, as the archbishop asserted in his *informe*, a great deal of pulque entered the city secretly and thus illegally "in Vessels, and small wineskins, in canoes, and hidden in other things" so as to avoid such oversight. Once in the city, he continued, pulque vendors could simply add hot water, and presumably other ingredients, to their pulque vats at will.[26] In part, this interest in the details of pulque production is strategically ethnographic, a motivation similar to that of Spanish missionaries such as Diego Durán and Bernardino de Sahagún, who dedicated their lives to documenting indigenous culture so as to facilitate evangelization and the Spanish colonial project.[27] Read against this totalizing desire, apparent gaps in

Spanish knowledge of—and control over—pulque production reveal the limits of colonial hegemony. Pulque "ethnographers" remained insecure, gripped by an incomprehension that was refracted back on indigenous producers themselves in the form of an essentialized cultural, even natural otherness. As the Royal University argued, "Because [pulque] passes through the hands of the Indians either during its production or during its transportation, [mixing] is unavoidable; and more so because what they most desire about it is its strength."[28] A pathologized Indian nature, an indigenous body thirsty only for drunken excess, was used to smooth over these epistemological fissures.

It was this unknown and unknowable *pulque mezclado*, and not its "pure" cousin, that Spanish clergy and colonial administrators were referring to when they criticized, as early as the first half of the sixteenth century, what they perceived as the indigenous population's heavy drinking.[29] Even after the 1692 uprising, most of the *informes* agreed about the healthful effects of *aguamiel* and white pulque, thought to cure common ailments as well as more serious epidemics like measles.[30] In his report, Martínez Falcón cited Doctor Francisco Hernández, who had served as the Crown's chief medical officer in New Spain, to demonstrate that pulque also "eases menstruation in women, softens the stomach, provokes urine, cleanses the kidneys and bladder, and cleanses the urinary cavities and passages."[31] Evidence came from not only Spanish physicians but also indigenous informants. Archbishop Aguiar y Seijas, who described mixed pulque in demonic terms, noted that "according to information that I have acquired from the most Learned Physicians as well as Indian Elders, *aguamiel*, or the pure and simple juice of the Maguey, is good and medicinal."[32] White pulque's medicinal properties were so widely accepted that they were acknowledged even by many of the authors who supported the blanket pulque prohibition (meant to eliminate both pure and mixed varieties). Thus, while attacking the drink for its causal relationship with sin, Friar Luzuriaga could still distinguish between its various types:

> *Aguamiel* is medicinal for some ills, and white pulque without roots for others: but this pulque with roots, is good for nothing, and bad for everything.[33]

For many pulque critics, additives did not simply turn the drink into a stronger and more concentrated version of the same substance. Rather, mixing was thought to fundamentally alter its nature, transforming—even "transubstantiating," in the words of the theologian Francisco Xavier Palavicino y Villarasa—it into something new and essentially different.[34] The mixture of two elements thus produced not a compound but an entirely new third element. As the Royal University wrote, "Mixture does not conserve the liquid's simple [nature] but alters it, making a third type (*especie*) of drink of an opposing, or different nature."[35] Similarly, Vetancurt opened his report with a description of "the conditions that make Pulque a liquid, and not a confection." He went on: "they mix it with roots and harmful ingredients, in order to make a brew (*brebaje*) from what is [naturally] water distilled from the Maguey."[36] Though not a scientist like Doctor Ximénez, Vetancurt mobilized an authoritative discourse of classification in order to mark, and by doing so produce, categorical difference. The transformation of "liquid" into "confection" and "water" into "brew" represents the corruption of that which is by nature good or indifferent. These changes were thought to overdetermine the uses to which the new substance could be put. A neutral substance can theoretically be used for many purposes, good or bad, but if a "brew" or "confection" is bad in essence, as Vetancurt suggested, then it can never be used for good—and must therefore be prohibited.[37]

The *informes* frequently drew on contemporary histories of precolonial customs regarding pulque as a means of justifying the prohibition. Among the Mexica, observed Vetancurt, the punishment for drunkenness ranged from demolishing the guilty party's house to public execution; women were to be stoned to death "like adulteresses." After describing this harsh treatment, he posed the rhetorical question: "If this is what the Gentiles did out of political interest, what should Christians do out of both political and spiritual [interests], in the service of God and his King?"[38] Regardless of the severity of the penalties for public intoxication before the arrival of the Spaniards, however, later indigenous commentators may not have shared this obsession with mixing. Where the *informes* go out of their way to identify the more or less bizarre elements that, when added to the drink, rendered it officially "mixed," the annals of Domingo de San Antón Muñón Chimalpahin Quauhtlehuanitzin paints a somewhat different picture. Writing at the end of the sixteenth century, Chimalpahin, as he is more commonly known, recorded in Nahuatl what he saw as the most important events taking place in Mexico City and the nearby Chalco region, his birthplace. Pulque makes an appearance as early as 1594, in an entry referencing "the people of Tacubaya, who make their living with white pulque (*yztac octli*)."[39] In the entry for the following year, Chimalpahin wrote:

> It was in December of the year 1595 that an epidemic of measles broke out, from which people died; the epidemic really raged. People were helped with white pulque; *eloquiltic tletlematzin* was drunk in white pulque (*beheloquiltic tletlematzin miya yn ipa[n] yztac octli*), with which it was cured. There were a very great many deaths; every day very many were buried.[40]

Here, as in many of the *informes*, white pulque is described as medicinal. (Although the "very great many deaths" imply that its effects may have been somewhat overestimated.) But I am more interested in what, for

Chimalpahin, does and does not constitute mixing. The operative phrase is "*eloquiltic tletlematzin* was drunk in white pulque." The translators suggest that the words *eloquiltic tletlematzin* "refer to specific herbs used for a variety of purposes."[41] Despite the fact that "herbs" appear frequently in the lists of "pernicious" ingredients, the mixture of these particular herbs with *pulque blanco* does not seem to alter the substance of the drink or transform it into the dreaded *pulque mezclado*. Chimalpahin preferred to call the drink *white pulque with herbs*, instead of "mixed pulque" or even just "pulque with herbs." That he never mentioned any other type of pulque or appears interested in developing his own list of mixture-producing ingredients suggests that Chimalpahin's primary interest lay in the drink's healing properties. But it also points to a subtle difference in the place that the category of the "mixed" occupied in his approach to the natural world. And the meaning of mixing, as we will see, extended far beyond the rim of the pulque mug.

MIXED PULQUE AND THE (RE)PRODUCTION OF SIN

The *informes* described mixed pulque as both a spiritual and temporal threat. Diego de la Cadena, a professor of theology at the Royal University, opened his report by declaring that the prohibition "will be of the best service to both Majesties: to Our Lord God, because of the very serious inconveniences, that occur in the Moral [realm]; and to the Catholic Majesty of Our Lord and King (may God protect him) because of the excessive and inevitable harms caused by [pulque] in the Political."[42] Most of the *informes*—all but three—were written by members of New Spain's clergy and therefore concern themselves primarily with the former. These reports constitute a laundry list of the Indians' greater and lesser sins, seemingly drawn less from personal experience or empirical evidence than from biblical references and other religious commentary—Saints Ambrose and Augustine figure prominently. Claims of renewed indigenous idolatry and sacrifice demonstrated, in the words of the Dominican friar Juan del Castillo, that alcohol "undoes the rustic and simple ways that the Indians had quickly adopted after their conquest and conversion."[43] Assertions of religious backsliding were articulated alongside other, somewhat contradictory claims that the indigenous population had in fact never abandoned its ancient religion. In his account of the uprising, for example, Sigüenza declared that "even today [the Indians have] not forgotten their ancient superstitions," and added parenthetically that "their most important deity" continued to be "the God of War."[44]

In either form, incomplete or imperfect conversion served as a powerful rhetorical device with which to attack pulque, while at the same time privileging the administrative perspective of the clergy responsible for these reports. Perhaps the most powerful argument *against* the pulque prohibition was the revenue that the sale of the pulque *asiento* (contract) provided the government. Many ecclesiastical authors sought to preempt this financial drawback by flatly asserting that the salvation of even a single soul was worth more than the hundreds of thousands of pesos gained by selling pulque permits. A wide variety of historical examples were given to demonstrate the Spanish crown's historical interest in evangelization over economics, including Philip II's costly invasion of Flanders and Philip IV's failed attempt to hold onto Portugal in 1640.[45]

But the reports did not limit their focus to the spiritual alone. Indeed, despite de la Cadena's analytical attempt to keep them separate, the temporal and spiritual worlds in many ways overlap—homicide can simultaneously constitute a mortal sin and a threat to political stability. Most important here were the "intimate" sins thought to take place in Mexico City's numerous pulquerías.[46] Critics frequently referred to the pulquería as a point of encounter where the city's many races were brought together by the pernicious drink. According to the minister of San Pablo parish, Bernabé Núñez de Paez, "with this Drink the Indians have built a friendship with the blacks and mulattos, who had always been their enemies; and with one another (*unos y otros*) they form a most perverse Plebe."[47] The composition of this plebe involved a simultaneously positive and negative movement: on one hand, the consolidation of a unified underclass; on the other, the disruption of the boundaries of identity, boundaries that elites clearly hoped to maintain and keep visible. For the Dean and Cabildo of Mexico City's cathedral, "another no less important problem with this lineage of vice which has so infested the plebe is that there is scarcely a Pulquería to be found that is not full of Blacks, Mulattoes, and other kinds of People (*otro genero de Gentes*) that would be shameful to mention." And those brought together by drink, they continued, "cannot be distinguished even by their customs."[48] What worried these authors, for whom lineage shaped moral behavior, was that identities would evade orderly classification: the transformation of what was "shameful to mention" into what was impossible to know.

Pulquerías were seen as dark, ambiguous spaces, where—not coincidentally—dark, ambiguous races met secretively to plot against their Spanish rulers. Archbishop Aguiar y Seijas described the seditious mix of blacks, mulattoes, mestizos, and Indians that "comes together by day, and especially at night, in rooms, alcoves, and hidden places" belonging to the pulquerías in order to "commit their unspeakable evils."[49] Among these "evils" the uprising would no doubt be counted, but the archbishop had more immediate concerns. "[I]t is not only the Indians who get drunk," he wrote, "but Women as well, and an equal amount of slaves, Blacks, Mestizos, Mulattoes, and a great many lower-class Spaniards—though not all of them, or as many, [get drunk] as much as the Indians."[50] Women are doubly implicated by the mechanics of this list: transformed into a racialized category, an additional ingredient thrown into the already dangerous social mixture of the pulquería, while simultaneously intersected by a far more insidious, biological form of mixing. Acknowledged as central actors in the production of race, women simultaneously come to serve as a marker of, even to embody race itself.[51] For Aguiar y Seijas, a reputed misogynist, singling out women for blame may have been inevitable.[52] But many of the *informes* joined in lamenting what the bishop-elect of Durango, don García de Legaspi Velasco, called "crimes of abominable sensuality." "It is inevitable that men and women will come together" in the pulquerías, he wrote, adding obliquely that "from this follow immediate problems that are easily understood."[53] Vetancurt, for his part, asserted that patrons commonly "offer each other their wives in a lustful exchange for [a mug of] Pulque."[54] Legitimate reproduction consecrated by marriage gave way to illegitimate, and likely cross-race, fornication.[55]

Within the shadowy pulquerías, out of reach of secular and ecclesiastical authorities, this convergence of men and women thus actualized yet another form of mixing. The friendly contact between Indians, blacks, mulattoes, and mestizos opened the door not only to cross-cultural conversation and conspiracy, but indeed, through the active participation of women, to "sensual" contact as well, facilitating the (re)production of ever increasing numbers of fractioned racial categories. In the minds of its critics, mixed pulque made these couplings, and the racial mixtures they produced, possible. At the same time, the (al)chemical processes that transformed *pulque blanco* into an entirely new substance echoed the unchecked sexuality of the pulquerías, which projected the possibility of new peoples and new kinds of people onto the future.[56] It was not just the salvation of the Indians' souls that mattered to these ecclesiastical authors—it was their belief that the dangers of mixing could not be contained within *pulque mezclado* but, through a sort of infusion if not consumption, would eventually penetrate the blood of the individual and the physiology of the social body, turning the city into a "Kingdom of mestizos, with [mixed] blood."[57]

MIXED PULQUE, MIXED PLEBE

Of all the *informes* presented to the viceroy, the one written by the full cloister of the Royal University of Mexico City deserves special attention. This is not only because of the prestige of its authors but also because it was the only one to be printed, which suggests that it may have been intended for wider distribution.[58] Packed with citations of classical and New World sources, from Herodotus and Aristotle to Solórzano and Torquemada, the University's report focused in particular on the question of governance. In the opening paragraph, as noted earlier, the authors established a causal link between mixing and social stability by citing a law from 1671 urging rulers "to avoid this mixture."[59] As in the other *informes*, the University's language of mixing applies equally to the composition of *pulque mezclado* and to the bodies of those thought to consume it. Deploying an optical neologism, they declared it "incredibly clear" (*ocularissimo*) that the origin of the uprising could be found in the Indians' "mixing (*mezclas*) with other members of the [Republic], blacks, mulattoes, and even Spaniards"—a fact, they continued, which "the ongoing trials against the participants in the riot will prove."[60]

If other *informes* only gestured at the spatiality of mixing, drawing in particular on the logic of the pulquería, the University built on this conceptualization of the Republic to read mixing as a concrete threat to the city. Like mixed pulque and its "mixed" consumers, Mexico City thus constituted an urban body suffering from a dangerous state of mixing that the University held responsible for the June 8 uprising. Foregrounding the corporeal horizon of their argument, the authors employed a reproductive metaphor to argue that "encounters with one another (*unos con otros*) in the pulquerías give birth to . . . death and other disorders":

> All legal thought prohibits unauthorized congregations and unconfirmed bodies: because this [city] of drinkers is not the entire City, it is not a monopoly (*monopolio*), but because it is of the entire plebe, it is *poliplebio*. What plotting will take place in these encounters? What robberies will be planned? And what else (*Y que que*)? It is not even necessary to say: the causes, and trajectory of the riot say enough.[61]

This dense passage situates the convergence of mixed racial bodies within the spatial dimensions of a concrete political unit. "What comes first," the University asserted, "is the cause of the City, and Republic."[62] But exactly what these polities may have to confront is not entirely clear. The University's rhetorical questions do not limit the possibilities to plotting (presumably on topics such as the injustice of the colonial regime) and robbery (presumably of government or Spanish property), but leave the door open with an open-ended "what else?": anything, however unimaginable, could conceivably take place. Perhaps the shock of insurrectionary violence was responsible for this formulation, which constitutes both a rhetorical narrowing and imaginative broadening of the authors' collective political horizon. Simultaneously addressing past and future, the logic of the University's argument has no need for precise link chains of cause and effect. Paradoxically, it was precisely the ambiguity of these unseen plots and unheard whispers that provided the best proof of their existence.[63]

Conspiracy, furthermore, emerges within a particular domain. As a counterpoint to the *monopolio* of the unitary city, the University coined and deployed a second neologism: the term *poliplebio*. Anna More has pointed to "a slippage between several meanings of the root 'poli"' in the interaction between these two words. On one hand, there is the "poli" of "poliplebio," which refers to the heterogeneous multitudes of the pulquerías. At the same time, there is the dual "poli" present in "monopolio." "Although the root of 'monopolio' is 'polein' or 'to sell,' the proximity of the question of the 'city' in this statement brings to mind the root 'polis.' Rather than a united city, a 'monopolio,' then, 'poliplebio' would indicate a plebeian city whose spread also effects a quasi-monopolization."[64] Within what the authors seem to imagine as a dense network of pulquerías, pulque drinkers constituted a plebeian underworld. This counterhegemonic "city of drinkers" functions conceptually via the metonym of the pulquería, whose transgressive space threatens to spread to the City/Republic. Much like the archbishop's concern with the obscurity of the pulquerías, the University's *poliplebio* remains similarly obscure and separate, yet at the same time effects a centrifugal movement, bleeding into and thereby contaminating the state's idealized *monopolio*. Indeed, its influence reached beyond the walls of the pulquerías and into public spaces. "In the pulquerías, in the plazas, in the streets, in the countryside," Friar Luzuriaga asserted, one could barely avoid stumbling over the monstrous bodies of the intoxicated citizens of this counter-city.[65] Furthermore, according to bishop-elect García de Legaspi, pulque stands permeated the organic city, "not only in its indigenous neighborhoods, but even in areas very close to its heart (*corazon*)."[66] In this view, urban space constitutes a body, like those chemical and biological bodies defined by mixing, at risk of contamination.

In the face of this threatening underworld, the University forcefully laid out the government's claim to political rule:

> The contagious man is not considered guilty, but even so because of the danger to others he is separated (*se aparta*) and exterminated.[67]

They continued:

> In the interest of public health even an innocent vassal can be exposed to death, and all vassals, for that matter, can be sent to war.[68]

The contagious man is a powerful metaphor. He represents at once victim and victimizer of mixing; his state is unintentional, but is nevertheless treated as if it were not. Like the mixed-blooded offspring of "sensual" contact in the pulquerías, mixture transforms him into a newly contaminated—and thus contaminating—agent. Death and war thus become the legitimate side effects of the state's imposition of order through purity, where the good of the *monopolio*, which stands in for the City/Republic, comes before that of its individual members. It is the question of governance, of what is to be done with the contagious man, that the slippage of categories between biological and social mixings is clarified: "He is separated and exterminated." In the context of the University's justification of state violence against "even an innocent vassal," the threat of extermination speaks for itself. More interesting, however, is the strategy of "separation." The *Diccionario de Autoridades* (1726) defines the verb "apartar" as follows:

> To separate, to divide one thing from another: like cattle, which are separated from one another (*uno de otro*), and likewise other types (*generos*) that are divided. Lat. *Separare, Dividere, Segregare*.[69]

Separation, division, segregation. In the case of the cattle, members of the same type are kept apart from each other. But the expression *unos y otros* is used frequently in the pulque *informes* to refer to the convergence of different types, racial types. For the University, the city, greater than the sum of inhabitants and the materials they consume, must be kept from mixing—it must be purified. The colonial state, then, must not only prohibit mixed pulque and by extension wipe the pulquerías off the map, but simultaneously redraw the lines of the city so as to redistribute its individual bodies into rigidly defined and bounded spaces and, as a consequence, legible identities.

CONCLUSION: PULQUE AND THE SEGREGATED CITY

By situating the plebe within a particular spatial domain, the University's *informe* contextualizes the viceroy's second policy response to the 1692 uprising: the segregation of the city. On July 1, about three weeks after the uprising, the viceroy asked Sigüenza to submit a proposal for dividing the city into separate Spanish and Indian sectors.[70] In his official report, submitted four days later, Sigüenza referenced Spanish historiographers such as Juan de Torquemada, Francisco López de Gómara, and Bernal Díaz del Castillo to prove that, at its foundation upon the ruins of Tenochtitlan, Mexico City had been laid out in segregated blocs, such that the Spanish population occupied the center or *traza* and Indians the *barrios* at the outskirts. In the words of Torquemada, which Sigüenza cited in the text, "this city does not mix (*no se mezcla*) with the Indians, rather they surround it on four sides, forming their own neighborhoods (*barrios*)."[71] Torquemada's history served to frame Sigüenza's assertion that this policy would in fact constitute a re-segregation, a return to Mexico City's (colonial) origins as laid out by Cortés.

The segregation proposal thus draws on what Mexican historian Edmundo O'Gorman has called the "principle of separation" instituted by the Spanish crown in the form of a spatial, legal, and administrative dichotomy between the so-called two republics: the *república de los españoles* and the *república de los indios*.[72] Some historians have read this policy as a "humanitarian" effort on the part of the Crown to prevent the exploitation of Indian communities at the hands of "pernicious" racial groups, including blacks, mestizos, and mulattoes.[73] These "others" were supposed to be incorporated into the Spanish republic, leaving Indian communities "pure" and protected in order to facilitate evangelization. Sigüenza's redeployment of the "principle of separation," however, inverts this original precedent: instead of protecting Indian villages from the intrusion of non-Indians, it serves to protect Spanish space from the penetration of Indians. By embedding identity in a restructured cityscape, this resegregation attempts to elide tensions between Spanish-born *peninsulares* and American-born *criollos* and consolidate, at least on a conceptual level, a unified "Spanish" (white) population at its sovereign center: to *monopolize* the city. As a structural-spatial politics of population, however, it simultaneously constitutes its opposite, what the Royal University so feared: a counterhegemonic *poliplebio* that comes to stand in for the Indian enemy identified by Sigüenza at the outset.

"[T]he hallmark of the Mexican plebe," writes Cope, "was its racially mixed nature." For Cope, this mixedness was expressed in the heterogeneity of a group that "included Indians, castizos, mestizos, mulattoes, blacks, and even poor Spaniards."[74] No doubt the plebe was composed of various racial groups, but this analysis captures only a small part of the multiple and interconnected mixings that permeated the natural, social, and administrative imaginaries of colonial elites, transgressing even such apparently solid categories as the human body. As the pulque *informes* suggest, the plebe's characteristic mixedness arose from not only its group heterogeneity, as Cope suggests, but also its particular positioning within the cityscape, as a group can be constituted only through spatial relations; the biologically "mixed" race of the individual bodies that composed that group, conceived through "sensual" contact in the pulquerías ("... castizos, mestizos, mulattoes..."); and, finally, the incorporation of certain foods seen to define those who consume them (as in the figure of the drunken Indian or the University's formulation of a "city of drinkers"). The plebe, in other words, was the most extreme manifestation of a more generalized concern.

In practice, the two prongs of the colonial state's response to the uprising were at best only marginally successful. Not only did the pulque prohibition fail to keep people from drinking, but in 1697 the government once again legalized *pulque mezclado*, reinitiated the pulque *asiento*, and decriminalized the pulquerías.[75] Evidently, theological arguments privileging the evangelizing mission over tax revenues could not, in the end, convince the cash-hungry state.[76] Nor did it help, as William Taylor notes, that "[s]ome of the wealthiest and most influential families in the city" were involved in the pulque business.[77] Similarly, the imposition of spatial and racial purity on the face of the city fared little better. Indigenous residents of the *traza* may have obeyed the segregation edict and moved out during several months, but soon thereafter began to return.[78] Nevertheless, we should not ignore these policies as little more than quixotic devices or psychological defense mechanisms designed by colonial elites to adjust "reality" to expectations in order to control their fear.[79] Although in material terms the imposition of a racialized order was a failure, in conceptual terms these policies and the discursive formations that shaped them generated a newly consolidated object of governance, a plebe-organism capable of being regulated and administered. An emerging population body whose natural dimensions and flows could be apprehended via increasingly abstract forms of data—it is no surprise that records of the 1691 doctrinal census played a key role in the discussion of segregation.[80]

Pulque, which stands at the intersection of Spanish colonialism and deeply "local" knowledges and practices, delineates both the space of the plebe as a social-group and sexual–individual convergence as well as the practices of consumption that gave these bodies meaning. Most importantly, the analysis of pulque advanced in the *informes* points to a common grid of intelligibility through which colonial elites perceived society at large: the impossibility of deciphering the constitutive elements of both pulque and plebe generated food and social bodies defined by indefinable mixing. In light of this specificity, we should be careful not to overgeneralize the relationship between the Spanish interest in indigenous foodways and the obsession with mixing that I have traced for Mexico City at the end of the seventeenth century. After all, not all indigenous alcohols, however dangerous, were considered "mixed." The Royal University's *informe*, for example, cites the Peruvian friar Bernardino de Cárdenas on the Indians' thirst for alcohol: "in Peru, a drink is made from ground maize that this Author calls *Chicha* . . . and it is intoxicating, and they establish little taverns [to sell] it."[81] While Cárdenas's critique of indigenous drinking is familiar, it does not lend itself to the spiraling attacks on mixing—chemical, biological, social, spatial—that were facilitated by the investigation of pulque in New Spain. This is not to say, of course, that mixing and race were unimportant outside Mexico, but simply that these concepts were imagined, articulated, and visualized in different ways.[82] Such comparisons, however, are beyond the scope of this essay. What I have tried to present here is but one localized figuration of the globalized contact zone, the way that local foodways were incorporated into and shaped Spanish colonial discourse and practices of governance, as not only nutritional or economic signifiers but also conceptual structures according to which the social world was organized and made legible.

NOTES

1. J. H. Elliott, *The Old World and the New, 1492–1650* (Cambridge: Cambridge University Press, 1970), 28.

2. For a critique of the concept of acculturation and an elaboration of the more nuanced transculturation, the key text, originally published in 1940, is Fernando Ortiz, *Contrapunteo cubano del tabaco y el azúcar*, ed. Enrico Mario Santí (Madrid: Cátedra, 2002). A more recent approach is Mary Louise Pratt's formulation of the "contact zone" in *Imperial Eyes: Travel Writing and Transculturation* (New York: Routledge, 1997), 6–7.

3. See, for example, Alfred Crosby, *The Columbian Exchange: Biological and Cultural Consequences of 1492* (Westport, CT: Greenwood, 1972); Sidney Mintz, *Sweetness and Power: The Place of Sugar in Modern History* (New York: Penguin Books, 1985); Nelson Foster and Linda S. Cordell, eds., *Chiles to Chocolate: Food the Americas Gave the World* (Tucson, AZ: University of Arizona Press, 1992); Jeffrey M. Pilcher, *Que Vivan Los Tamales! Food and the Making of Mexican Identity* (Albuquerque: University of New Mexico Press, 1998), chap. 2; Marcy Norton, "Tasting Empire: Chocolate and the European Internalization of Mesoamerican Aesthetics," *The American Historical Review* 111, no. 3 (June 2006): 660–691; and Norton, *Sacred Gifts, Profane Pleasures: A History of Tobacco and Chocolate in the Atlantic World* (Ithaca, NY: Cornell University Press, 2008). Norton's excellent work deals with the "assimilation" of

tobacco and chocolate in colonial context, but primarily as part of an argument about how these products were inserted into the global economy. In a more local vein, John E. Kicza's study of the late colonial pulque industry in New Spain traces the process by which Spanish producers increasingly took control of the production of this indigenous commodity. But, for Kicza, pulque holds little cultural or political significance or specificity; *any* product native to the Americas (such as cacao or maize) could just as easily fill its role. Pulque thus serves as an empty economic signifier, just another site for Spanish capital accumulation. I am interested in the way pulque in particular offered colonial elites both a site for state intervention and a language with which to articulate the politics of that intervention. Kicza, "The Pulque Trade of Late Colonial Mexico City," *The Americas* 37, no. 2 (1980): 193–221.

4. The relationship between food and colonial governance in the Americas has received less scholarly attention. One interesting exception comes from Enrique Rodríguez-Alegría, who uses archaeological remains and historical documents to examine eating practices as a form of political strategy for Spanish elites. See Rodríguez-Alegría, "Eating Like an Indian: Negotiating Social Relations in the Spanish Colonies," *Current Anthropology* 46 (2005): 551–73. Also see Sophie D. Coe, *America's First Cuisines* (Austin, TX: University of Texas Press, 1994), chap. 16; and John C. Super, *Food, Conquest, and Colonization in Sixteenth-Century Spanish America* (Albuquerque: University of New Mexico Press, 1988).

5. Recent scholarship on the events of the uprising includes R. Douglas Cope, *The Limits of Racial Domination: Plebeian Society in Colonial Mexico City, 1660–1720* (Madison, WI: University of Wisconsin Press, 1994), chap. 6; Natalia Silva Prada, *La política de una rebelión: Los indígenas frente al tumulto de 1692 en la Ciudad de México* (Mexico City: El Colegio de México, 2007); and Pilar Gonzalbo Aizpuru, "El nacimiento del miedo, 1692: Indios y españoles en la ciudad de México," *Revista de Indias* 68, no. 244 (2008): 9–34. Beginning in 1691, central Mexico was hit by a "dual agricultural crisis" (a shortage of both wheat and maize) that caused grain prices to spike. While viceregal officials were sent to procure grains from the surrounding areas, high prices and distribution problems impeded a solution. In the end, the city's granary (*albóndiga*) was left empty. See Cope, *Limits of Racial Domination*, 128–134; and Gonzalbo Aizpuru, "El nacimiento del miedo," 14–15.

6. Father Joseph de la Barrera wrote of the Indians' "so entirely unexpected audacity in the most principal court of this Kingdom." Joseph de la Barrera to Conde de Galve, Archivo General de Indias (hereafter AGI), Mexico 333, fol. 471v. Unless otherwise noted, all translations are mine.

7. "Those who most persisted in their complaints were the Indians, the most ungrateful, thankless, grumbling, and restless people that God ever created." Carlos de Sigüenza y Góngora, "Letter of Don Carlos de Sigüenza to Admiral Pez Recounting the Incidents of the Corn Riot in Mexico City, June 8, 1692," in Irving Leonard, *Don Carlos de Sigüenza y Góngora: A Mexican Savant of the Seventeenth Century* (Berkeley, CA: University of California Press, 1929), 244. According to Irving Leonard, Sigüenza served as "a sort of official historian" for the Viceroy Conde de Galve and his description of the uprising constituted "a semi-official report of the affair, possibly made at the behest of the viceroy." See Leonard, *Sigüenza y Góngora*, 105, 112. For a detailed account of Sigüenza's relationship with the viceroy, see Iván Escamilla González, "El siglo de oro vindicado: Carlos de Sigüenza y Góngora, el Conde de Galve y el tumulto de 1692," in *Carlos de Sigüenza y Góngora: Homenaje 1700–2000*, ed. Alicia Mayer (Mexico City: UNAM, 2002), II, 179–203. Cope traces the development of this "official" narrative about the uprising, which he calls the "treacherous Indians" explanation, in *Limits of Racial Domination*, 126–27.

8. Sigüenza, "Letter to Admiral Pez," 275; translation altered. A decade earlier, Sigüenza had already written of the "DETESTABLE PULQUE" that was "the cause and origin of so much damage" and whose use he called "in no way indifferent, but always sinful." See Sigüenza, *Parayso Occidental, plantado, y cultivado por la liberal benefica mano de los muy Catholicos, y poderosos Reyes de España Nuestros Señores en su magnifico Real Convento de Jesus Maria de Mexico* (1684), fol. IXr, http://www.cervantesvirtual.com/servlet/SirveObras/12585075434593728876657/index.htm (accessed July 2009).

9. Sigüenza, "Letter to Admiral Pez," 275; see also Antonio de Robles, *Diario de sucesos notables* (Mexico City: Editorial Porrua, 1946), II, 257.

10. Robles, *Diario*, II, 264.

11. Robles, *Diario*, II, 264.

12. Robles, *Diario*, II, 265.

13. By rendering either pulque or its prohibition "absolute." See, for example, Leonard, *Sigüenza y Góngora*, 133; as well as recent essays like Cope, *Limits of Racial Domination*, 127; Silva Prada, *La política de una rebelión*, 498; and Gonzalbo Aizpuru, "El nacimiento del miedo," 25–27. Tim Mitchell uses

scare-quotes to call into question the legitimacy of the category of white (medicinal) pulque: after the 1692 prohibition, he writes, "legal sales of 'medicinal' *pulque* slaked the thirst of Indians and poor Creoles alike." Mitchell, *Intoxicated Identities: Alcohol's Power in Mexican History and Culture* (New York: Routledge, 2004), 24. Notable exceptions are José Jesús Hernández Palomo, *La renta del pulque en la Nueva España, 1663–1810* (Seville: Escuela de Estudios Hispano-Americanos, 1979); and William B. Taylor, *Drinking, Homicide, and Rebellion in Colonial Mexican Villages* (Stanford, CA: Stanford University Press, 1979), chap. 2. For a critique of scholarly overreliance on Sigüenza's text, see Mabel Moraña, "El 'tumulto de indios' de 1692 en los pliegues de la fiesta barroca: Historiografía, subversión popular y agencia criolla en el México colonial," *Agencias criollas: La ambigüedad 'colonial' en las letras hispanoamericanas*, ed. José Antonio Mazzotti (Pittsburgh, PA: Biblioteca de América, 2000), 161–175. Running parallel to the pulque debates, seventeenth-century debates about chocolate as medicine or food highlight the shifting and multivalent significance of food and drink in Europe. See Ken Albala, "The Use and Abuse of Chocolate in Seventeenth-Century Medical Theory," *Food and Foodways* 15 (2007): 53–74.

14. Juan de Luzuriaga to Conde de Galve, AGI Mexico 333, fol. 338r.

15. The University's *informe* was the only one that was printed. See the *Informe que la Real Universidad, y Claustro Pleno de ella de la Ciudad de Mexico de esta Nueva España haze a el Excellentissimo Señor Virrey de ella en conformidad de orden de su Excelencia de 3 de Iulio de este año 1692 sobre los inconvenientes de la bebida de el Pulque* (Mexico City, 1692), fol. 1r.

16. "[S]ex . . . was at the pivot of the two axes along which developed the entire political technology of life. On the one hand, it was tied to the disciplines of the body: the harnessing, intensification, and distribution of forces, the adjustment and economy of energies. On the other hand, it was applied to the regulation of populations, through all the far-reaching effects of its activity." Michel Foucault, *The History of Sexuality, Vol. 1: An Introduction*, trans. Robert Hurley (New York: Vintage Books, 1978), 145. This is not to say that colonial elites were uninterested in regulating sexuality. Patricia Seed traces a shift in the institutional site of social control regarding marriage in colonial Mexico from the church in the sixteenth and seventeenth centuries to the state in the eighteenth. See Seed, *To Love, Honor, and Obey in Colonial Mexico: Conflicts over Marriage Choice, 1574–1821* (Stanford, CA: Stanford University Press, 1988). On sixteenth-century approaches to "remedying" indigenous and mestizo women (and in some cases men) in *conventos* and *colegios*, see Kathryn Burns, *Colonial Habits: Convents and the Spiritual Economy of Cuzco, Peru* (Durham, NC: Duke University Press, 1999), chap. 1; and Jacqueline Holler, *Escogidas Plantas: Nuns and Beatas in Mexico City, 1531–1601* (New York: Columbia University Press, 2005). Ann Laura Stoler's important work on the regulation of the intimate in the Dutch East Indies has resituated Foucault's approach to race within a colonial context. See Stoler, *Carnal Knowledge and Imperial Power: Race and the Intimate in Colonial Rule* (Berkeley, CA: University of California Press, 2002).

17. Cf. Cope, *Limits of Racial Domination*, 22: "The hallmark of the Mexican plebe was its racially mixed nature. Mexico's lower class included Indians, castizos, mestizos, mulattoes, blacks, and even poor Spaniards." I return to Cope's analysis in the conclusion.

18. In the colonial period, the source of the word "pulque" was itself mysterious: Durán suggested that, like "maize," it came from the Caribbean islands; Clavijero, writing in the eighteenth century, countered that it was originally an Araucan (Chile) word, though he admitted that "it is difficult to say how this name came to Mexico." See Durán, *Historia de las Indias de Nueva España* (Mexico City: Editora Nacional, 1951), II, 240; Francisco Javier Clavijero, *Historia antigua de Mégico*, trans. José Joaquín de Mora (London: R. Ackermann, 1826), I, 393.

19. Ayuntamiento to Conde de Galve, AGI Mexico 333, fol. 322v. If the plebe took on racialized qualities that had previously been attributed to the Indian, as Cope suggests, it was the study of indigenous culture itself—in this case, pulque—that provided colonial elites with the discursive formation necessary to define, and thereby constitute, this plebeian body as such. Cope, *Limits of Racial Domination*, 22–23.

20. According to the Dominican missionary Diego Durán, pulque was considered divine and used solemnly and with much devotion in religious ceremonies. See Durán, *Historia de las Indias*, II, 237–238. Pulque was "the sacred milk of the inexhaustible breasts of Mayahuel, goddess of the maguey, prototype of the generous mother. Mayahuel was represented as She with Four Hundred (that is to say, innumerable) Breasts. . . . It was the last taste in the mouths of the captive warriors tethered to fight on the gladiatorial stone, as it was the first in the mouths of infants introduced to public ceremonial life, when pulque was drunk to full inebriation." Inga Clendinnen, *The Aztecs: An Interpretation* (Cambridge: Cambridge University Press, 1991), 245. Also see Taylor, *Drinking, Homicide, and Rebellion*, chap. 2.

21. Indeed, pulque's alcohol content (approximately 4 percent) is quite low, significantly less than that of Spanish wine. Taylor, *Drinking, Homicide, and Rebellion*, 31.

22. Francisco Antonio Ximénez to Conde de Galve, AGI Mexico 333, fol. 540v.

23. Franciso Xavier Palavicino y Villarasa to Conde de Galve, AGI Mexico 333, fol. 528r; Francisco Martínez Falcón to Conde de Galve, AGI Mexico 333, fol. 414v; Obispo de Valladolid to Conde de Galve, AGI Mexico 333, fol. 283v; and Cayetano Francisco de Torres, "Virtudes maravillosas del Pulque, medicamento universal, ó Polychresto," Biblioteca Nacional de México (BN), MS 23, fol. 4v. Hernández Palomo gives a detailed description of maguey cultivation and pulque production in the colonial period in *La renta del pulque*, 14–30. Some of the *informes* disagreed with this classification of pulque's stages, which follows the *informe* written by Doctor Ximénez. Friar Antonio Guridi, the minister of the indigenous parish of Santiago Tlatelolco, for example, wrote only of *aguamiel* on one hand, and a generalized "pulque" on the other, blurring the white and mixed varieties together. See Antonio Guridi to Conde de Galve, AGI Mexico 333, fol. 496r–497r. I follow Doctor Ximénez here because his *informe*, which was specifically cited and adopted by the Council of the Indies, best seems to represent the conventional wisdom of the moment. See Consejo de Indias to Conde de Galve, AGI Mexico 333, fol. 590r–592v.

24. Francisco Martínez Falcón to Conde de Galve, AGI Mexico 333, fols. 406r-v. This root may have been *ocpatli*, although it seems unlikely that Martínez Falcón would have been unaware of something so commonly mentioned in other *informes*, such as Antonio Guridi to Conde de Galve, AGI Mexico 333, fol. 496v.

25. Augustín de Vetancurt to Conde de Galve, AGI Mexico 333, fol. 499r.

26. This was part of the archbishop's effort to calculate the number of sins caused by pulque in Mexico City. By multiplying the number of mules entering the city by the number of *arrobas* each one could carry, he determined that some five million *arrobas* of pulque entered the city each year. Next, he figured that each *arroba* would generate two "sins of drunkenness," thus reaching the total of ten million sins of drunkenness per year. At this point, however, he was forced to give up, because the quantity of other sins caused by drunkenness was so high that "only God can count them." Francisco de Aguiar y Seijas to Conde de Galve, AGI Mexico 333, fols. 272v–273r.

27. Tzvetan Todorov, *The Conquest of America: The Question of the Other*, trans. Richard Howard (Norman, OK: University of Oklahoma Press, 1999), 202–42; José Rabasa, *Inventing America: Spanish Historiography and the Formation of Eurocentrism* (Norman, OK: University of Oklahoma Press, 1993), chap. 4, esp. 125–130, 151–164.

28. *Informe que la Real Universidad*, fol. 1v.

29. Taylor argues that these critiques reveal differences between Spanish and Indian drinking cultures or practices rather than in the relative quantity consumed. See Taylor, *Drinking, Homicide, and Rebellion*, 41. *Pulque blanco* was the only kind legally permitted during the colonial period. Hernández Palomo, *La renta del pulque*, 31–33.

30. Hernández Palomo, *La renta del pulque*, 10–13.

31. Martínez Falcón to Conde de Galve, AGI Mexico 333, fol. 407r. On the life and writings of Francisco Hernández, as well as their diffusion in Europe, see Hernández, *The Mexican Treasury: The Writings of Dr. Francisco Hernández*, ed. Simon Varey and trans. Simon Varey, Rafael Chabrán, and Cynthia L. Chamberlin (Stanford, CA: Stanford University Press, 2000), 3–25.

32. Aguiar y Seijas to Conde de Galve, AGI Mexico 333, fol. 269r. In fact, much like the church ethnographers such as Bernardino de Sahagún, Spanish doctors like Francisco Hernández drew heavily on indigenous knowledge to produce their findings. Philip II instructed Hernández to "consult, wheresoever you go, all the doctors, medicine men, herbalists, Indians, and other persons with knowledge in such matters [i.e., medicinal uses of native plants and animals]." See "The Instructions of Philip II to Dr. Francisco Hernández," in *The Mexican Treasury*, 46.

33. Juan de Luzuriaga to Conde de Galve, AGI Mexico 333, fol. 337v.

34. Francisco Xaviar Palavicino to Conde de Galve, AGI Mexico 333, fol. 525r.

35. *Informe que la Real Universidad*, fol. 4v. Also see Aguiar y Seijas to Conde de Galve, AGI Mexico 333, fol. 267r.

36. Augustín de Vetancurt to Conde de Galve, AGI Mexico 333, fol. 499r.

37. For example, Antonio Girón, minister of Santa Cruz parish, argued that pulque should not be considered indifferent "because all things that uniformly induce physical or moral necessity towards an action, cannot be called indifferent [with regard to] the good or the bad." Girón to Conde de Galve, AGI Mexico 333, fol. 520r.

38. Augustín de Vetancurt to Conde de Galve, AGI Mexico 333, fols. 501v–502r. Such claims are problematic, as they rely on the recollections of elite indigenous informants at least a half-century after the fact. Lockhart suggests that historians have "too readily accepted idealized and self-serving posterior statements that hardly anyone drank pulque before the conquest." See James Lockhart, *The Nahuas After the Conquest: A Social and Cultural History of the Indians of Central Mexico, Sixteenth through Eighteenth Centuries* (Stanford, CA: Stanford University Press, 1992), 112. Also see Taylor, *Drinking, Homicide, and Rebellion*, chap. 2.

39. Don Domingo de San Antón Muñón Chimalpahin Quauhtlehuanitzin. *Annals of His Time*, eds. and trans. James Lockhart, Susan Schroeder, and Doris Namala (Stanford, CA: Stanford University Press, 2006), 51. It is notable that the translators do not know what to do with "iztac octli." In a footnote, they write, "It is not clear to us if this means simply pulque in general, or if white pulque is a special kind. Molina gives white wine for *iztac octli*." But Molina also gives "vino" (wine) for "octli" (pulque); as we saw above, in Doctor Ximénez's reference to "Wine medicine," it was common practice to refer to *pulque* in Spanish as "vino." It is, therefore, highly unlikely that Chimalpahin was writing about Spanish wine, white or otherwise.

40. Chimalpahin, *Annals*, 55.

41. "*Eloquiltic* seems to be an adjectival form based on *elotl* (*elote* in Spanish), a green ear of corn on the plant, and *quilitl*, any of a variety of green plants of the type used for salads. *Tlemaitl* is a sort of ladle to carry fire in and probably could refer to a ladle or spoon more generally." The translators go on to question, once again, "whether *iztac octli* could be white wine." See Chimalpahin, *Annals*, 54–55n3. Rémi Siméon defines "eloquiltic" as a medicinal plant used to treat pleurisy. Siméon, *Diccionario de la lengua náhuatl o mexicana*, trans. Josefina Oliva de Coll (Mexico City: Siglo XXI, 2004), 147.

42. Diego de la Cadena to Conde de Galve, AGI Mexico 333, fol. 399r.

43. Juan del Castillo to Conde de Galve, AGI Mexico 333, fol. 386v.

44. Sigüenza, "Letter to Admiral Pez," 246; translation altered.

45. Miguel de Estrada to Conde de Galve, AGI Mexico 333, fols. 493r-v.

46. Cf. Stoler, *Carnal Knowledge*, 9–13.

47. Bernabé Núñez de Paez to Conde de Galve, AGI Mexico 333, fol. 463r.

48. Dean y Cavildo to Conde de Galve, AGI Mexico 333, fol. 315v.

49. Aguiar y Seijas to Conde de Galve, AGI Mexico 333, fol. 271v.

50. Aguiar y Seijas to Conde de Galve, AGI Mexico 333, fol. 273r; my emphasis.

51. Cf. Kathleen Ross, *The Baroque Narrative of Carlos de Sigüenza y Góngora: A New World Paradise* (Cambridge: Cambridge University Press, 1993), 11: "How women behave sexually will define the order of colonial society and maintain the separation of the Spanish, Indian, and African races. Mixed-race people—*castas*—upset this neat order. Women, then, are much more then incidental to the baroque era in Spanish America and its literary expression; they are central actors as the encounter of Old and New Worlds moves into its second century."

52. "A twisted Catholic puritan, he had a pathological aversion for women, to whom he imputed all the evils against which the Church inveighed. According to his biographer, he regarded his myopic vision as a special boon since it prevented him from seeing members of the less homely sex. If, through some mischance, a woman crossed his threshold, he promptly ordered the bricks torn up and replaced upon which sacrilegious feet had trod." Irving Leonard, *Baroque Times in Old Mexico: Seventeenth-Century Persons, Places, and Practices* (Ann Arbor, MI: University of Michigan Press, 1959), 160. We should take Leonard's words with more than a grain of salt, as he does not entertain the possibility of other, more nuanced readings of these colonial documents.

53. García de Legaspi Velasco to Conde de Galve, AGI Mexico 333, fol. 308r, 309r.

54. Agustín de Vetancurrt to Conde de Galve, AGI Mexico 333, fol. 499v. In his *Teatro Mexicano*, published one year after the prohibition was lifted in 1697, Vetancurt would once again deploy this language. Pulque, he wrote, makes drinkers commit "innumerable offenses against God" including "incest with even their own Mothers. . . . They trade wives with each other (*unos y otros*), and if one buys another a drink he is paid back in a lustful exchange with that man's wife; and from this, [come] robberies, homicides, dances, and superstitious idolatries, calling *pulque* the water of God, as if it were blessed." Agustín de Vetancurt, *Teatro Mexicano: Descripción breve de los sucesos ejemplares de la Nueva España en el Nuevo Mundo Occidental de las Indias* (Madrid: Porrúa Turanzas, 1960), I, 442–443.

55. Cf. Asunción Lavrin, "Sexuality in Colonial Mexico: A Church Dilemma," in *Sexuality and Marriage in Colonial Latin America*, ed. Asunción Lavrin (Lincoln, NE: University of Nebraska Press, 1989), 47–92, esp. 57: "Confronting the church at the beginning of the seventeenth century was a

situation of lax personal relationships and sexual interethnic encounters among the so-called lesser social elements."

56. Cf. Stuart B. Schwartz and Frank Salomon, "New Peoples and New Kinds of People: Adaptation, Readjustment, and Ethnogenesis in South American Indigenous Societies (Colonial Era)," *The Cambridge History of the Native Peoples of the Americas, Vol. III, Part 2*, eds. Frank Salomon and Stuart B. Schwartz (Cambridge: Cambridge University Pres, 1999), 443–501; and Cope, *Limits of Racial Domination*, 4. These new racial categories would soon after be depicted visually in the eighteenth-century genre of *casta* paintings. These paintings depict cross-race couples and their offspring, mapping the genealogical progression of *mestizaje* or racial mixing. "It is no coincidence that casta paintings were created only a few years after the famous riot of 1692 in Mexico City." See Ilona Katzew, *Casta Painting: Images of Race in Eighteenth-Century Mexico* (New Haven, CT: Yale University Press, 2004), 202.

57. Ayuntamiento to Conde de Galve, AGI Mexico 333, fol. 322r.

58. There are at least two copies of the University's printed report. One is located in Seville, Spain at the AGI Mexico 333, fols. 566r–584v. The other is in the Fondo Reservado of the BN in Mexico City. The opinion of at least one of the twenty-six signatories was so respected that he was also asked to produce his own separate *informe*. See Joseph Vidal de Figueroa to Conde de Galve, AGI Mexico 333, fols. 376r–383r.

59. *Informe que la Real Universidad*, fol. 1r.

60. *Informe que la Real Universidad*, fol. 10r.

61. *Informe que la Real Universidad*, fol. 10r.

62. *Informe que la Real Universidad*, fol. 15v.

63. Cf. Guha's discussion of rumor and insurgency: "Ambiguity . . . is indeed what makes rumour a mobile and explosive agent of insurgency, and it is a function precisely of those distinctive features which constitute its originality—namely, its anonymity and transitivity." Ranajit Guha, *Elementary Aspects of Peasant Insurgency in Colonial India* (Durham, NC: Duke University Press, 1999), 260.

64. Anna More, "Colonial Baroque: Carlos de Sigüenza y Góngora and the Post-Colonization of New Spain" (Ph.D. diss., University of California, Berkeley, 2003), 215.

65. Juan de Luzuriaga to Conde de Galve, AGI Mexico 333, fol. 338r.

66. García de Legaspi Velasco to Conde de Galve, AGI Mexico 333, fol. 309r.

67. *Informe que la Real Universidad*, fol. 14r.

68. *Informe que la Real Universidad*, fol. 15v.

69. *Diccionario de Autoridades* (Madrid: Real Academia Española, 1726), 327, http://buscon.rae.es/ntlle/SrvltGUILoginNtlle (accessed July 2009).

70. Sigüenza's segregation proposal is located in Mexico City at the Archivo General de la Nación (AGN) *Historia* 413, fols. 4r–5r. In the interest of simplicity, I will refer to the version published by "Sobre los incovenientes de vivir los indios en el centro de la ciudad," *Boletín del Archivo General de la Nación* 9, no. 1 (January-March 1938): 1–33.

71. "Sobre los inconvenientes," 6.

72. See Edmundo O'Gorman, "Reflexiones sobre la distribución urbana colonial de la ciudad de México," in *Seis estudios históricos de tema mexicano* (Xalapa, Mexico: Universidad Veracruzana, 1960), 11–40. Others use the stronger term "segregation" instead. See Magnus Mörner, "La política de segregación en la Audiencia de Guatemala," *Revista de Indias* 24, nos. 95–96 (1964): 137–151; and Mörner and Charles Gibson, "Diego Muñoz Camargo and the Segregation Policy of the Spanish Crown," *Hispanic American Historical Review* 42, no. 4 (November 1962): 558–568. More recently, scholars working with primary sources written in Nahuatl have suggested that the separation of the two "republics" had more to do with the practical exigencies of colonial rule: Spanish colonialism was built atop the already existing structures of indigenous governance. See Lockhart, *The Nahuas*, 26–30.

73. Mörner and Gibson, "Diego Muñoz Camargo," 558.

74. Cope, *Limits of Racial Domination*, 22.

75. Hernández Palomo, *La renta del pulque*, 78–80.

76. The "very important objective of maintaining the Armada de Barlovento" was apparently a central reason for reversing the prohibition. See Consejo de Indias to Conde de Galve, AGI Mexico 333, fol. 590r. Also see Hernández Palomo, *La renta del pulque*, 80–84.

77. Taylor, *Drinking, Homicide, and Rebellion*, 68. Even some of the *informes* condemned the greed of the Spanish owners of the maguey plantations. Archbishop Aguiar y Seijas, for example, wrote

harshly of the "Spanish Haciendas measuring eight, ten, and twelve thousand feet [and] dedicated entirely to maguey." Aguiar y Seijas to Conde de Galve, AGI Mexico 333, fol. 270r.

78. Cope, *Limits of Racial Domination*, 179–80n56.

79. As in Gonzalbo Aizpuru, "El nacimiento del miedo," 10, 21.

80. "Sobre los inconvenientes," 17, 22; O'Gorman, "Reflexiones sobre la distribución urbana," 28. Cf. Foucault, *History of Sexuality*, 139–140.

81. *Informe que la Real Universidad*, fols. 5v–6r.

82. Race was named and depicted with different typologies, terminologies, and representational devices in colonial Mexico and Peru. Terminology for racial identity in South America tended to be based explicitly on "race fractions" or relative quantities of blood (e.g., *cuarterón*, *tercerón*, etc.), while in Mexico these categories were rarely used. Similarly, with very few exceptions, *casta* paintings were specific to New Spain, often incorporating specifically Mexican text and imagery. See Irene Silverblatt, *Modern Inquisitions: Peru and the Colonial Origins of the Civilized World* (Durham, NC: Duke University Press, 2004), 124–127; Isidoro Moreno Navarro, "Un aspecto del mestizaje americano: El problema de la terminología," *Revista española de antropología americana* 4 (1969): 201–218; and Katzew, *Casta Painting*, chap. 2.

REFERENCES

Albala, Ken. 2007. The Use and Abuse of Chocolate in Seventeenth-Century Medical Theory. *Food and Foodways* 15: 53–74.

Burns, Kathryn. 1999. *Colonial Habits: Convents and the Spiritual Economy of Cuzco, Peru*. Durham: Duke University Press.

Chimalpahin Quauhtlehuanitzin, Domingo de San Antón Muñón. 2006. *Annals of His Time*. Eds. and trans. James Lockhart, Susan Schroeder, and Doris Namala. Stanford: Stanford University Press.

Clavijero, Francisco Javier. 1826. *Historia antigua de Mégico*. Trans. José Joaquín de Mora. London: R. Ackermann.

Clendinnen, Inga. 1991. *The Aztecs: An Interpretation*. Cambridge: Cambridge University Press.

Coe, Sophie D. 1994. *America's First Cuisines*. Austin, TX: University of Texas Press.

Cope, R. Douglas. 1994. *The Limits of Racial Domination: Plebeian Society in Colonial Mexico City, 1660–1720*. Madison, WI: University of Wisconsin Press.

Crosby, Alfred. 1972. *The Columbian Exchange: Biological and Cultural Consequences of 1492*. Westport, CT: Greenwood.

Diccionario de Autoridades [1726–1737]. Ed. Real Academia Española. Retrieved 27 July 2009 from http://buscon.rae.es/ntlle/SrvltGUILoginNtlle

Durán, Diego. 1951. *Historia de las Indias de Nueva España y islas de Tierra Firme*. Mexico City: Editora Nacional.

Elliott, John Huxtable. 1970. *The Old World and the New, 1492–1650*. Cambridge: Cambridge University Press.

Escamilla González, Iván. 2002. "El siglo de oro vindicado: Carlos de Sigüenza y Góngora, el Conde de Galve y el tumulto de 1692." *Carlos de Sigüenza y Góngora: Homenaje 1700–2000*. Ed. Alicia Mayer. Mexico City: UNAM, II, 179–203.

Foster, Nelson, and Linda S. Cordell, eds. 1992. *Chiles to Chocolate: Food the Americas Gave the World*. Tucson, AZ: University of Arizona Press.

Foucault, Michel. 1978. *The History of Sexuality, Vol. 1: An Introduction*. Trans. Robert Hurley. New York: Vintage Books.

Gonzalbo Aizpuru, Pilar. 2008. "El nacimiento del miedo, 1692: Indios y españoles en la ciudad de México." *Revista de Indias* 68.244: 9–34.

Guha, Ranajit. 1999. *Elementary Aspects of Peasant Insurgency in Colonial India*. Durham, NC: Duke University Press.

Hernández, Francisco. 2000. *The Mexican Treasury: The Writings of Dr. Francisco Hernández*. Ed. Simon Varey. Trans. Simon Varey, Rafael Chabrán, and Cynthia L. Chamberlin. Stanford, CA: Stanford University Press.

Hernández Palomo, José Jesús. 1979. *La Renta del Pulque en la Nueva España, 1663–1610*. Seville: Escuela de Estudios Hispano-Americanos.

Holler, Jacqueline. 2005. *Escogidas Plantas: Nuns and Beatas in Mexico City, 1531–1601*. New York: Columbia University Press.

Informe que la Real Universidad, y Claustro Pleno de ella de la Ciudad de Mexico de esta Nueva España haze a el Excellentissimo Señor Virrey de ella en conformidad de orden de su Excelencia de 3 de Iulio de este año 1692 sobre los inconvenientes de la bebida de el Pulque. Mexico City. 1692.

Katzew, Ilona. 2004. *Casta Painting: Images of Race in Eighteenth-Century Mexico*. New Haven, CT: Yale University Press.

Kicza, John E. 1980. The Pulque Trade of Late Colonial Mexico City. *The Americas* 37.2: 193–221.

Lavrin, Asunción. 1989. "Sexuality in Colonial Mexico: A Church Dilemma." *Sexuality and Marriage in Colonial Latin America*. Ed. Asunción Lavrin. Lincoln, NE: University of Nebraska Press. 47–92.

Leonard, Irving. 1959. *Baroque Times in Old Mexico: Seventeenth-Century Persons, Places, and Practices*. Ann Arbor, MI: University of Michigan Press.

———. 1929. *Don Carlos de Sigüenza y Góngora: A Mexican Savant of the Seventeenth Century*. Berkeley, CA: University of California Press.

Lockhart, James. 1992. *The Nahuas After the Conquest: A Social and Cultural History of the Indians of Central Mexico, Sixteenth Through Eighteenth Centuries*. Stanford, CA: Stanford University Press.

Mintz, Sidney. 1985. *Sweetness and Power: The Place of Sugar in Modern History*. New York: Penguin Books.

Mitchell, Tim. 2004. *Intoxicated Identities: Alcohol's Power in Mexican History and Culture*. New York: Routledge.

Molina, Alonso de. 2004. *Vocabulario en lengua castellana y mexicana*. Ed. Miguel León-Portilla. Mexico City: Editorial Porrúa.

Moraña, Mabel. 2000. "El 'tumulto de indios' de 1692 en los pliegues de la fiesta barroca: Historiografía, subversión popular y agencia criolla en el México colonial." *Agencias criollas: La ambigüedad 'colonial' en las letras hispanoamericanas*. Ed. José Antonio Mazzotti. Pittsburgh, PA: Biblioteca de América, 161–75.

More, Anna. 2003. "Colonial Baroque: Carlos de Sigüenza y Góngora and the Post-Colonization of New Spain." Ph.D. diss.: University of California, Berkeley.

Moreno Navarro, Isidoro. 1969. Un aspecto del mestizaje americano: El problema de la terminología. *Revista española de antropología americana* 4: 201–18.

Mörner, Magnus. 1964. La política de segregación en la Audiencia de Guatemala. *Revista deIndias* 24.95–96: 137–51.

Mörner, Magnus and Charles Gibson. 1962. Diego Muñoz Camargo and the Segregation Policy of the Spanish Crown. *Hispanic American Historical Review* 42.4: 558–68.

Norton, Marcy. 2008. *Sacred Gifts, Profane Pleasures: A History of Tobacco and Chocolate in the Atlantic World*. Ithaca, NY: Cornell University Press.

———. 2006. Tasting Empire: Chocolate and the European Internalization of Mesoamerican Aesthetics. *The American Historical Review* 111.3: 660–691.

O'Gorman, Edmundo. 1960. "Reflexiones sobre la distribución urbana colonial de la ciudad de México." *Seis Estudios Históricos de Tema Mexicano*. Xalapa, Mexico: Universidad Veracruzana, 11–40.

Ortiz, Fernando. 2002. *Contrapunteo cubano del tabaco y el azúcar*. Ed. Enrico Mario Santí. Madrid: Cátedra.

Pilcher, Jeffrey M. 1998. *Que Vivan Los Tamales! Food and the Making of Mexican Identity*. Albuquerque: University of New Mexico Press.

Pratt, Mary Louise. 1997. *Imperial Eyes: Travel Writing and Transculturation*. New York: Routledge.

Rabasa, José. 1993. *Inventing America: Spanish Historiography and the Formation of Eurocentrism*. Norman, OK: University of Oklahoma Press.

Robles, Antonio de. 1946. *Diario de sucesos notables*. Mexico City: Editorial Porrua.

Rodríguez-Alegría, Enrique. 2005. Eating Like an Indian: Negotiating Social Relations in the Spanish Colonies. *Current Anthropology* 46: 551–73.

Ross, Kathleen. 1993. *The Baroque Narrative of Carlos de Sigüenza y Góngora: A New World Paradise*. Cambridge: Cambridge University Press.

Schwartz, Stuart B. and Frank Salomon. 1999. "New Peoples and New Kinds of People: Adaptation, Readjustment, and Ethnogenesis in South American Indigenous Societies (Colonial Era)." *The Cambridge History of the Native Peoples of the Americas, Vol. III: South America, Part* 2. Eds. Frank Salomon and Stuart B. Schwartz. Cambridge: Cambridge University Press, 443–501.

Seed, Patricia. 1988. *To Love, Honor, and Obey in Colonial Mexico: Conflicts over Marriage Choice, 1574–1821*. Stanford, CA: Stanford University Press.

Sigüenza y Góngora, Carlos de. 1929. "Letter of Don Carlos de Sigüenza to Admiral Pez Recounting the Incidents of the Corn Riot in Mexico City, June 8, 1692." Irving Leonard. *Don Carlos de Sigüenza y Góngora: A Mexican Savant of the Seventeenth Century*. Berkeley, CA: University of California Press, 210–77.

———. 1684. *Parayso Occidental, plantado, y cultivado por la liberal benefica mano de los muy Catholicos, y poderosos Reyes de España Nuestros Señores en su magnifico Real Convento de Jesus Maria de Mexico*. Mexico City: Juan de Ribero. Retrieved 27 July 2009 from http://www.cervantesvirtual.com/servlet/SirveObras/12585075434593728876657/index.htm

Silverblatt, Irene. 2004. *Modern Inquisitions: Peru and the Colonial Origins of the Civilized World*. Durham, NC: Duke University Press.

Siméon, Rémi. 2004. *Diccionario de la lengua náhuatl o mexicana*. Trans. Josefina Oliva de Coll. Mexico City: Siglo XXI.

Silva Prada, Natalia. 2007. *La política de una rebelión: Los indígenas frente al tumulto de 1692 en la Ciudad de México*. Mexico City: El Colegio de México.

"Sobre los incovenientes de vivir los indios en el centro de la ciudad." 1938. *Boletín del Archivo General de la Nación* 9.1: 1–33.

Stoler, Ann Laura. 2002. *Carnal Knowledge and Imperial Power: Race and the Intimate in Colonial Rule*. Berkeley, CA: University of California Press.

Super, John C. 1988. *Food, Conquest, and Colonization in Sixteenth-Century Spanish America*. Albuquerque: University of New Mexico Press.

Taylor, William B. 1979. *Drinking, Homicide, and Rebellion in Colonial Mexican Villages*. Stanford, CA: Stanford University Press.

Todorov, Tzvetan. 1999. *The Conquest of America: The Question of the Other*. Trans. Richard Howard. Norman, OK: University of Oklahoma Press.

Vetancurt, Agustín de. 1960. *Teatro Mexicano: Descripción breve de los sucesos ejemplares de la Nueva España en el Nuevo Mundo Occidental de las Indias*. Madrid: Porrúa Turanzas.

"To Make a Curry the India Way": Tracking the Meaning of Curry Across Eighteenth-Century Communities

STEPHANIE R. MARONEY
University of California, Davis, California, USA

With attention to the cultural mobility of local and global foodstuffs, this study examines the movement of curry as a product of England's colonization of India. The concept of a curry was developed by the British East India Company while stationed in India. Members of the EIC would describe any saucy Indian dish as a "curry," and when these men returned to England, they brought back their desire for Indian food. The movement of curry helped to shape its definition as a colonial product of India incorporated into English cuisine. By tracking curry and curry powder from its inception as an East India Company staple to the cookbooks and kitchens of eighteenth century Britain, this study shows how the distinct locality of curry changed its meaning over time.

Alan Davidson in the *Oxford Companion to Food* tentatively confirms that curry comes from the south Indian Tamil word *kari* (a spiced sauce poured over rice), first used by the Portuguese, who introduced the chili plant to India in the sixteenth century; however, the English use of the word came to describe any spicy dish with a thick sauce or gravy that came from any part of India.[1] Curry is a colonial foodstuff, whose history provides an interesting perspective on the complex colonial relations between Britain and India. It is difficult to classify a dish that is neither Indian nor British; the meaning of curry is many—its various definitions depend on time, place, history, and geography. Tracking the movement of curry by focusing on three communities of curry eaters shows that how, when, and by whom it was eaten changed its cultural meaning.

Rather than purely recount the history of curry or use it as a vehicle for a larger theoretical argument, as other writers have done, curry can be analyzed through the various localities where it was consumed.[2] Rather than insist on the authentic Indianness of curry, or argue for its naturalization and assimilation into British cuisine, its meaning is continuously changed and affected by the community which consumes it. Movement, or mobility, is a more productive way to conceptualize curry's history. Mobility here is defined as the movement from one location to another with specific material conditions shaping the meaning and values associated with the food—a meaning that is always in flux and under revision. This is not a question of evolution, which implies a progress or a single entity evolving, but a shifting set of expectations and meanings as curry moves from one location to another, and yet another.

By looking at three communities of people consuming curry in different times and places—the British in India, the EIC community in England, and English domestic cooks—I explore how curry is eaten from group to group. Each group interprets and uses curry differently, building layers of meaning—like a recipe passed down through the generations. Ultimately, there are many different curries. By examining the movement of curry, my argument is a contribution about how food practices move from one "local" to another—a cultural explanation for the many iterations of curry, curried, and curry powder. Curry is a case study that provides evidence for how complicated the processes are in the mobility of foodways.

Curry was a staple of daily life and enjoyed by members of the East India Company (EIC) living in India in the eighteenth century. When these men returned home to England, they reproduced the curries they enjoyed abroad in coffeehouses or had them prepared by their own wives and mothers. The EIC community in England attempted to replicate the "real Indian curries" that they ate while living abroad. Gradually, the greater metropolitan English middle-class adopted curry and were exposed to the dish through eighteenth- and nineteenth-century cookbooks. It was in these cookbooks that English people, particularly women, previously unfamiliar with or uncertain of Indian food and culture could experiment with the tastes and flavors of far away.

Although the use of cookbooks as texts is open to a multitude of interpretations and can be subject to over-reading and ambiguity, as Janet Theophano explains, "There is much to be learned from reading a cookbook besides how to prepare food."[3] Cookbooks and recipes have been commonly overlooked as primary documents, and the stories they tell reveal the author's interpretation of their communities and the "visions they have of society and culture."[4] Arjun Appadurai affirms that cookbooks "tell cultural tales," in that they "reflect shifts in the boundaries of edibility, the proprieties of the culinary process, the logic of meals [. . .] and the structure of domestic ideologies."[5] Like other social texts, cookbooks and recipes can define what is culturally acceptable or taboo, and also determine what is and is not a part of any culture's cuisine. And for many authors of eighteenth- and nineteenth-century English cookbooks, the preface, table of contents, and individual recipes were means to establish a British culinary sensibility and style.

A REAL INDIAN CURRY

A scene in William Thackeray's *Vanity Fair* neatly sets the stage for tracking the movement of curry. Set during the Napoleonic Wars (1803–1815), *Vanity Fair* contains one of the fullest depictions of an English family sitting down to a curry dinner in England. Seated at the Sedley family's fictional table is each community that I identify as contributing to the shifting meaning of curry. Joseph Sedley, an East India Company tax collector, has returned from India and joins his family and guest Miss Rebecca Sharp to celebrate his homecoming:

> Now we have heard how Mrs. Sedley had prepared a fine curry for her son, just as he liked it, and in the course of dinner a portion of this dish was offered to Rebecca. 'What is it?' said she, turning an appealing look to Mr. Joseph. 'Capital,' said he. His mouth was full of it; his face quite red with the delightful exercise of gobbling. 'Mother, it's as good as my own curries in India.'
> 'Oh, I must try some, if it is an Indian dish,' said Miss Rebecca. 'I'm sure everything must be good that comes from there.'
> 'Give Miss Sharp some curry, my dear,' said Mr. Sedley, laughing. Rebecca had never tasted the dish before. 'Do you find it as good as everything else from India?' said Mr. Sedley.
> 'Oh, excellent!' said Rebecca, who was suffering tortures with the cayenne pepper. 'Try a chili with it, Miss Sharp,' said Joseph, really interested.
> 'A chili,' said Rebecca, gasping [. . .] and put one into her mouth. It was hotter than the curry [. . .] 'Water, for Heaven's sake, water!' she cried. Mr. Sedley burst out laughing. [. . .] 'They are real Indian, I assure you,' said he.[6]

Speaking through a mouth filled with food, Joseph Sedley expresses his joy and pleasure at "gobbling" his mother's curry, even comparing it to some of his own in India. For the EIC officer, this curry elicits a memory of and a fondness for a specific time and place. For the most part, an EIC officer in Sedley's position would have had his curries prepared by Indian cooks, who would not have served a singular "curry," but rather, would have brought a diversity of dishes with a variety of names to his English table. Sedley has come to think of himself as an expert on all things Indian, so much so that while he applauds his mother's "capital" curry, he does say later in the novel that although the "curry was capital [. . .] perhaps there was *not* enough citron juice in it."[7]

Sedley's mother represents the larger community of those obliquely related to the East India Company, who prepare curry dinners in England possibly for the sake of indulging their sons' and husbands' nostalgia. Outside of fiction, the British in India were relatively successful in convincing their friends and families in England of the delights of Indian food. Lizzie Collingham relates how family members in England were eager to hear about the adventures and "exotic lives" of their sons and brothers in India, and these men "often enclosed recipes in letters."[8] Likewise, into the nineteenth century, wives of EIC members who had spent time in India with their husbands returned to England and instructed their cooks how to prepare a "real Indian curry." As these men returned home, they brought with them a desire for the foods and flavors of India.

Miss Rebecca Sharp is the obvious EIC outsider. She has not yet embraced curry, but (at that moment in the novel) belongs to the burgeoning middle class of which curry becomes increasingly popular. Becky "suffers tortures with the cayenne," while Joseph's palate is accustomed to the overly spiced and absurdly hot EIC-inspired creation. Becky's pleas for water reveal that the larger British public was unaccustomed to spicy food at this time. This passage in Thackeray's novel gives evidence of a non-EIC-member's reaction to curry, and situates it as a relatively unknown dish outside of that community.

The story of curry in England really begins in India with members of the East India Company. The British in India, generally, incorporated Indian ingredients into their English diet thus forming a new kind of Anglo-Indian cuisine. Replicating a proper English diet in India proved unsuccessful and unhealthy; tinned and imported goods from Europe were expensive to ship, and frequently lacked the nutritional benefits of fresh fruits, vegetables, dairy, and meat.[9] Compared to canned goods, indigenous foodstuffs were significantly cheaper and healthier. Cookbooks targeted toward the British in India often urged them "to eat 'more of the country,' to eat 'native' fruits and vegetables, fish, and meat."[10]

There is no dish called "curry" that was eaten by Indians in Indian homes during the eighteenth and nineteenth centuries. However, a version of the more contemporary dish of curry was eaten regularly by East India Company officers, who appropriated the local Indian food culture. The British in India used the phrase "curry and rice" to describe just about every Indian dish brought to their table. They typically lumped the wide variety of Indian food into either "curries" or "pillaus," and incorporated regional food varieties into dishes served in their homes without much regard for each ingredient's specific use within Indian cuisine.[11] For the EIC community, curry was a part of company culture and figured prominently in their daily diets. Moreover, it was a foodstuff that helped to define their experience of India.

BRINGING CURRY HOME

Along with newly acquired fortunes and possessions, returned East India Company members brought back to England a desire for curry. Men who returned rich from their exploits in India were commonly called nabobs, an English "corruption of the word nawab, meaning a governor or ruler of a district."[12] James Holzman describes how the nabob household "adapted native conditions to their own convenience," and he identifies some "distinctive ways of life" that "made some impression upon contemporary England."[13] Of these, Holzman distinguishes their "partiality for curry and Madeira" as the most obvious difference from "the lives of ordinary country gentlemen."[14] In the late eighteenth century, curry began to appear on coffeehouses menus that had become popular meeting grounds for returned EIC members. Coffeehouses helped cultivate a curry-eating population in England, and these establishments incited in the retired EIC officers a feeling of nostalgia for their time in India.

The coffeehouse crowd was largely nabob, although less wealthy sailors, merchants, and other maritime clientele could indulge their taste for curry at seaside ports and dockside restaurants. In 1810, Dean Mahomet, an Indian entrepreneur who emigrated to Europe in 1784, opened the Hindostanee Coffee-House in Portman Square, an eating house targeting a specific clientele of "Europeans who had worked or lived in India, men he [Mahomet] called 'Indian gentlemen.'"[15] Mahomet courted the EIC curry-eaters in an advertisement for the Hindostanee Coffee-House that promised the "greatest epicures to be unequalled to any curries ever made in England."[16] Mahomet decorated his coffeehouse with bamboo-cane chairs and paintings of Indian scenery, and he included a separate smoking room complete with hookahs and Indian spices, oils, and tobacco. Charles Stewart, a notorious patron who was rumored to have "16 Indian wives and to have bathed in the Ganges every morning when in Calcutta," referred to Mahomet's coffeehouse as the "Hooka Club."[17] Despite some favorable reviews in the *Epicure's Almanack* (1815), the Hindostanee Coffee-House met with financial difficulties—partly due to competition from more well-established rival coffeehouses, but also because the wealthy nabobs and elite of the Portman Square neighborhood could choose to have their own Indian dishes prepared at home.

What EIC members ate in London, prepared by coffeehouse chefs and, more increasingly, by women who did not participate in the experience abroad, was a different kind of curry than what they consumed in India. It was a re-creation of India—a dish made without the readily available spices, ingredients, and native cooks of India. In order for curry to move out of coffeehouse circles, it had to leave the all-male world of the EIC and enter English women's domestic sphere. While at home, families of returned EIC members—not unlike the Sedley family—were able to simulate the foods and flavors of India.

The larger English public was also able to do this by preparing the recipes found in increasingly popular cookbooks. Although members of the EIC are ultimately responsible for curry's presence in England, cookbook recipes helped to cultivate the taste and accessibility of curry and defined

To make a **Currey** *the* **India** *way.*

TAKE two Fowls or Rabbits, cut them into ſmall Pieces, and three or four ſmall Onions, peeled and cut very ſmall, thirty Pepper Corns, and a large Spoonful of Rice, Brown ſome Coriander Seeds over the Fire in a clear Shovel, and beat them to Powder, take a Tea Spoonful of Salt, and mix all well together with the Meat, put all together into a Sauce-pan or Stew-pan, with a Pint of Water, let it ſtew ſoftly till the Meat is enough, then put in a Piece of freſh Butter, about as big as a large Walnut, ſhake it well together, and when it is ſmooth and of a fine Thickneſs, diſh it up, and ſend it to Table; if the Sauce be too thick, add a little more Water before it is done, and more Salt if it wants it. You are to obſerve the Sauce muſt be pretty thick.

FIGURE 1 Hannah Glasse, "To Make a Currey the India Way."[19]

how a curry in England should be made. It was through these recipes that curry was transformed into something other than nabob food. Cookbook recipes broke apart the association of curry with East India Company culture, and both domesticated and anglicized the dish. Curry was presented as an Indian staple that was easy to prepare and economical to produce. Troy Bickham argues that curry was "neither too exotic nor too complicated to prepare,"[18] which positions the dish as an accessible new way to cook Indian food in English homes.

The first known recipe for curry in an English cookbook appears in the first edition of Hannah Glasse's *The Art of Cookery* in 1747 (Figure 1). The simplicity of this recipe, and even the title, presents the dish as fairly simple to prepare without any traditionally Indian spices or unfamiliar cooking techniques. This is not the curry of Joseph Sedley—the curry that burned Becky's lips and had her pleading for water. Alan Davidson remarks wryly of the transposition that has taken place in Glasse's curry recipe: "What once had been an Indian sauce to go with rice has become an English stew with a little rice in it."[20] Glasse makes the dish familiar and comfortable for English cooks, who would recognize an "English stew with a little rice in it." By using few ingredients and following her promise of recipes "plain and easy," Glasse increases curry's appeal to the English middle-class as an economic and familiar dish.

Glasse's curry recipe appears in the same way throughout the second (1747) and third (1748) editions of *The Art of Cookery*. However in 1751, as her book goes into its fourth printing, Glasse modifies the recipe in interesting ways (Figure 2).

This recipe is a virtual transformation: chicken is the specified meat of choice (the index refers to making "a currey of chickens the Indian way"), and Glasse has introduced new spices into the recipe. The most important additions to the ingredients of the 1751 recipe are in the curry spice mix: turmeric and ginger add a new depth to the literal and symbolic meanings of the dish. Coriander is removed from this recipe and replaced with turmeric, a root that contributes a dull flavor but exotic color. In Glasse's 1747 recipe, it is not clear what differentiates her curry from any other stewed rabbit/fowl dish. The main ingredients are not unique to the recipe and certainly the spices do not set it apart from any other rice and meat stew. In the 1751 edition, Glasse includes turmeric in the curry recipe (its only appearance in *The Art of Cookery*), which gives this curry its distinctive orange color and visually marks the dish as different from typical English fare.

Hannah Glasse's 1751 chicken curry must have been quite successful as the recipe appears in identical form in subsequent cookbooks from other authors. Mary Cole's *The Lady's Complete Guide* (1788) and the 1794 edition of Maximilian Hazlemore's *Domestic Economy* (which cites Cole as the source of the recipe) both use Glasse's recipe for "Currey the Indian Way."[22] Lifting recipes from other cookbooks was fairly standard practice during this period. Historian Gilly Lehmann notes that when she was compiling *The Art of Cookery, Made Plain and Easy*, Glasse took "342 of her 972 receipts from other books, most notably from the 1743 edition of *The Lady's Companion*."[23] Copying a specific curry recipe could suggest that other cookbook authors wanted to include a curry in their collections, but were not yet sure how to construct the dish in new ways. While Glasse's curry recipe emerged as the new authority, some cooks created their own blends of curry, typically using variations of turmeric, coriander, pepper, ginger, and cayenne.

These English curry recipes did not much resemble dishes in Indian cuisine. Rather, these recipes were modified based on the availability of English products. Apples replaced mangoes; lemon juice was substituted for tamarinds; cucumbers for bitter gourds, and butter instead of ghee. Over time, the English ingredients became regarded as components for a good curry rather than a substitution for the ingredients in Indian cookery, and the standardized spice blend of English curry powder was sprinkled onto any dish to make it "Indian food."

To make a Currey *the* Indian *Way.*

TAKE two ſmall Chickens, skin them and cut them as for a Fricaſey, waſh them clean, and ſtew them in about a Quart of Water, for about five Minutes, then ſtrain off the Liquor and put the Chickens in a clean Diſh; take three large Onions, chop them ſmall and fry them in about two Ounces of Butter, then put in the Chickens and fry them together till they are Brown, take a Quarter of an Ounce of Turmerick, a large Spoonful of Ginger and beat Pepper together, and a little Salt to your Palate, ſtrew all theſe Ingredients over the Chickens whilſt it is frying; then pour in the Liquor, and let it ſtew about Half an Hour, then put in a Quarter of a Pint of Cream, and the Juice of two Lemons, and ſerve it up. The Ginger, Pepper and Turmerick muſt be beat very fine.

FIGURE 2 Hannah Glasse, "The Make a Currey the Indian Way."[21]

A SMALL TABLE SPOONFUL OF CURRY POWDER

While the origins of curry powder are unknown, David Burton supports the conclusion that it was "invented in the seventeenth century as an export commodity for East India Company employees to take or send back to England."[24] While there is no evidence that the date is accurate, it is reasonable to state that curry powder was designed to be exported from India and not used within the subcontinent. From its origins, curry powder was a supposedly Indian commodity exported to Europe.

In 1784, a listing appeared in *The Morning Herald and Daily Advertiser* specifically directed at "Persons of Rank, Traders to all Nabobs, and Servants," advertised the "invaluable rich ingredient called curry powder."[25] This ad is the earliest known description of ready-mix curry powder in print and capitalizes on the nabobs' acquired tastes of India by targeting them as the prime purchasers. Tillman Nechtman, in his essay "Nabobs Revisited," notes how the advertisement marks the nabobs as the "community responsible for curry's presence in Britain [. . .] [and] answerable for introducing it to their nation."[26] More than a "valuable ingredient," curry powder is presented in this ad as the cornerstone for Indian cookery, of which all the "celebrated East-India[n] dishes [. . .] are made." The advertisement then encourages the reader to visit Sorlie's Perfumery Warehouse and receive "directions on how to use it [curry powder] by which any person can make up a dish of Curry."[27] Curry powder is advertised as an integral part of authentic Indian cuisine and as the stuff of which those real Indian curries are made.

More than an innocuous mixture of spices, curry powder came to England as a commercialized colonial export marketed to the nabob and EIC community. But curry powder moved out of the EIC circles, and was gradually incorporated into English cuisine, in the form of a convenient and pre-ground commercial powder available on store shelves around 1780. English cooks used curry powder as they saw fit, employing it in a variety of "un-Indian" ways, as a means of anglicizing Indian cooking methods to suit English culture. Curry powder was mixed with flour and used as a sauce thickener, whereas Indian sauces were thickened with ground almonds, pastes, or coconut milk. Where readers of cookbooks were previously instructed to hand-grind and mix their own powders, they were now directed to simply add several spoonfuls of curry powder to their dishes.

In 1773, Charlotte Mason published *The Lady's Assistant for Regulating and Supplying Her Table,* including one of the earliest curry recipes calling for "curree powder." Mason's recipe for "Curree of Chickens" directs the reader to douse "two large spoonfuls of curree powder" over frying chicken, add the "liquor the chickens were boiled in [and] let all stew till they are tender."[28] Other popular recipes making use of ready-made curry powders are Susanna Kellet's 1780 *A Complete Collection of Cookery Receipts*, whose "A Curry of Chickens" recipe requires pepper, salt, cayenne, "a small table spoonful of curry powder" and "two small teaspoonfuls of turmerick [sic] to colour."[29] Kellet's recipe is interesting because it uses turmeric specifically "to color," or to visually mark the dish as different from "traditional" English food. Presumably, there would already be turmeric in the curry powder, so to add two more teaspoons would make the dish very orange and exotic looking. Curry powder also appears in Mrs. Frazer's 1791 curry chicken recipe in *The Practice of Cookery, Pastry, Pickling, Preserving, &c.*, which nearly replicates Hannah Glasse's in 1751, but whereas Glasse instructs the reader to toast and pound turmeric, ginger, and pepper, Frazer simply states: "take a small table spoonful of currey."[30]

Richard Briggs' 1794 recipe for "Currey of Chickens" in *The English Art of Cookery* specifically directs the reader to "get a bottle of currey powder" and add liberally to the frying chicken. Briggs also suggests the use of cayenne pepper "as sometimes the currey powder is not hot enough."[31] The overemphasis on spicy, hot curry is a direct throwback to the EIC's painfully hot curries.

Briggs' recipe is also important in that it calls for a bottle of curry powder. Some cookbooks included recipes for homemade curry powder, and it is not unlikely that frugal housewives were blending their own spices and making their own powders. Since Briggs instructs his reader to "get a bottle of curry powder," he is most likely referring to the pre-made, commercially available version. Gilly Lehmann sees the commercialization of food products such as curry powder as a "spread of metropolitan fashions." Cooks could purchase the ready-made curry powder, pickles, and catsups that "appeared so frequently in their [cooking] manuals."[32] Cookbooks and household manuals were integral in disseminating England's colonial encounters and metropolitan fashions through products such as commercial curry powder, and also in anglicizing foreign foods such as curry.

Hannah Glasse's early attempts to present a real Indian curry in her 1747 and 1751 recipes instructed readers to roast and hand-grind the ingredients—a process much closer to Indian spice preparation. But a later editor of Glasse's cookbook succumbs to the sheer utilitarianism of curry powder, as evidenced by the recipe in the 1796 edition of *The Art of Cookery* (roughly its 22nd edition). The 1796 edition is sold with Glasse's original preface, but contains a letter from the male editor, who promises that the new recipes are "much improved." What Glasse called "Currey the Indian Way" is now "Another Way to make a Curry; easier, and much approved." Apparently, "easier" and "much approved" means that the recipe now calls for "two large spoonfuls of curry powder" and cayenne (Figure 3).

This recipe has changed drastically from Hannah Glasse's first attempt at curry in 1747; it calls for the heat of cayenne, commercialized ready-made curry powder, "thick gravy," and even a few chopped pickles. From 1747 to 1796, Glasse's curry recipe was altered and adapted as curry gained popularity throughout English kitchens. This is not the coffeehouse curries of retired EIC officers, nor is it an attempt to replicate the Indian-made dishes that those men ate abroad. Rather, this curry is suited for English tastes and English kitchens, and this recipe has become a familiar dish to readers of English cookbooks.

Women in the nineteenth century modified curry recipes, experimented with their own curry spice blends, and applied them to various English dishes (curried eggs, fish, pie). English women played a key role in the anglicization of curry powder, and took this staple of EIC food culture and made it their own. In a change from the "manly" curries of the EIC, women's experiences and opinions reformed the meaning of curry powder, and its increased use by women in English kitchens made it a familiar condiment. Curry powder made it possible to prepare curry quickly and easily without actually cooking Indian food in the proper sense. Any dish could be curried just by adding a tablespoon of yellow powder. But because English women relied heavily on the availability of pre-ground and bottled, commercially available blends, these powders tended to be standardized mixtures that easily went stale and were often cut with ground rice or flour. Even dangerous traces of lead were found in curry powders and cayenne in order to heighten the red color.[34] Despite the inferior quality, cost, and apparent health risks, bottled curry powders exploded on the market and made their way into many English kitchens.

Women's magazines and periodicals were filled with recipe ideas and cooking tips, as well as entries related to curry and curry powder. Nupur Chaudhuri studies women's role in the popularization of curry and curry powder by looking at magazines such as *Queen* and *EDM*. Chaudhuri tracks the acceptance of curry by middle-class English housewives, who developed a specific opinion of and taste for curry powder through cookbook recipes and women's periodicals. Women often complained that curry was too hot and, wanting to better enjoy the dish, sought out ways to impart more flavor and less heat. Curious about the process of making curry powder, women wrote in requesting modifications of existing curry recipes; one reader asked *Queen* if anyone could "recommend me a curry powder possessing the Indian flavour, without the excessive heat, by which all

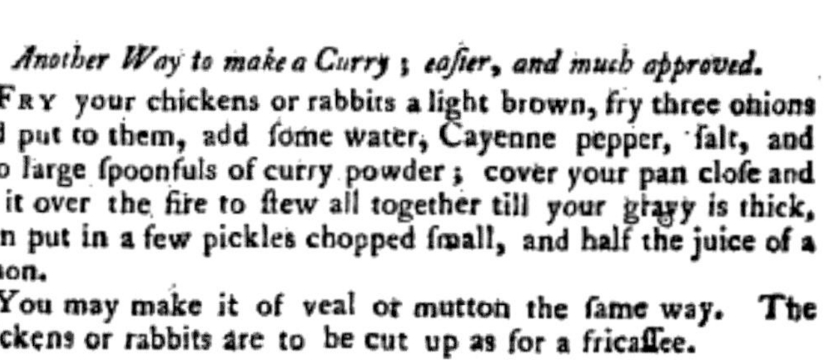
Another Way to make a Curry; eafier, and much approved.

FRY your chickens or rabbits a light brown, fry three onions and put to them, add fome water, Cayenne pepper, falt, and two large fpoonfuls of curry powder; cover your pan clofe and fet it over the fire to ftew all together till your gravy is thick, then put in a few pickles chopped fmall, and half the juice of a lemon.

You may make it of veal or mutton the fame way. The chickens or rabbits are to be cut up as for a fricaffee.

FIGURE 3 Hannah Glasse, "Another Way to Make a Curry; Easier, and Much Approved."[33]

powders, I have ever tested in England are spoilt."[35] Curry recipes appearing in the mid- to late nineteenth century were modified on account of women's preferences—many removed the excessive amounts of cayenne and substituted laborious hand-roasted and ground spices for bottled curry powder.

Commercial powders were marketed to English women as a nutritious and economic addition to their family's daily diet. Isabella Beeton, in her successful 1861 book *Mrs. Beeton's Book of Household Management*, included the following note under her recipe for "Indian Curry-Powder":

> Note.—We have given this recipe for curry-powder, as some persons prefer to make it at home; but that purchased at any respectable shop is, generally speaking, far superior, and, taking all things into consideration, very frequently more economical.[36]

Isabella Beeton, and other cookbook authors, shaped a discourse about curry powder, which was focused on economics, convenience, and domestic utility. English women (who cooked from either cookbooks or shared recipes) became the community responsible for defining the meaning and composition of curry. Curry moved from the Indian homes of EIC officers and into English cookbooks, kitchens, and shops.

CONCLUSION

From curry to curry powder, this food history demonstrates how the mobility of foodstuffs from one location or community to another presents an opportunity for examining changing cultural values through foodways. Curry was introduced to England as an Indian dish, and the culinary representation of Britain's colonization of India. It was a foodstuff that was practically synonymous with East India Company culture. Curry was the daily meal for EIC members in India, and when they returned to England, they recreated that experience in coffeehouses steeped in nostalgia.

Cookbook recipes for curry seemed to incorporate England's colonial encounter with India through curry, and balanced women's interest in cooking Indian food with the practicality of kitchen economics. Curry moved out of London coffeehouses and onto grocery shelves, where the commercialization of ready-made curry powder helped to cultivate and popularize the taste for curry in the English culinary landscape. The inclusion of name-brand, commercial curry powders in cookbooks and household manuals, as well as reviews attesting to their authenticity, turned India's local food culture into a commodity constructed through colonialism.

By the late nineteenth century, curry powder had become a familiar ingredient in English kitchens. Curry had become anglicized so completely that recipes now appeared in the English cooking sections of Victorian cookbooks, as evidenced here by the author of *Modern Domestic Cookery*:

> Curry, which was formerly a dish almost exclusively for the table of those who had made a long residence in India, is now so completely naturalized, that few dinners are thought complete unless there is one of the table.[37]

NOTES

1. Alan Davidson, "Curry," *The Oxford Companion to Food* (Oxford: Oxford University Press, 1999), 235.

2. Curry has received a surprising amount of critical attention, and it has been addressed in largely two different ways: the debate over whether curry is an English or Indian foodstuff, and the use of curry as an example for larger arguments about imperialism and nationalism. Perhaps the two most influential treatments of curry are Lizzie Collingham's book *Curry: A Tale of Cooks and Conquerors* (New York: Oxford University Press, 2006) and Susan Zlotnick's essay "Domesticating Imperialism: Curry and Cookbooks in Victorian England" (*Frontiers* 16.2/3, 1996: 51–68). While both authors have presented sound and—in the case of Collingham's *Curry*—almost exhaustive studies, they approach curry from different angles. Collingham more or less adheres to the is-curry-English-or-Indian debate, and she tells the story of curry (and other Indian, Anglo-Indian, and British foods) from a wholly historical perspective. Zlotnick embraces the second scenario, situating her argument of curry in women's domestic identity. She shows through the example of curry how Victorian women did the domesticating work of the Empire. Neither author exclusively examines curry as a foodstuff, nor focuses primarily on its local and global foodways.

3. Janet Theophano, *Eat My Words: Reading Women's Lives Through the Cookbooks They Wrote* (New York: Palgrave Macmillan, 2003), 6.

4. Theophano, *Eat My Words*, 3.

5. Arjun Appadurai, "How to Make a National Cuisine: Cookbooks in Contemporary India," in *Food and Culture: A Reader,* 2nd edition, eds. Carole Counihan and Penny Van Esterik (New York: Routledge, 2008), 289.

6. William Makepeace Thackeray, *Vanity Fair* [1840] (New York: Penguin, 2003), 30–31.

7. Thackeray, *Vanity Fair*, 34 (emphasis in original).

8. Collingham, *Curry*, 133.

9. Helen Pike Bauer, "Eating in the Contact Zone," in *Consuming Culture in the Long Nineteenth Century*, eds. Tamara S. Wagner and Narin Hassan (Lanham, MD: Lexington Books, 2007), 95.

10. Mary Procida, "Feeding the Imperial Appetite: Imperial Knowledge and Anglo-Indian Domesticity," *Journal of Women's History* 15.2 (2003), 141.

11. See Collingham, *Curry*, 109–10, 115, 130.

12. Collingham, *Curry*, 130.

13. James Holzman, *The Nabobs in England: A Study of the Returned Anglo-Indian, 1760–1785* (New York: Holzman, 1926), 90.

14. Holzman, *The Nabobs in England*, 78.

15. Michael H. Fisher, *The First Indian Author in English: Dean Mahomed (1759–1851) in India, Ireland, and England* (Delhi: Oxford University Press, 1996), 257.

16. From the (London) *Times*, 27 March 1811; quoted in Fisher, *The First Indian Author in English*, 258.

17. Collingham, *Curry*, 129.

18. Troy Bickham, "Eating the Empire: Intersections of Food, Cookery, and Imperialism in Eighteenth-Century Britain," *Past and Present* 198 (2008), 104.

19. Hannah Glasse, *The Art of Cookery, Made Plain and Easy* (London: Author, 1747), 52. Image accessed through Eighteenth Century Collections Online.

20. Alan Davidson, "Curry Powder," *The Oxford Companion to Food* (Oxford: Oxford University Press, 1999), 236.

21. Hannah Glasse, *The Art of Cookery, Made Plain and Easy ... With Additions*, 4th edition (London: Author, 1751), 101. Images accessed through Eighteenth Century Collections Online.

22. Mary Cole, *The Lady's Complete Guide; or Cookery in All Its Branches* (London: G. Kearsley, 1788), 191; Maximilian Hazelmore, *Domestic Economy; or, a Complete System of English Housekeeping* (London: J. Creswick & Co., 1794), 118.

23. Gilly Lehmann, *The British Housewife: Cookery Books, Cooking, and Society in Eighteenth-Century Britain* (Totnes, UK: Prospect Books, 2003), 110.

24. Burton, *The Raj at Table: A Culinary History of the British in India* (London: Faber & Faber, 1994), 74.

25. *The Morning Herald and Daily Advertiser*, 4 May 1784.

26. Tillman W. Nechtman, "Nabobs Revisited: A Cultural History of British Imperialism and the Indian Question in Late Eighteenth-Century Britain," *History Compass* 4.4 (2006), 655.

27. *The Morning Herald and Daily Advertiser*, 4 May 1784.

28. Charlotte Mason, *The Lady's Assistant for Regulating and Supplying her Table* (London: J. Walter, 1773), 245.

29. Susanna Kellet, Elizabeth Kellet, and Mary Kellet, *A Complete Collection of Cookery Receipts* (Newcastle-upon-Tyne: T. Saint, 1780), 28–29.

30. Mrs. Frazer, *The Practice of Cookery, Pastry, Pickling, Preserving, &c.* (Edinburgh: Peter Hill, T. Cadell, 1791), 69.

31. Richard Briggs, *The English Art of Cookery,* 3rd edition (London: G.G. and J. Robinson, 1794), 245–246.

32. Lehmann, *The British Housewife*, 257.

33. Hannah Glasse, *The Art of Cookery Made Plain and Easy, in which are included, one hundred new receipts, not inserted in any former edition. With a copious index* (London: printed for T. Longman, B. Law, J. Johnson, G. G. and J. Robinson, H. Gardner [and 19 others], 1796), 129.

34. Arthur Hill Hassan's *Adulterations Detected; or, Plain Instructions for the Discovery of Frauds*, published in many editions throughout the 1850s, identified dangerous levels of lead and vermillion in cayenne pepper—one of the main ingredients in bottled British curry powders. Also, articles in the *Dublin Review* (Ed. Nicholas Patrick Wiseman, 1855), *The Lancet* (vol. 2, 1852), *Chambers' Encyclopedia* (1865) and other publications quoted Hassan's findings or introduced their own.

35. From *Queen* 6 January 1886; quoted in Nupur Chaudhuri, "Shawls, Jewelry, Curry, and Rice in Victorian Britain," in *Western Women and Imperialism: Complicity and Resistance*, eds. Nupur Chaudhuri and Margaret Strobel (Bloomington, IN: Indiana University Press, 1992), 239.

36. Isabella Beeton, *Mrs. Beeton's Book of Household Management* [1861] (Oxford, UK: Oxford University Press, 2000), 133.

37. *Modern Domestic Cookery, Based on the Well-Known Work of Mrs. Rundell* (London: John Murray, 1851), 311.

The "Coffee Doctors": The Language of Taste and the Rise of Rwanda's Specialty Bean Value

JENNY ELAINE GOLDSTEIN
Department of Geography, University of California, Los Angeles, California, USA

The emergence of Rwanda's specialty coffee sector during the early twenty-first century has brought high-end Rwandan coffee to the shelves of coffee retailers across the United States, Europe, and Japan. While a variety of factors have influenced the rapid development of Rwanda's specialty coffee industry, one of the most significant has been the training of domestic coffee tasters. Known as cuppers, these taste professionals act as a unique link in this global foodway and help enable perception of locally based flavors through marketplace mechanisms. The Rwandan cupper is not simply another middleman in a very long commodity chain. Rather, she or he plays a new role in transforming a generic cash-crop commodity into locality-based luxury item. This new role highlights the language and standards used to differentiate coffees in producing countries for international niche markets.

With ideal climatic and topographic conditions for growing the heirloom "Bourbon" varietal of *Coffea arabica*, Rwanda is naturally well positioned to produce high-quality coffee. Rwandan coffee does indeed have many environmental factors working in its favor, yet those alone fail to explain why, after a century of production, the Rwandan brew suddenly "tastes better."[1] While coffee exported from Rwanda was once marked only by a crude letter grade indicating size and degree of visible defects, an increasing volume of coffee is now leaving the country distinguished by point of origin or purported taste. Those familiar with Rwandan coffee at both the origin and consumption ends of this complex and global foodway also claim that these beans are in fact of higher "quality" than ever before, with distinctive flavors for which coffee drinkers are willing to pay more, thus increasing potential profits for Rwandan coffee growers. As a result, Rwandan coffee catapulted from being virtually unknown within the "specialty" sector of the global coffee industry to attracting attention and praise from high-end United States, European, and Japanese coffee companies within the first decade of the twenty-first century.

Rwanda's shift towards exporting coffee bound for niche markets, differentiated by locality and taste attributes, is enabled by a multitude of global dynamics and characterizes a general turn towards quality improvement throughout the coffee industry worldwide. In an international coffee market long plagued by oversupply, the perception that growers are often only remunerated a small fraction of the cost of a commercial cup of coffee has become commonplace among self-identifying socially conscious consumers. This perceived economic contradiction has been partially responsible for the rise of niche coffees in recent decades, as well as the diversification and differentiation of the specialty coffee industry. Niche coffees offer consumers perceived taste improvements over mass-produced coffee blends, thus increasing the price consumers are willing to pay and in some instances guaranteeing larger profits for coffee producers in the developing world. Strategies through which niche coffees are created vary among coffee producing countries; Fair Trade certification is one widely recognized option being pursued by some exporters and importers. Rwanda is unique, however, in its recent embrace of a different quality improvement mechanism, namely the training of domestic coffee tasters, or cuppers as they are known in the industry.

I argue that domestic coffee cuppers—a new type of middlemen—have altered local coffee production dynamics and drawn international attention to, and even helped produce, the taste attributes of coffee beans grown and processed in Rwanda. Through their tasting practices, Rwandan coffee cuppers are partially responsible for the rise of place-based coffee differentiation and the corresponding creation of certain material qualities in the beans themselves. This paper shows how Rwandan coffee cuppers are doctoring coffee beans on a microscale for global markets and how producing coffee that "tastes good" requires work that is not only driven by perceptions of consumer demand but is also inherently political. It also raises questions as to whether Rwanda's implementation of a coffee cupping program is relying on *local* taste to an extent that producers in this exporting country are able to capture more of their coffee's financial value within a global foodway.

This research is based on ethnographic fieldwork including participant-observation and semistructured interviews conducted in Rwanda in 2008 at three coffee cupping laboratories, coffee processing centers, and in the national Sustaining Partnerships to Enhance Rural Enterprise and Development (SPREAD) project office in Kigali.[2] I contextualize the rise of Rwandan specialty coffee within an industry that, historically, was solely state-regulated and quantity-oriented. Rwandan cuppers are also part of a reorganization of the traditional coffee commodity chain in which tasting, or cupping, has typically been practiced only by importers, roasters, and consumers, or as a final quality control check at the point of exportation. The rationale behind this focuses on shifting some control to those involved with coffee production in Rwanda over the potential to capture profits within the coffee market. Led by the United States Agency for International Development (USAID), the rhetoric accompanying this agricultural development program focuses on improving the lives and incomes of coffee producers, and more broadly, on reducing poverty in this largely rural country. Although this article does not quantify the extent to which Rwandan coffee growers' livelihoods have been impacted by this quality improvement program, I explain how *some* farmers are receiving additional financial premiums as a result and suggest that the creation of high-value coffee beans in Rwanda may lead to additional financial risk. I also discuss the various types of quality defined by the international coffee industry, and I describe the cuppers' daily work routine. In addition to tasting coffee, they collaborate with processing center managers and facilitate sample collection for international coffee buyers, drawing the buyers' attention to coffees from certain parts of the country over others. Finally, by examining the Rwandan cuppers' encounters with others in the industry and the drink itself, this article raises valuable questions about the use of tasting as a standardizing practice within the global coffee-based foodway.

FROM COLONIAL CROP TO DEVELOPMENT DARLING

Coffee cultivation was first encouraged in Rwanda by missionaries during German colonial rule, who distributed seeds and bushes in 1905. Subsequently, the Belgian mandate administrators in the 1920s demanded that peasants uproot edible crops and replace them with the Bourbon variety of *Coffea arabica*. Brazil had recently turned to large-scale coffee production and threatened to control the world market and drive down the global commodity price. Europeans perceived Brazil's actions as a threat to colonial economies and power structures, which depended on stable coffee prices. The Belgian and British governments implemented systems of coerced labor and directed East African colonies to expand production. By the 1950s, tropical Africa's coffee exports rivaled Latin America and Indonesia (Kamola 2007; Clarence-Smith and Topik 2003; Pendergrast 1999).

Coffee-producing countries, including Rwanda, unsuccessfully attempted to raise commodity prices during the 1960s by forming a cartel. Consuming countries responded to these attempts by creating the United Nations-mandated International Coffee Agreement (ICA), which was signed in 1962 by the United States government, the United States coffee industry (which composed the largest body of importers), Latin American coffee producing countries, and some African nation-states such as Rwanda. The terms were set largely by consumers, including the United States, which also backed Brazil's military junta. The agreement imposed price controls and import and export quotas on 43 exporting countries and 24 importing countries in an attempt to bolster prices paid to producers in response to a depressed global commodity market drowning in over-supply, and effectively governed 99% of the global coffee market (Daviron and Ponte 2005; Clarence-Smith and Topik 2003; Pendergrast 1999).

In tension with shifting regulations of global coffee markets, the internal organization of Rwanda's coffee industry evolved during this period as well. In 1956, at the urging of Hutu elites, a European-led Catholic organization donated one hectare of land to Hutu farmers for the establishment of a coffee cooperative called TRAFIPRO (*travail fidélité progrès*). Though couched in terms of economic development aid for farmers, this organization also intended to establish economic leadership opportunities for Hutu businessmen within a coffee sector long-dominated by Tutsi. Hutus were growing increasingly frustrated with their marginalized political–economic status. Though they composed only 20% of the population, the colonial regime had given Tutsi favored political standing throughout their occupation. By 1958, with global coffee prices relatively high, TRAFIPRO was generating profit for its members, both urban and rural, although many of its original Hutu board members had been replaced with Tutsi (Kamola 2007; Scherrer 2002).

Following independence from Belgium in 1961, Rwandan President Kayibanda, a Hutu, continued to enforce laws surrounding coffee production, including punishment for those who neglected coffee plant maintenance and intercropped coffee with subsistence foods (Verwimp 2003). OCIR-Café (*Office des Cultures Industrielles du Rwanda*), a government board, was founded in 1964 to oversee all coffee exports and manage relations with international coffee traders. President Kayibanda also turned TRAFIPRO's existing countrywide network into a state-run marketing and exporting company that operated coffee purchasing stores throughout the country. But by the late 1960s, TRAFIPRO emerged at the center of a regional dispute as Hutu from the northern regions became suspicious that TRAFIPRO was favoring southern Hutu coffee producers, particularly those in Gitarama prefecture, Kayibanda's home region (Kamola 2007; Verwimp 2003). Kayibanda's minister of defense, Habyarimana, accused TRAFIPRO of diverting profits to Kayibanda's favored political associates. Meanwhile, Habyarimana seized power in a *coup d'état* in 1973 and closed down TRAFIPRO shortly thereafter, in the face of mounting debts and widespread corruption (Scherrer 2002; Uvin 1998).

Habyarimana's regime immediately created a government-run coffee monopsony called Rwandex, which controlled purchasing from farmers, marketing, and exportation from Kigali until the 1980s. The government purchased all coffee grown in the country at federally subsidized prices, processed the coffee minimally and sold it, as a homogenous commodity, to coffee conglomerates worldwide. The internal organization of the restructured coffee industry strongly favored Hutu producers from the northern Gisenyi and Ruhengeri prefectures, the area around Habyarimana's homeland. Because of its abundant rainfall and high altitude these provinces were considered especially ideal for growing coffee and Habyarimana gave the predominantly Hutu producers in this region extra economic incentive to increase plantings, at the expense of farmers in the southern Gitarama and Butare prefectures.

After several decades of relatively high and stable prices, coffee commodity markets declined sharply in 1985 because of global glut. The largest producers feared the imminent dismantling of the International Coffee Agreement, prompting massive sell-offs of coffee by mid-1989. This caused the Arabica "C" market price per pound to drop from $1.80 to $1.00 within one month. Consensus held that the international commodity regulatory institution had failed. Rwanda's export earnings from coffee declined from 14 billion RwF to 5 billion RwF in 1986 alone. The government attempted to maintain the subsidized prices paid to growers resulting in a spiral of debt. Rwandan loyalty to President Habyarimana rested on his regime's ability to sustain domestic incomes by purchasing coffee through Rwandex. As the commodity, or "C," price for coffee continued to decline and Habyarimana could no longer pay subsidized prices, unrest began to grow among the largely Hutu peasant class (Kamola 2007; Verwimp 2001).

Over a million Rwandans, predominantly Tutsi, were murdered between April and July of 1994. While discussion of the various causes of the genocide are beyond the scope of this article, the widely accepted account of the violence pitted Hutu extremists against Tutsi and moderate Hutu. Hundreds of thousands of refugees fled to present-day Democratic Republic of Congo, Tanzania, and Uganda; many of the Hutu extremists who had carried out the genocide fled to the Democratic Republic of Congo as well. The Tutsi-led opposition group Rwandan Patriotic Front, led by general Paul Kagame, planned a counterattack from Uganda and quelled the chaos during the summer of 1994. Kagame claimed leadership immediately following the genocide, appointed himself president in 2000, and ran unopposed in national elections in 2003. He was re-elected in 2010 with over 90% of the vote, despite widespread international criticism that the elections were not genuinely democratic.[3]

The genocide of 1994 nearly halted the Rwandan economy and coffee exports slowed to a trickle in the years immediately following the civil war. International aid money flooded the country through the late 1990s, mostly in the form of food donations and basic health services. Kagame has strongly tied post-genocide ethnic reconciliation and poverty reduction to economic development (Kagame 2009; Zorbas 2004). Determined not to repeat neighboring countries dependence on international aid such as food donations, Kagame instead encouraged the donor community to invest in the agricultural and service-sector business enterprises. Kagame's "Vision 2020" plan, for example, includes increasing export-oriented, high-value agricultural production in addition to building national infrastructure and creating private-sector urban industry as a means to economic stability by 2020 (Vision 2020 2000). USAID, the William J. Clinton Foundation, the Bill and Melinda Gates Foundation, and private donors have all followed suit, investing millions of dollars in the Rwandan coffee industry during the first decade of the twenty-first century.[4] But Kagame's relationships with high-profile development agencies and his ambition to turn Rwanda into the economic powerhouse of East Africa have also brought wider scrutiny from policy makers and scholars. Many have criticized Kagame's government for strongly repressing dissenting political opinion, and preventing freedom of press, and have raised questions as to whether Rwanda's rapid economic growth can be sustained within a questionably democratic political regime (Zorbas 2004; Pottier 2002).

Nevertheless, in addition to money, business investors have brought fresh ideas about how Rwanda's post-genocide economy should be developed. Citing Rwanda's ideal climate and unique coffee plant varietal as the natural basis for high-value coffee for export, policymakers and international coffee buyers recommended improving the material quality of Rwandan coffee via processing methods as a path to enter the global specialty market. Other trade-related options, such as Fair Trade certification for coffee and tea, were also considered as a means to agricultural economic development. But such models have largely been set aside in Rwanda in favor of investing in industry-related infrastructure, such as roads and processing centers, and in the domestic coffee cupping program. Notably, Kagame also sought out relations with the CEO of Starbucks Coffee beginning in 2007, citing Starbucks as an ideal partner for Rwanda's coffee industry and inviting the company to open farmer support centers, cupping laboratories and cafes in the country.[5] Because coffee is one of Rwanda's few exportable resources, the twenty-first century quality improvement of Rwanda's coffee also represents a rebranding of the country's image in the international eye. By marketing Rwandan "farmers as artisans" and their coffee's taste attributes as unique, Kagame hopes Rwanda will be recognized for something other than violence and thus attract further business investment in the service sectors as well as bolster agricultural export growth.

International Monetary Fund and World Bank policies, and affiliated international development agencies, have a long history of utilizing agricultural export markets as a means to elevating farmers' incomes in Africa (Dolan 2005; Diop et al. 2005; Elias and Carney 2004; Payer 1979). But poverty reduction in Rwanda, particularly in rural areas, has taken on additional significance vis-à-vis the plan for national unity and reconciliation that Kagame has instituted post-genocide. As Zorbas (2004) explains, tying poverty reduction to national unity suggests that the genocidal violence was perpetrated by socioeconomic dynamics. While this debate cannot be adequately dissected here, the belief that agricultural export markets may lead to poverty reduction and societal reconciliation in Rwanda operates as an additional justification for development agency investments in tangible interventions, such as coffee quality improvement programs.[6]

GEOGRAPHICAL DIMENSIONS

Rwanda today has a population hovering around 10 million and is projected to rise to between 13 and 16 million by 2020. It is the most densely populated country in sub-Saharan Africa, with an average of 340 inhabitants per square kilometer. Although 90 percent of the population today lives in rural areas, an additional four to seven million inhabitants would increase the country's population density to that of a uniformly urban-like settlement pattern. Nearly all rural inhabitants are involved in agricultural production, which comprises 40 percent of the national gross domestic product (Rwanda Development Indicators 2008). Rwanda has minimal natural resources other than agricultural products and is, therefore, largely dependent on coffee and tea exports in addition to a small but growing service sector, largely based in Kigali, and employing only a small fraction of the population.

The average inhabitable hectare of land is divided among nine Rwandans; two-thirds of Rwandan households own less than one-quarter hectare of land, and only 6 percent of households own more than half of a hectare (Rwanda Development Indicators 2008). Most of Rwanda's land cover includes terrain that is extremely steep, particularly in the western half of the country. These western provinces receive higher rainfall than those in the east, making them more suitable for rain-fed agriculture and, therefore, the more desirable. The three most densely populated provinces—Ruhengeri, Gisenyi, and Cyangugu—all lie on the border of Lake Kivu and across Rwanda's steepest mountains, where the majority of the coffee is grown. Coffee is cultivated primarily by smallholder farmers at altitudes ranging from 1200 to 1800 meters in a majority of provinces, with the average coffee farmer owning 165 plants.[7] Tea is also a major export commodity but is largely grown on large government-owned plantations. Nearly all smallholders grow a combination of crops for export and for personal consumption or sale at local markets, from which they earn a small income to supplement seasonal earnings from coffee. The vast majority of cultivable land in Rwanda is given to food crops for subsistence, such as cassava and plantains. Most coffee plants are not intercropped with other plant species, however, nor are they grown under tree canopies as is typical throughout Latin America and other parts of East Africa. Most coffee cultivation is organic by default, since most farmers are unable to afford inputs, such as pesticides and fertilizers.

Coffea arabica is the only species of coffee grown in Rwanda. It is harvested between March and July. Ripening occurs later in the season at higher altitudes; the higher the contrast between daytime and nighttime temperatures (as occurs at higher altitudes), the more concentrated the sugars of the coffee plant become. Harvesting cherries later in the season—in May or June as opposed to March—also presumes the sugars, and thus flavors, have had more time to develop. Because Rwanda is landlocked and exporting coffee via air is too costly, coffee is trucked to Mombasa, Kenya, where it is then shipped overseas.

Export production of green coffee is generally between 20,000 and 30,000 tons per year, though the exact amount fluctuates depending on rainfall and other climatic variables. In 2008, Rwanda exported 22,000 tons of green, or unroasted, coffee, worth US$46.9 million.[8] Coffee is grown on just 3% of cultivable land but comprises between 40–80% of the total value of agricultural production.[9] Coffee and tea are Rwanda's two largest exports by both volume and earnings, though the exact percentage of earnings fluctuates year to year. Rwanda is a small player in global terms, and is not among the top 20 coffee producing countries by export value or volume.[10] But as a percentage of total GDP, Rwanda depends more heavily on coffee exports than the top three producers, Brazil, Vietnam, and Indonesia.

GLOBAL DEMAND FOR SPECIALTY COFFEE

Specialty coffee is defined loosely as coffee of "high quality." It is almost exclusively derived from the species *Coffea arabica*, which grows only at high altitudes in the tropics and is mellower in flavor than its high-yielding counterpart, *Coffea robusta*. Arabica coffee accounts for around 60% of global production but a larger percentage of revenue; the largest coffee conglomerates incorporate both species of coffee into their blends (Linton 2004). Often, specialty coffee has limited availability on the production side, and/or carries value-laden flavoring, packaging, or branding on the consumption side (Ponte 2002; Pendergrast 1999). U.S.-based companies, such as Starbucks, deal within the specialty sector while coffee marketed under labels such as Folger's or Maxwell House is not specialty. These brands are imported and roasted by one of the four largest international coffee conglomerates—Sara Lee, Proctor and Gamble, Nestlé, and Phillip Morris, which source large quantities at the lowest prices (Daviron and Ponte 2005; Linton 2004). Specialty coffee importers will often pay a premium for coffee with certain quality attributes and pass the premiums on to consumers who are willing to pay upwards of US$2 per cup of specialty brew or US$12 per pound of roasted coffee beans.

The majority of the world's coffee is still traded through global commodity markets and its value is underwritten by the New York and London

Coffee Exchanges. In 2008, the average price for Arabica coffee sold on the New York Coffee Exchange was $1.38 per pound.[11] Though the price paid to coffee growers in producing countries varies and fluctuates widely, the average grower in Rwanda producing for this commodity market received around 30 U.S. cents per pound of green coffee beans throughout the early 2000s.[12] But higher-priced specialty coffee has been steadily rising in demand and production: it accounted for 15% of green coffee imports into the United States in 2000 but roughly 40% of U.S.-based coffee sales.[13] The global demand for specialty coffee is projected to be growing between 5–20% per year, with demand increasing in newer markets such as China and Eastern Europe (Raynolds 2007; Daviron and Ponte 2005).

Origin-oriented specialty coffee drinkers choose from a global map. Certain countries, such as Colombia, or micro-regions, such as Ethiopia's Sidamo and Guatemala's Antigua, have successfully created recognizable brands based on place-names. By marketing consistent and unique flavor attributes, coffee beans from these areas are tied to *terroir* conditions—ecological and production-based—though without the state-regulated Appellation d'Origine Controlee or similar labels required by European wine producers (Guthman 2007; Barham 2003). Beyond place-based marketing, there also exist differences in coffee production methods. Organically and shade-grown, fairly traded and bird-friendly: each of these coffee growing and trading standards uses certification and labeling practices to make certain favorable aspects of the production and distribution process visible to the consumer. Ecological labeling has been particularly popular in Latin America, where conventional coffee is often grown in forests or on plantations where pesticide spraying is common. In East Africa, and particularly in Rwanda, coffee is less commonly grown in complex forest regimes or on plantations than it is by small landholders, rendering many such certifications irrelevant.

Each form of labeling is arguably an amalgam of well-articulated marketing and an attempt to link coffee drinkers to otherwise anonymous places and methods of coffee production—all of which become the basis for raising the economic value of a coffee above the "C" price set by fluctuating commodity exchanges. These options and many others also represent the coffee industry's differentiation over the past few decades, perhaps more than any other commodity industry of similar global value.[14]

Consumers are key players in the global coffee market, but they are not catalyzing the drive towards quality improvement as much as they are maintaining and encouraging the specialty sector's quality differentiation through purchasing habits. As Linton (2004) explains, producers and roasters must create the initial demand for a particular characteristic imbued within the coffee by marketing its social value, such as is the case with fair trade coffee. Consumers maintain the demand once they are introduced to and convinced of the coffee's value; only then are they willing to pay a premium price for those embedded values. Yet paradoxically, as consumers at one end of a long foodway have been paying more than ever for endless varieties of specialty coffee with varying social significance attached, coffee growers' opportunities to receive a parcel of the financial premiums from an intensely competitive market remain few.

SUCCESSES AND LIMITATIONS OF MARKETING SCHEMES

Trade has long been proposed by development scholars as one path to development in the global south (Moyo 2009; Payer 1979). The concept of fair trade has emerged as one tactic to overcome economic and social disparities between the producers of agricultural commodities and consumers of imported agro-food products. Particularly within the specialty coffee industry, fair trade schemes have sought to bring transparency to the exchanges embedded in global commodity chains and pass capital back to marginalized coffee producers, imbuing the tangible commodity with symbolic value. Some scholars have shown its relative success among coffee growers to be uneven at best (Bacon 2008; Jaffee 2007; Goodman 2004). Among the major criticisms of fair trade certification as an approach to increasing the capital passed on to coffee growers is its inability to address fundamental problems of global supply. This has been interpreted crudely as too much quantity and not enough material quality (Linton 2004). The few extra cents of price premium passed on to coffee farmers is created through symbolic value, marketed to consumers as concern for social justice or the environment (Renard 2005; Linton 2004; Goodman 2004).

Though fair trade, along with other coffee labeling schemes such as organic and Rainforest Alliance, have raised global awareness of the social and environmental conditions under which coffee is grown, it has failed to incentivize coffee farmers to produce coffees with higher material quality. Coffees bearing variously the fair trade or organic label are often criticized as mediocre in quality (Linton 2008). Because certification schemes fail to create or regulate material quality, there is little incentive for farmers to produce a higher-quality coffee than that which is already certified. Opportunities for farmers to gather premiums even higher than those offered to them through labeling certifications remain limited. The minimum price guaranteed for cooperatives meeting the fair trade criteria was $1.26 per pound of washed Arabica in 2008, or $.05 per pound higher than the "C" price, whichever is higher.[15] Similarly, a cooperative is encouraged to produce and sell as much as they can through fair trade or other certification, which does not address the global problem of coffee oversupply. Nor does it account for the difficulty many specialty importers have in finding large enough quantities with high material quality to supply an increasingly differentiated consumer market. In other words, fair trade has attempted to work through ideas about market structure and governance using alternative trading regimes but fails ultimately to offer an economically sustainable approach to increasing the value generated by producers. If the price of "C" coffee were to plummet well below $1.26, as it did during the coffee crisis of the early 2000s, Fair Trade would provide a buffer for producers to mitigate their losses. When the price of "C" coffee is relatively high, as it was from 2005–2010, fair trade certification provides little additional income to producers and is often not worth the higher production costs.

With a focus on "just" labor practices, fair trade certification also obliges all interested farmers to form democratically organized cooperatives. The formation of cooperatives allows farmers to manage their own processing and marketing, and thus eliminate some of the profit-capturing middlemen operating between the growers and importers. There are a few highly sought-after coffees from Rwanda that are produced by cooperatives, such as Bufcafe, which has won numerous awards in the country's Golden Cup and Cup of Excellence competitions. But to some extent fair trade's mandatory cooperative structure conflicts with the current organization of farmers contributing to Rwanda's coffee sector. In Rwanda, approximately one-third of processing centers are cooperatively managed while the rest are owned and managed primarily by private Rwandan investors, considered by some Western coffee buyers to be more efficient at brokering purchasing contracts.[16] Since 2001 the rapid growth of privately owned washing stations has also enabled farmers in remote areas to sell their coffee beans for processing. A mandate for cooperative formation and fair trade certification might have delayed or inhibited washing station construction, which is at odds with the objectives of government, non-governmental organizations, and donors, specifically investment in tangible infrastructure and entrepreneurial ventures with potential for high capital return.

COFFEE QUALITY: MATERIAL AND SYMBOLIC

To understand how coffee quality may be improved, it is important to differentiate types of quality as they are produced and exchanged within the country of origin.[17] Daviron and Ponte (2005) propose one particularly useful set of definitions on quality in *The Coffee Paradox*. They divide quality into material, symbolic, and in-person; each type of quality is based on attributes either inherent to the bean or adhered to the bean as it is transferred within the commodity chain from farmers via processors, exporters, importers and roasters, to consumers. Symbolic quality attributes refer to immeasurable or immaterial characteristics such as the trade-marking, branding, and reputation of coffee. Sustainability labels such as fair trade, organic, shade-grown, and other certifications add symbolic value, indicating to the consumer that the coffee has social and environmental worth that extends beyond the material coffee bean itself. Coffee that is sold to consumers as a blend of beans from varying origins carries symbolic value marketed by the roaster, often evocative of a type of a company's roasting style or imagery that may or may not directly reflect the origin, or material quality, of the beans themselves.

Material quality attributes, which coffee cuppers seek to discern, "are often seen as intrinsic, objective, and embedded in the coffee bean" (Daviron and Ponte 2005: 34) and encompass chemical, biochemical, and physical characteristics that can be measured objectively through technology and/or the human senses. Sensory perception, especially taste and smell, determines the material quality of beans traded within the specialty industry. Exporters often taste the brewed coffee beans before they leave the country of origin to check for off-flavors that may signal the presence of molds or mildews; coffee that fails to meet basic taste standards may not be exported. Similarly, importers and roasters taste and smell purchased brewed coffee samples to check for defects and gage the most appropriate roasting length of a particular batch. By contrast, coffee not designated as specialty but destined for mainstream commodity markets is evaluated by quality control inspectors who check only for visible, as opposed to flavor-based, defects at points of exportation and importation. Coffee is also evaluated by size and shape, with these visual designations determining varying grades, such as A, B, or C quality.[18] In Rwanda, coffee of inferior quality is consolidated from around the country and sorted according to grade in large warehouses in Kigali before export. The government-run OCIR-Café coordinates consolidation and sorting, pays processors for beans, and sells the product on the coffee commodity market. This coffee, evaluated by size and shape alone, is likely to be purchased by one of the world's large coffee conglomerates. Taste characteristics such as sweetness, flavor, and acidity of the beans are never included in this commodity transaction.

Additional material attributes figure prominently into other market transactions, particularly within the specialty sector. The coffee plant varietal, agro-ecological growing conditions and processing methods all contribute to certain material attributes of coffee. Such specific material attributes may not be measured by sight alone, but rather through tasting practices. Beans of potentially superior material quality, therefore, undergo many rounds of tasting, or "cupping," traditionally undertaken by importers and roasters rather than by producers within the country of origin. And whereas countries with long-established and globally recognized coffee identities, such as Colombia, Brazil, Indonesia, and Ethiopia, have long employed cuppers, more often than not they are employees of export companies, and usually do not collaborate directly with coffee growers and processors.

In Rwanda, cupping is increasingly a state-endorsed enactment of direct collaboration between producers and processors. By shifting the discernment of flavor characteristics and the subsequent marketing of unique, consistent, and localized flavors to the countries where coffee originates, Daviron and Ponte (2005) argue that material quality can be tied to symbolic quality at origin and thus increase the farmers' share of coffee revenues. As they describe:

> "...market power [is] not simply...controlling market share, but...the ability to define the 'identity' of a coffee—in other words, the ability to set the language and the reference values that determine production norms and quality standards." (Daviron and Ponte 2005: ix).

In one respect, this means that material quality attributes, such as flavor from a specific region, have the potential to become the basis for symbolic value, similar to state-regulated appellations or place-based branding in the wine industry. Industry actors can thus shift the value creation to the point of origin; differentiation and identity definition moves away from the consumer, toward the producer. Training Rwandan cuppers to discern and improve quality as part of the coffee production process offers coffee producers the opportunity for increased market share. Notwithstanding the fact that Rwandan coffee is increasingly differentiated by local Rwandan places and production methods, I argue that the language of discernment and quality is far from indigenous.

RAPID CONSTRUCTION: RWANDA'S COFFEE INFRASTRUCTURE RISES

In 2001, there were no coffee-washing stations in Rwanda; by the end of 2008, there were 120 washing stations and over 4,000 tons out of 22,000 total tons of exported coffee was fully washed and thus destined for the specialty market rather than the "C" market.[19] Some of the washing stations are funded by government agencies, some are financed through USAID-sponsored organizations, and others by private international investors. In addition to funding washing station construction, some organizations distribute bicycles to coffee growers so they can reach processing centers more rapidly, thereby decreasing the chance that material quality of the beans would start to disintegrate before they are washed.[20]

"Coffee washing" refers to the water process whereby the exterior of the coffee "cherry" is removed from the bean. Unwashed processing, the alternative and older production method, relies on sun-drying before the cherry hull is removed.[21] Washed coffee is of little extra value to importer-roasters who are looking to purchase large quantities rather than source a specific type of quality. But coffee washing is a necessary processing step for coffee from most producing countries to gain entrance to the specialty market.[22] "Fully washed" refers to the end process whereby coffee cherries later sold have been floated in large, shallow water tanks to reveal density. Higher-density, and thus fully formed beans—which are actually the seed of the coffee plant's fruit—sink while the floating cherries are skimmed off. The red exterior of the coffee cherries are removed by a depulping machine and the remaining portion is then left to ferment in water for up to 12 hours, at which point the remaining layers surrounding the coffee bean becomes soggy enough to remove. The beans are then spread out on drying tables or racks (either shaded or unshaded) for up to three days to dry, and the visibly defective beans are removed by hand. Beans at this stage are called "parchment" because of the thin papery skin covering the coffee bean. This processed parchment, or "green" coffee, is kept separated in lots according to the day on which they are harvested, though any given day's lot can contain hundreds of farmers' harvested cherries.

Four regional farmer support centers, each containing a cupping laboratory, have also been constructed by the Sustaining Partnerships for Rural Enterprise and Agribusiness Development (SPREAD) project, which receives funding from USAID. The regional cupping laboratories are located in four geographically distinct locations: one is in the capital city of Kigali, while the other three are situated at higher altitudes in regions where coffee growing is extensive—Butare prefecture in the south, Gisenyi in the north, and Cyangugu in the west. The laboratories collect coffee samples, separated by day of harvest and processing center, which are tasted by Rwanda's trained cuppers daily and the findings are reported to the coffee washing station owners. These laboratories were not built to be economically sustainable but instead act as nascent training centers where both cuppers and farmers learn how to produce and detect quality and defects. Some companies, such as Starbucks, have begun to build their own cupping laboratories and some washing stations are planning to have cupping laboratories on site in the future. Though coffee roasting is generally done within the country of consumption, cuppers have also been trained by visiting American and European coffee buyers to roast samples for tasting so the batches closely mimic the coffee that will be sold to consumers.

CAREER COFFEE CUPPING

The coffee cuppers are a significant node in the long chain of quality discernment and value creation within the specialty coffee industry stretching from Rwanda's coffee farms to high-end coffee shops in the United States, Europe, and Japan. Although all coffee-producing countries employ coffee cuppers, they most often work as quality controllers at the final point of exportation, checking for defects and corroborating coffee shipments with export orders. In Rwanda, however, three dozen cuppers have been trained by American coffee buyers to taste coffee as part of the production process itself: not only are they stewards of quality control but they are also involved in the *production* of material quality.[23] They act as intermediaries between coffee-washing station owners, cooperative boards and international coffee buyers seeking unique and consistent taste profiles. In this sense, the cuppers act as links to place and taste, highlighting the superior coffee-growing microregions within Rwanda for coffee buyers and, ultimately, consumers.

Kigali's coffee cupping laboratory is down a dusty hill from the OCIR-Café offices and inside a cavernous warehouse where coffee sorters grade tons of beans destined for the "C" market, and through an unmarked doorway. I would arrive early in the morning to find the cuppers quietly brewing their morning black tea. Coffee has never been a popular drink among Rwandans, nor is there any sign of its adoption as an everyday beverage by professional coffee tasters. One particular morning Nathalie was already consulting with the director of one coffee cooperative on his recently sampled beans when I arrived.[24] Nathalie's criticism of the man's beans was that they had a "lack of body in mouthfeel." Her diagnosis was that the green coffee beans had been exposed to too much afternoon sun on the drying racks at the washing station. "These beans were good, very good," says Nathalie. "They are sweet, citrus… but they lack body. It's because of the drying process."

At coffee-growing origin, domestic cupping is more than a matter of gustatory significance. Rwanda's more than 30 cuppers are well-paid coffee professionals, many of whom work five days a week at one of the four cupping laboratories. They play an important role in facilitating coffee sample selection as international buyers only visit the country for a few days at a time, and a few times per year. Cuppers also offer feedback to processing station managers on how to improve their coffee quality through relatively simple changes in production methods such as removing defective beans, harvesting cherries at proper ripeness and drying the parchment adequately. These variations in processing are all discerned through thorough and systematic tasting.

Most of the cuppers working in Rwanda today were trained by a small selection of American coffee buyers, who are also professional cuppers, in 2003 and 2004. Training has continued over the subsequent years as more coffee buyers have a presence in the country and more Rwandans seek to become cuppers. The majority of Rwandan cuppers are in their 20s and early 30s, are equally male and female, and are often pursuing some form of higher education, particularly in business administration programs in Kigali. Many of them were born outside of Rwanda and returned with their families after the civil war; a few also grew up in coffee-producing households and are active in coffee growing as well as cupping.[25] There is no rule stipulating who can be trained as a cupper, although having previous exposure to the coffee industry increases the likelihood that they will be well-positioned for training. There is currently too little work available for all of the trained cuppers to be employed full-time. Some of them are employed elsewhere but assist with larger-scale cupping endeavors such as preparing for 2008's and

2010's national Cup of Excellence competition, in which coffees from regions throughout Rwanda were ranked by an international jury and sold at auction. Others hope to find jobs when privately owned cupping laboratories open. Those who have secured full-time positions in one of the national cupping labs hold prestigious jobs and could be considered part of the small but slowly emerging middle class in Kigali.

STANDARDIZED TASTING ROUTINES

The cuppers begin their day by organizing the previous day's roasted samples stored in cubbies around the lab: three, four, even five dozen small bags of coffee beans are laid out on a long table without chairs that is roughly chest-height for most of the cuppers. Each sample has a numerical code that corresponds to a washing station and harvest date, which are kept anonymous on the cupping table. A laboratory assistant, who won't participate in that round of cupping, is generally present to code each batch. A day's work includes cupping samples from either from a single washing station, separated by harvest date, or from multiple washing stations but harvested around the same time. They first set out colorful plastic plates, each holding a cup of freshly roasted beans. Each sample of beans is ground and measured into three different glass cups, which allows the cuppers to check for consistency within lots. They'll sniff each cup of dry grounds, making notes on the initial aromas. Then the assistant pours hot water slowly over each cup of grounds from a large, silver kettle. One cupper will circulate around the table, breaking and pushing aside the crust of the grounds as each cup is brewing, which allows the cuppers to sniff the escaping brewed aromas. Before the crust of the grounds is broken, the cups look murky enough to be holding muddy water. He or she then spoons off the foam and any floating grounds (the remaining grounds have settled to the bottom) after precisely four minutes. The three or four cuppers make their way around the table, slurping a spoonful of each cup's brew using a soup spoon with a sharply angled handle, pausing after spitting out each mouthful into plastic cups to jot down notes on their clipboards. Because flavors change somewhat dramatically as coffee cools, the cuppers usually work through each round of samples twice, once while they are still hot and again after the coffee has cooled slightly. Hot coffee also masks imperfections that the cuppers want to uncover; imperfections and defects become more apparent as the temperature falls. They work quietly, rarely speaking to one another during cupping, the silence in the lab broken only by the sound of slurping. After perhaps 30 or 40 minutes, each cupper will retreat to the sides of the room to manually compute scores for each sample and expand on any notes they've taken. On a particularly busy day during harvest season, the cuppers might work their way through three tables' worth of samples before lunchtime.

Cuppers quantify flavor and aroma following the guidelines of the internationally recognized Specialty Coffee Association of America's (SCAA) Coffee Quality Institute.[26] Cleanliness, sweetness, acidity, mouthfeel, flavor, aftertaste, and balance are all considered to be measurable attributes and are assigned a score from one to eight.[27] They use standardized scoring sheets, listing each of these categories, distributed by SCAA. The scores from each category are added, points subtracted for defects, and a final score assigned; final scores generally range from between 70—unexceptional, low-grade coffee—to 100. Washed coffee is typically expected to score above 80; scores above 86 are acceptable to the highest-end coffee buyers, who generally pay at least double the coffee commodity price, often much more. Finally, one cupper will enter all the day's scores, along with any qualitative notes, into a cumulative logbook that contains data on each washing station.

Rwandan cuppers have also acquired a new language of taste to describe flavor and aroma, not dissimilar from that used in the wine industry. Because aroma, and, to a certain extent flavor, are deemed to be unquantifiable, cuppers are expected to provide notes, in English, on a coffee's dominant qualitative, material attributes, although English is many of the cuppers' third language, following Kinyarwanda and French. Some of the cuppers speak English well enough to communicate with visiting international coffee buyers: some know only enough words in English to describe the coffees. All prefer to speak to one another in Kinyarwanda. Additionally, the cuppers sometimes act as translators during meetings between coffee buyers and processing station owners, some of whom don't speak English. Their language of description often corresponds to flavors and aromas with which most Rwandans were previously unfamiliar—e.g., blueberry and violet. Few of the flavors are indigenous, or even readily available in their natural form, in East Africa. American coffee buyers and consultants have imported samples of many foods, as well as sets of perfume-like aroma vials, to help cuppers build a kind of taste-memory from which they can draw their more subjective assessments of the coffees.

Nathalie sends Jean-Paul, the cooperative representative, out with a list of all the day-lots harvested in April and May and processed at a washing station in the northern part of the country, and a corresponding list of scores. She explained to me after he left that "if the beans aren't dry enough, they can be sent back. If they are too dry, it's too late … There is no tool to measure moisture content," Nathalie retorts with a hint of remorse, that "the farmers, they just taste the beans!" Like Nathalie, all the cuppers employed at the laboratories act as the "coffee doctors," offering advice to washing station owners or cooperative directors who come seeking quality quantification and tips on how to improve their beans. They are also the "referees," as Nathalie called them, providing a crucial link between processing and exportation and, ultimately, between producers and consumers. "If you don't know, if you don't cup," explained Nathalie, "you can't improve. You can't change the processing," referring to the fact that few farmers or washing station owners taste their own coffee. Without tasting, they believe, there is no way of knowing a coffee's value. Without knowing the value, quality improvement and the potential for increased income it brings with it, is futile. Nathalie and her boyfriend, Joseph, a long-time cupper who started his own cupping consulting business, seemed incredulous that some of the washing station owners have yet to believe this. "They have to understand the value of the cuppers," Nathalie said vigorously with Joseph nodding at her side, "because we make the value."

During one particular round of cupping, a selection of samples from Gitarama province, just west of Kigali, was separated not only by the day of harvest but also by an assigned grade: a single day's harvest separated into grade A_1 and grade A_2. Specialty coffee buyers would have been interested only in the beans graded A_1, indicating beans that are uniformly sized and shaped. Over one hundred farmers may have contributed to any given day's harvest, making it impossible to identify the location of the coffee beyond the washing station, presuming that cherries were grown within a roughly ten-kilometer radius. But in the cupping lab, all possible imperfections must be unveiled within individual day lots. One particular selection of day lots included two dozen samples from a single washing station. I cupped one day's lot harvested on 30 May that tasted harsh and tangy on my tongue, lingering like lemon pith. Another day lot from the same washing station but harvested on 9 June was chalky and watery, full of tannins and lacking in body. This became clear when I tasted a spoonful of a day lot from 22 May that, by comparison, tasted wholly familiar to my palate. The cuppers and I were only vaguely able to articulate in words why this particular sample was the most paradigmatic of the selection on the table, using phrases such as "full-bodied," "clean," and "nice acidity." But each cupper gave it a score of 90 or above. Such a high score was perhaps more descriptive than the linguistic phrases, as it gave context to this sample in relation to the quality of the others on the table. Qualitative descriptors, by contrast, are rarely comparative.

When the cuppers offer feedback to processing center managers in the midst of the coffee harvesting season, their analyses can alter production methods at the washing stations and on growers' properties. For example, coffee cherry ripening occurs later at higher altitudes; the higher the contrast between daytime and nighttime temperatures, as occurs at higher altitudes, the more concentrated the sugars of the coffee plant become and thus produce, at least in theory, more flavor development. Harvesting cherries later in the season also presumes the sugars have had more time to develop, but as with all stages of coffee processing, a few underripe or diseased beans could throw off an otherwise fully ripened batch. The cuppers detect ripeness even before they taste the coffee—aromas reminiscent of popcorn emanating from the roasting machines indicate the presence of underripe beans, while beans that smell medicinal, or like black tar, during roasting are overripe. Additionally, beans that continuously pop during roasting usually mean that the coffee was left to dry too long in the sun. The cuppers then deliver their diagnoses on these material attributes to processing center managers, or sometimes to groups of growers directly, encouraging them to sort their cherries more carefully before washing them or harvest more frequently—every week as opposed to every other week. Harvesting ripe cherries and drying the parchment properly are two of the biggest concerns of high-end coffee buyers, who repeatedly emphasize that taking these steps is the only way to produce coffee that they will be interested in buying. As one coffee buyer wrote in a guestbook after seeing green cherries mixed in with the bright red ones at a washing station that had produced coffees he had particularly admired: "Ripe cherry is the only solution." No purchasing contract was made there that day. When the coffee buyers are not present to look over everyone's shoulder, the cuppers step in to remind producers that the quality of their beans *can* be improved and thus sold at a higher price than the "C" market offers. The only final proof of "quality improvement," however, is determined at the cupping table.

Coffee buyers from the United States, and increasingly Europe and Japan, eventually form contracts with washing stations to purchase meticulously processed beans from the most prized microregions of Rwanda. Such quality batches, which are marketed by importing companies under a processing center, cooperative, or region name, comprise the minority of Rwandan coffee exports. But the prices these buyers are willing to pay are roughly 200% more than growers receive when they sell their beans on the commodity market; they are also higher than the prices certification schemes such as fair trade offer. Not all coffee farmers in Rwanda receive such high prices, and farmers able to secure contracts with the high-end importers do not receive such prices for their entire harvest. But meticulously processed and sorted beans that undergo multiple rounds of tasting by Rwandan cuppers, represent a growing percentage of many farmers' total production and also of the entire Rwandan coffee market.

An element of risk involved in entering contracts with high-end buyers based on material taste attributes should also be considered. Although some of these buyers offer multi-year contracts with producers, most prefer to purchase beans on a year-to-year basis, based on cupping results of sample lots. The buyers may look to a previous year's supplier initially, only to discover that the coffee no longer has the same taste attributes. Because the buyers, and increasingly the cuppers as well, demand that growers put more labor into harvesting, processing, and sorting their beans without guaranteeing payment ahead of time, many producers are reluctant to become involved with such buyers, choosing to forego the possibility of both profit and loss. Many coffee companies hunting for Rwanda's most prized beans also write their own trading guidelines and some encourage a high degree of price transparency for all actors in the commodity chain. Unlike in fair trade, the highest-end buyers want growers to receive financial premiums for their highest-quality beans directly, rather than distribute premiums to cooperative boards or processing center owners. This may minimize the risk of corruption that sometimes affects coffee cooperatives and private processing centers. But growers receiving premiums directly may also forego the opportunity for social and/or environmental improvement projects whereas fair trade guidelines mandate that premiums earned through certification fund long-term projects, such as schools or additional coffee processing infrastructure, that benefit the community at large (Linton 2008b).[28] In addition, because these trading practices, often called "Direct Trade" or relationship-based trade, are not standardized across companies nor regulated by third parties, as certification schemes are, growers still rely on processing center owners and managers to negotiate prices and guidelines with buyers on their behalf. They also depend heavily on these middlemen, and the cuppers as well, to communicate knowledge about the value of their coffee in the marketplace. The leverage growers ultimately have to insist on a "fair" price from buyers depends significantly on the scores and qualitative assessments their beans receive in the cupping laboratories.

CONCLUSION

In recent years, market-based, U.S.-led development programs have emphasized "quality improvement" in agricultural sectors as a key component of successful economic development. Coffee cupping—a standardized tasting practice—has been implemented in Rwanda as part of the country's, and a broader international, turn towards coffee quality improvement. The doctoring done by Rwanda's cadre of American-trained cuppers and their ancillary communities shows that the international search for coffee that "tastes good" *and* has authentic ties to specific regions has implications far beyond the cupping laboratories. In particular, I suggest that the cuppers' collaboration with international coffee buyers, processing center managers, and growers has altered production dynamics at washing stations and on the farms where coffee is grown. The coffee cupping laboratories and the cuppers' work gives legitimacy to taste attributes and thus, to the prices offered for certain beans. Furthermore, coffee cupping in Rwanda plays an instrumental role in differentiating localities on the ground, laying the foundation for single-origin branding based on the perception of authentic and consistent flavor attributes, and corresponding financial value. Some Rwandan coffee growers are well positioned to earn more than what the commodity market or certification schemes offer as a result of the feedback they receive from cuppers and the subsequent deals brokered with high-end coffee companies. But the extent to which these profitable contracts offer long-term economic stability or complete protection from global market fluctuations remains questionable. More research is certainly needed to determine precisely what effects this quality improvement program has had on farmers' incomes and livelihoods in Rwanda.

Additionally, given the contentious history and regional patronage of government-run coffee organizations in Rwanda, careful attention needs to be paid to current state involvement in the coffee sector. Although President Kagame has stressed the need for free market trade for agricultural exports, the government agency OCIR-Café still oversees a large proportion of domestic coffee production. Many cooperatives and processing center managers are forming relationships directly with international buyers and thus bypassing much of OCIR-Café's close oversight. But if, as evidence from the cupping laboratory shows, coffee bean quality is largely determined by processing and tasting in the domestic cupping laboratories, can we trust that farmers in all regions can access this infrastructure and, subsequently, high-value markets? This also raises questions of whether the cuppers themselves are involved in patronage relationships and whether they are free to fairly consider coffees from all subregions. While those working within the coffee industry in Rwanda have stressed that coffee is evaluated solely on the basis of its taste attributes, alternative political–economic motives should be considered in future research.

Finally, coffee cupping is predicated on an increasingly standardized and global language of taste, which enables the Rwandan cuppers to facilitate communication within an otherwise opaque foodway. The proliferation of American-based coffee tasting practices to Rwanda has made it possible to objectify and quantify flavor as a means to economic, and coffee quality, development. But it also raises questions as to how, and by whom the terms of coffee "quality," and increasingly authenticity, are being defined. One coffee consultant working in Rwanda told me that Japan has a rapidly growing specialty coffee import market. With their beverage discernment already honed by hundreds of years of tea drinking and ceremony, and an emerging appreciation for origin-designated wines, it is not surprising that the Japanese are interested in buying the same high-end Rwandan coffees destined for the United States and Europe. Japanese buyers seek the same high quality—materially and symbolically—Rwandan coffee as their Western counterparts, yet different. Japanese taste preferences for sweetness, acidity, and bitterness diverge from that of Westerners. Would the Japanese be looking for wholly different flavor profiles in Rwandan coffee, and is it necessary for them to train their own cuppers? Would they use the same American-based scoring rubric or the same English-language derived qualitative descriptors? The implications of these questions hold more than gustatory significance. As suggested earlier in this paper, market power derives from the ability to determine the language through which a coffee's quality, and thus identity, is defined. These production-based cuppers have helped codify the quality standards of one transnational foodway and have the potential to do so for other importing countries, with the incentive of increased profits for coffee growers. But the extent to which the cuppers can translate taste development into sustained economic development may depend on their future ability to define in their own terms what constitutes quality, and authentically Rwandan, coffee.

NOTES

1. See Alex Renton, "Jack Sprat: Fair trade food—it just tastes better" *The Times*, February 13, 2009, http://www.timesonline.co.uk/tol/life_and_style/food_and_drink/article5718241.ece. For contrasting opinions, see Rwanda Blue Bourbon at http://urbansemiotic.com/2006/03/30/starbucks-whole-bean-coffee-review/

2. The author has no financial or contractual affiliation with the organizations and companies contacted during this research. Funding for this project was provided by the University of California, Los Angeles graduate student support. Generous thanks to the many coffee experts who offered their time and thoughts towards this project, both in the United States and in Rwanda.

3. Though Kagame won both the 2003 and 2010 elections with over 90% of the national vote, many domestic and international critics doubt the extent to which these elections were actually democratic as his government prevented many opponents from running. Also see Human Rights Watch at http://www.hrw.org/africa/rwanda for more criticism of Kagame's regime.

4. See the William J. Clinton Foundation at http://www.clintonfoundation.org/what-we-do/clinton-hunter-development-initiative/i/success-story-rwandan-farmers-coffee and the Gates Foundation at http://www.gatesfoundation.org/learning/Pages/progress-report-technoserve-business-training-coffee-farmers-africa.aspx for more on business development funding in the Rwandan coffee industry.

5. M. Allison, "Starbucks to Open Center for Coffee Farmers in Rwanda," *The Seattle Times*, Business and Technology, 4 December 2007.

6. Nongovernmental organizations (NGOs), such as Technoserve, as well as USAID, have been instrumental in making these recommendations. Many NGOs working to revitalize Rwanda's coffee industry receive funding from large donor institutions, such as the Gates Foundation.

7. National Institute of Statistics of Rwanda, http://statistics.gov.rw

8. http://rwandacafe.com/index

9. See article at http://www.busiweek.com/index.php?option=com_content&task=view&id=903&Itemid=1

10. 9 Food and Agriculture Indicators, Rwanda (2006). United Nations Food and Agriculture Organization. Retrieved 24 January 2009 from http://www.fao.org

11. http://www.fao.org

12. Prices Paid to Growers in Current Terms, U.S. cents per lb. (2004–2007). International Coffee Organization. Retrieved 8 December 2008 from http://www.ico.org/asp/display7.asp

13. This figure might be higher than actual, taking into account profit generated by retailers though mixing with milk for espresso drinks (Daviron and Ponte 2005).

14. At the beginning of the 21st century, coffee was the second-most-valuable traded commodity on international markets, following oil (Pendergrast 1999).

15. For more on fair trade price premiums, see http://www.transfairusa.org/content/resources/faq-advanced.php#minimum

16. Personal interview with multiple industry personnel. Kigali, Rwanda, 2008.

17. For a broader discussion of quality as evaluated by consumers, see Daviron and Ponte (2005), Renard (2005). Given the scope of this article, quality will be referred to as it pertains to producing countries.

18. Within these designations, A-quality beans are the most uniform in size and shape while C-quality are visibly misshapen and of varying sizes (Daviron and Ponte 2005)

19. The SPREAD Annual Report Draft (2007). Kigali, United States Agency for International Development: 1–33. Retrieved 8 May 2008 from http://www.spreadproject.org. In 2008, there were 120 washing stations in Rwanda.

20. Bikes to Rwanda is one nonprofit organization working to lease bicycles to coffee farmers.

21. For countries with a drier climate, dry-processed coffee is generally considered to be a better production method; for countries such as Rwanda with an abundant water supply and a wetter climate, washing the coffee is a crucial step in producing a higher-quality coffee bean.

22. The extent to which this type of processing is practiced or considered necessary varies by country, but in Rwanda, all coffee that will be sold on the specialty market must be fully washed.

23. Funding to train the cuppers between 2006 and 2011 has been provided by the SPREAD project under the guidance of Texas A&M University; between 2002 and 2005 funding was provided by a similar project, Partnerships to Enhance Agriculture in Rwanda through Linkages (PEARL), sponsored by Michigan State University.

24. All personal names have been changed to protect confidentiality.

25. The fact that a person living in Rwanda today was born in a neighboring country and returned with their family after the civil war often indicates that their parents had fled the country during the first waves of Tutsi expulsion in the 1960s.

26. See http://www.coffeeinstitute.org/ for information on specific guidelines the Specialty Coffee Association of America uses to determine quality within the coffee industry.

27. There are a few different scoring rubrics; this description corresponds to the one used in preparation for the Cup of Excellence competition.

28. See also Fair Trade guidelines at http://www.transfairusa.org

REFERENCES

Bacon, C. M. 2008. Are sustainable coffee certifications enough to secure farmer livelihoods? The millennium development goals and Nicaragua's fair trade co-operatives. *Globalizations* 5: 259–274.

Barham, E. 2002. Towards a theory of values-based labeling. *Agriculture and Human Values* 19: 349–360.

Barham, E. 2003. Translating terroir: The global challenge of French AOC labeling. *Journal of Rural Studies* 19: 127–138.

Bigagaza, J., Abong, C., and Mukarubuga, C. 2002. *Land Scarcity, Distribution, and Conflict in Rwanda. Scarcity and Surfeit: The Ecology of Africa's conflicts.* J. Lind, Sturman, K. (eds.). South Africa: Institute for Security Studies, 51–82.

Bourdieu, P. 1984. *Distinction: A Social Critique of the Judgment of Taste.* Cambridge, MA: Harvard University Press.

Bowen, S. and Zapata, A. V. 2009. Geographical indications, terroir, and socioeconomic and ecological sustainability: The case of tequila. *Journal of Rural Studies*, 25, 108–119.

Busch, L. 2000. The moral economy of grades and standards. *Journal of Rural Studies* 16: 273–283.

Clarence-Smith, W. G. and Topik, S. 2003. *The Global Coffee Economy in Africa, Asia, and Latin America,* 1500–1989. New York: Cambridge University Press.

Daviron, B. and Ponte, S. 2005. *The Coffee Paradox: Global Markets, Commodity Trade and the Elusive Promise of Development.* New York: Zed Books Ltd.

Diop, N., P. Brenton, et al. 2005. *Trade Costs, Export Development, and Poverty in Rwanda.* World Bank Policy Research Working Paper No. 3784.

Dolan, C. S. 2008. In the mists of development: Fair trade in Kenyan tea fields. *Globalizations* 5: 305–318.

——— 2005. Benevolent intent? The development encounter in Kenya's horticulture industry. *Journal of Asian and African Studies* 40: 411–438.

Elias, M. and J. Carney. 2004. *Shea Butter, Globalization, and Women of Burkina Faso*. In *A Companion to Feminist Geography*. Seager, J. and Nelson, L. (eds.) Oxford, England: Basil Blackwell, 93–108.

Freidberg, S. 2004. *French Beans and Food Scares: Culture and Commerce in an Anxious Age*. New York: Oxford University Press.

Gereffi, G. et al. 2005. The governance of global value chains. *Review of International Political Economy* 12(1): 78–97.

Goodman, M. K. 2004. Reading fair trade: Political ecological imaginary and the moral economy of fair trade foods. *Political Geography* 23: 891–915.

Guthman, J. 2007. The Polanyian way? Voluntary food labels as neoliberal governance. In *Antipode* 39: 456–478.

Jaffee, D. 2007. *Brewing Justice: Fair Trade Coffee, Sustainability, and Survival*. Berkeley, CA: University of California Press.

Kagame, P. 2009. *The Backbone of a New Rwanda*. In *the River They Swim: Essays From Around the World on Enterprise Solutions to Poverty*, Fairbanks, M. et al. (eds.) West Conshohocken, PA: Templeton Press, 11–15.

Kamola, I. 2007. The global coffee economy and the production of genocide in Rwanda. *Third World Quarterly* 28(3): 571–592.

Korsmeyer, C. 1999. *Making Sense of Taste: Food and Philosophy*. Ithaca, NY: Cornell University Press.

Levi, M. and Linton, A. 2003. Fair trade: A cup at a time? *Politics and Society* 31(3): 407–432.

Linton, A. 2008a. Ethical trade initiatives. *Globalizations* 5(2): 227–229.

——— 2008b. A niche for sustainability? Fair labor and environmentally sound practices in the specialty coffee industry. *Globalizations* 5(2): 231–245.

Linton, A. et al. 2004. A taste of trade justice: marketing global social responsibility via Fair Trade coffee. *Globalizations* 1(2): 223–246.

Loveridge, S., Mpyisi, E., and Weber, M. 2002. Farm-level perspectives in Rwanda's coffee chain coordination challenge. In *Agricultural Policy Synthesis: Rwanda Food Security Research Project/MINAGRI*, Michigan State University, 2E: 1–6.

Loveridge, S., Nyarwaya, J. B., and Shingiro, E. 2003. Decaffeinated? Situation, trends, and prospects for smallholder coffee production in Rwanda. *Agricultural Policy Synthesis: Rwanda Food Security Research Project/MINAGRI*, Michigan State University, 5E: 1–5.

Moyo, D. 2009. *Dead Aid: Why Aid Is Not Working and How There Is a Better Way for Africa*. New York: Farrar, Straus, and Giroux.

Muradian, R. and Pelupessy, W. 2005. Governing the coffee chain: The role of voluntary regulatory systems. *World Development* 33(12): 2029–2044.

Payer, C. 1979. The World Bank and the small farmers. *Journal of Peace Research* 16(4): 293–312.

Pendergrast, M. 1999. *Uncommon Grounds: The History of Coffee and How It Transformed Our World*. New York: Basic Books.

Ponte, S. 2002. The "Latte Revolution"? Regulation, markets, and consumption in the global coffee chain. *World Development* 30(7): 1099–1122.

Pottier, J. 2002. *Re-Imagining Rwanda: Conflict, Survival, and Disinformation in the Late Twentieth Century*. New York: Cambridge University Press.

Raynolds, L. 2002. Consumer/producer links in fair trade coffee networks. *Sociologia Ruralis* 42(4): 404–424.

Raynolds, L., Murray, D., and Heller, A. 2007. Regulating sustainability in the coffee sector: A comparative analysis of third-party environmental and social certification initiatives. *Agriculture and Human Values* 24: 147–163.

Renard, M. C. 1999. The interstices of globalization: The example of fair coffee. *Sociologia Ruralis* 39(4): 484–500.

——— 2003. Fair trade: Quality, market, and conventions. *Journal of Rural Studies* 19: 87–96.

——— 2005. Quality certification, regulation, and power in fair trade. *Journal of Rural Studies* 21: 419–431.

Roussel, B. and F. Verdeaux. 2007. Natural patrimony and local communities in Ethiopia: Advantages and limitations of a system of geographical indications. *Africa* 77: 130–150.

Rwanda Vision 2020 Plan. 2000. Kigali, Rwanda: Ministry of Finance and Economic Planning. Retrieved 1 February 2009 from www.gesci.org/assets/files/Rwanda_Vision_2020.pdf

Rwanda Development Indicators—006. 2008. Kigali, Rwanda: National Institute of Statistics. Retrieved 4 June 2009 from http://www.statistics.gov.rw

Scherrer, C. 2002. *Genocide and Crisis in Central Africa: Conflict Roots, Mass Violence, and Regional War.* Westport, CT: Praeger Publishers.

Storey, A. 1999. Economics and ethnic conflict: Structural adjustment in Rwanda. *Development Policy Review* 17(1): 43–63.

Tardif-Douglin, D., Ngirumwami, J. L., Shaffer, J., Murekezi, A., and Kampayana, T. 1996. *Finding the balance between agricultural and trade policy: Rwanda coffee policy in flux.* East Lansing, Michigan State University, Department of Agricultural Economics. Working Paper No. 59: 1–29.

Uvin, P. 1998. *Aiding Violence: The Development Enterprise in Rwanda.* West Hartford, CT: Kumarian Press.

Verwimp, P. 2000. Development ideology, the peasantry, and genocide: Rwanda represented in Habyarimana's speeches. *Journal of Genocide Research* 2: 325–361.

Verwimp, P. 2003. The political economy of coffee, dictatorship, and genocide. *European Journal of Political Economy* 19: 161–181.

Zorbas, E. 2004. Reconciliation in post-genocide Rwanda. *African Journal of Legal Studies* 1(1): 29–52.

Fast Food and Nutritional Perceptions in the Age of "Globesity": Perspectives from the Provincial Philippines

TY MATEJOWSKY

Department of Anthropology, UCF Brevard Campus, Cocoa, Florida, USA

As the influence of corporate fast food expands outside of the U.S. and Europe, many of the health problems previously associated with Western eating habits and nutritional regimes are beginning to proliferate across the developing world. Significantly, their rise serves as a troubling indicator of the "globesity" that threatens to overwhelm existing health care systems worldwide. To better understand the role of fast food cuisine in this accelerating trend, this article examines prevailing fast food consumption patterns and nutritional perceptions in the contemporary Philippines. Data from a 2005 consumer survey completed by over 160 college students in a provincial Philippine city provide insights into how this style of cuisine is now conceptualized and utilized locally amongst young adults. No less significant, survey findings also establish a basis from which tentative conclusions can be drawn about fast food's growing impact on health and health behaviors in moderate and low income countries.

A proliferation of health problems previously associated with Western eating habits and nutritional regimes in the developing world has in many ways paralleled the rising influence of corporate fast food outside of the U.S. and Europe (Hawkes 2002; Mydans 2003; Prentice 2006). Diverse urban populations throughout Africa, Asia, Latin America, and elsewhere are now experiencing sharp increases in medical conditions like obesity, cardiovascular disease, and Type 2 diabetes, as corporate chain restaurants promoting diets rich in calories, saturated fat, salt, and sugar continue their rapid global spread (Gill 2006; Popkin et al. 2002; Rosenthal 2008; Schlosser 2001: 240–243; Ulizaszek 2007).

Significantly, these chronic disorders stand poised to rival those stemming from hunger and undernutrition as major public health challenges for developing nations if preventative action is not soon taken (Stix 2007). More broadly, their rise serves as a troubling indicator of the looming "globesity" that threatens to overwhelm existing health care systems worldwide, place additional strains on already stressed government coffers, and diminish the overall quality of life for communities across the socioeconomic spectrum in both developed and less developed societies (Prentice 2006).

The World Health Organization (WHO), which first called attention to this impending crisis in the 1990s, initially estimated that over 115 million of the approximately 300 million adults suffering from obesity-related problems lived in developing societies (Kim & Popkin 2006). More recent figures suggest that the obesity gap separating industrialized nations from their less affluent counterparts is steadily narrowing, with poorer countries comprising an increasing share of the world's chronically overweight (Stix 2007). In fact, obesity rates in many developing societies are now approaching those of Western industrialized nations (Popkin & Gordon-Larsen 2004).

> According to the Food and Agricultural Organization (FAO) of the United Nations: "A 1999 United Nations study found obesity in all developing regions, and growing rapidly, even in countries where hunger exists. In China, the number of overweight people jumped from less than 10 percent to 15 percent in just three years. In Brazil and Colombia, the figure hovers around 40 percent—a level comparable to a number of European countries. Even sub-Saharan Africa, where most of the world's hungry live, is seeing an increase in obesity, especially among urban women. In all regions, obesity seems to grow as income increases" (International Obesity Task Force 2008).

While such demographic changes seemed almost inconceivable a generation ago, their recent emergence illustrates how processes of globalization and modernization can have less than optimal health outcomes for affected populations. Rising obesity and obesity-related conditions in low and moderate income nations, especially in urban areas, are problems largely arising from a rapid nutrition transition (Popkin & Gordon-Larsen 2004). This trend is characterized by a shift away from unvaried diets of traditional and often simple foods towards more varied diets chiefly based on unhealthy, animal-source, and processed foods containing high concentrations of sugar and fat (Popkin et al. 2002). The increased internationalization and commercialization of the global food trade has played prominent role in nutrition transition across Asia and elsewhere around the world (Nugent 2005; Pingali 2007; Popkin & Gordon-Larsen 2004).

With the number of people currently overweight surpassing those suffering from undernutrition worldwide by some 500 million (Stix 2007), a significant transformation in the health and dietary practices of developing populations appears all but irreversible. In fact, it is anticipated that within the next decade the total number of people classified as overweight or obese will effectively double (Nugent 2005). Most of this growth will occur in the urban centers of poor countries. Factors underlying this rising trend of overnutrition are essentially the same as those driving up obesity rates in the developed West: namely, the spread of sedentary lifestyles, a general lack of exercise, increased technological dependency, insufficient or seemingly contradictory nutrition information, and the now wide availability of high-fat, energy-dense, micronutrient-poor foods (Popkin & Gordon-Larsen 2004; Ulizaszek 2007; WHO 2008). Left unchecked, the sweeping changes wrought by this newly globalized nutritional regime suggest a rather bleak future for the health and well-being of most low and moderate income countries.

CORPORATE FAST FOOD AND "GLOBESITY"

Without overestimating corporate fast food's causative role in this burgeoning trend, it appears that the relationship between industry encroachment into non-Western markets and rising globesity is more than just correlational (Smith 2006:201–202). If anything, multinational chains like McDonald's have helped introduce and popularize new dietary practices across the developing world that not only undermine traditional foodways but also figure prominently in an aggregate shift towards overnutrition (Hawkes 2002; Pingali 2007). Their spread has also given rise to an increasing number of indigenous fast food chains—the Philippines' Jollibee, Brazil's Bob's, and Guatemala's Pollo Campero, among others—whose extensive knowledge of native palates and preferences offers real advantages in cultivating and sustaining local customer bases (Stein 2007).

The proliferation of Western and Western-style chain restaurants in diverse cultural settings across developing societies arguably stands as one of globalization's most vivid metaphors (ibid.). Aggressive marketing, especially the indigenization of corporate fast food's standardized menu and service format to better accommodate local tastes and preferences, contributes significantly to the industry's far-reaching influence (Matejowsky 2006; Watson 1997). The billions of dollars spent on advertising and overseas expansion fosters new consumer expectations about appropriate dietary choices at the local level (Hawkes 2002). The special cultural relevance now associated with national and multinational fast food brands as indicators of social status, material affluence, and modern taste, in part, perpetuates this cuisine's popularity in what was once called the Third World (Matejowsky 2007; Yan 2000:211–212).

Possibly no less significant are prevailing beliefs about global and local fast food's dietary value and overall wholesomeness *vis-à-vis* more traditional fare (Yan 1997:44–45). As foreign markets took off in East Asia and neighboring regions in the 1980s, it was quickly noted that part of the appeal of American-style fast food for some overseas consumers centered on its perceived nutritional qualities. Rather than being viewed as unhealthy or nutritionally deficient, this style of cuisine was often considered to be—if not actively conducive to physical health—then certainly not detrimental to one's general well-being. Such assumptions were based primarily on the standardized preparation scheme that most national and multinational chain restaurants follow (Yan 2000:211). The efficiency and regimentation of this culinary approach reinforces notions that American-style fast food is generally superior to indigenous cuisine since it is "scientifically designed." In other words, its menu items provide daily essentials such as water, sugar, fat, protein, starch, and vitamins and meet rigorous industry standards for quality and hygiene (Yan 1997:44–45). Corporate fast food's reliance on advanced kitchen technology and pre-cooked/ready-made servings only serves to bolster this view. By comparison, traditional native cooking styles appear all but quaint, with recipes and ingredients seemingly at odds with the scientific principles of modern quick-service eateries. Notably, the comparative expense of American-style fast food adds to the sense that diners are getting ample nutritional value for their money.

As concerns about fast food, public health, and corporate responsibility continue to spur debate in the U.S., Europe, and other developed nations, such issues have generated much less attention elsewhere (Hawkes 2002; Smith 2006:155–156; 175–179). The apparent lack of scrutiny directed towards national and multinational fast food's negative health consequences in moderate and low income countries is surely understandable given the industry's previously limited market presence and the medical urgencies related to persistent hunger and undernutrition. At the outset of the 21st century, it appears that governments and health services of less affluent societies are struggling to realign focus and resources away from longstanding health problems towards the challenges of an impending obesity crisis (Stix 2007). With fast food consumption so inextricably linked to aggregate weight gains in the industrialized West, it is clear that any effective strategy for arresting rising obesity rates in developing countries must take into account the influence of corporate fast food (Pingali 2007; WHO 2002).

OBJECTIVES AND OVERVIEW

Understanding of corporate fast food's growing impact on indigenous health and health behaviors becomes more deeply resonant when examined at the community level. Accordingly, this article considers the various ways this style of cuisine is now conceptualized and its influence mediated amongst college students within a specific developing locality. Paying particular attention to consumer practices and attitudes amid ongoing rivalries between national and multinational restaurant chains, this research offers insights into (1) how local young adults living in provincial areas perceive corporate fast food cuisine with regards to diet, nutrition, and hunger satisfaction, and (2) how prevailing consumption patterns and nutritional perceptions figure into emerging health trends within developing societies. Findings from this work are primarily data driven. They not only augment knowledge of globalization's diverse outcomes within developing milieus, they also challenge popular assumptions about the hegemony of Western fast food brands and the underlying dynamics of local health, health behaviors, and food economics.

Before describing the effects of corporate fast food within the examined locality, I will trace the rise of quick-service eateries countrywide, examine those chains at the forefront of fast food expansion, and relate these developments to recent national health trends. Following this I will present research findings gathered during an intensive 2005 ethnographic field session. Notably, the collected data enhance this study's empirical soundness by operationalizing fast food practices and attitudes amongst young adults in developing contexts. More significantly, it helps delineate some of the underarticulated beliefs that this subset of local consumers has about diet, nutrition, and health *vis-à-vis* corporate fast food cuisine. Finally, I will synthesize major research findings and offer some closing comments on the interplay between corporate fast food, global health, and local nutritional perceptions.

FAST FOOD IN THE PHILIPPINES

To better understand the sometimes complex interplay between corporate fast food and nutritional perceptions in developing contexts, this paper focuses on recent trends in the Philippines. The country presents an ideal setting for this type of research, as its political economy has been steadily transformed by processes of globalization and neoliberalism over recent decades. Among other changes wrought by this new market climate is the rise of a largely urbanized and brand-savvy middle class, comprising about one-fifth of the country's 96 million inhabitants (Virola 2007). With a clear capacity for capital accumulation and mass consumption, this influential segment of Philippine society has helped spur growth in a variety of local retail sectors, including a now-thriving fast food scene (AC Nielsen 2004). By 2000, there were approximately 2,000 national and multinational fast food restaurants operating nationwide, with some 60 million regular patrons (Business Asia 2000). Significantly, these consumers spent considerable amounts of money on fast food even when they had little disposable income (ibid).

Unquestionably, fast food appetites have grown substantially countrywide following McDonald's official launch in Metro-Manila some 25 years ago. Since this time numerous transnational chains including A&W, Burger King, Dunkin' Donuts, Domino's, KFC, Pizza Hut, Kenny Rogers' Roasters, and Wendy's have opened outlets across the islands, giving many Filipinos their first taste of quick-service eateries. Their high-profile and international allure has sparked considerable interest in American-style fast food at the local level (AC Nielsen 2004). This continuing fascination, however, has not always translated into widespread success for multinational brands.

Western chains have experienced less than optimal results within the nation's booming fast food trade (Wilson 2004). Even global powerhouse McDonald's has encountered its share of setbacks trying to establish a viable market presence in the Philippines. Notably, the country remains one of the few territories where the Golden Arches do not dominate fast food retailing (*Economist* 2002). Given its lead in most other foreign markets, McDonald's uneven performance in the Philippines stands as much as an anomaly as it does an embarrassment for the company (Conde 2005; Wilson 2004). Homegrown outfits like Chowking (Chinese fast food), Greenwich Pizza, and, most especially, Jollibee (hamburgers, French fries, fried chicken, spaghetti, and various desserts) have fared much better than their Western counterparts in cultivating and sustaining consumer followings amongst Filipinos. The success of domestic brands over foreign chains is partly reflected in the number of outlets they have operating nationwide. In 2004, there were 467 Jollibee eateries in the Philippines, while McDonald's had only 240 restaurants. Similarly, Chowking maintained 245 outlets across the islands, nearly twice as many as its closest Chinese food competitor, and Greenwich Pizza topped rival Pizza Hut by over 100 locations with 217 restaurants (Wilson 2004).

Jollibee, which essentially operates like a Filipino version of McDonald's with comparatively priced products (see Appendices 1 and 2 for McDonald's and Jollibee stationary menus) and similar amenities, currently maintains a commanding 55 per cent share of the Philippines' fast food market with some 600 outlets countrywide, outnumbering rival McDonald's by over 300 stores. For 2006, the company posted upwards of P2.146 billion in net income, exceeding the previous year's high of P1.69 billion. Jollibee's system-wide sales—which gauge all the sales to consumers and franchised stores—rose by 13.5 percent, while net income as a per cent of revenue grew from 5.8 percent in 2005 to 6.4 percent in 2006 (Cuevas 2007). Such earnings have, in turn, helped Jollibee consolidate its lead with the recent purchase of once rival domestic chains Greenwich Pizza (240 Philippine locations as of 2007) and Chowking (375 Philippine locations as 2007).

Notably, Jollibee is now ranked as one of Southeast Asia's most profitable corporations with over 1,655 franchises, branches, and subsidiaries spread across the Asia-Pacific and beyond (Conde 2005). Interestingly, much of Jollibee's success comes from emulating the innovative standards and techniques that McDonald's pioneered in the U.S. decades ago. This borrowing, coupled with aggressive marketing and constantly updated Filipino-influenced menus, has allowed Jollibee to reign supreme for almost 25 years as the Philippines' top fast food player (Matejowsky 2008).

HEALTH AND OBESITY IN THE PHILIPPINES

Against this backdrop of corporate fast food expansion, another trend has steadily gained momentum nationwide. The Philippines' health profile is becoming increasingly complex as obesity and obesity-related conditions exert new pressure on existing public health systems (Adair 2004). Overweight and obesity rates have edged noticeably upwards over recent years as the effects of newfound economic prosperity began taking root locally (FAO 2001:15–18).

Recent WHO age-standardized estimates for overweight and obesity amongst males and females aged 15+ years in the Philippines from 2002 through 2015 appear rather disconcerting healthwise, particularly for females (WHO 2008). Projected figures for 2002 suggest that the proportion of Filipinos with body mass index (BMI) categories of overweight, classified as a BMI higher than 25 (Gibson 2005), is 21.7% for males and 25.4% for females. Three years later in 2005 these figures increase only slightly for males to 21.9%, while those for females notably rise to 28.5%. By 2010, the anticipated prevalence of overweight Filipinos stands at 22.2% for males and 33.6% for females. Significantly, by 2015, the projected estimate for overweight males is 22.5%, reflecting only a 0.8% increase from 2002, while the percentage of overweight females is 38.8, a 13.4% jump from 2002 (WHO 2008).

When attention turns to obesity, defined as a BMI of over 30 (Gibson 2005), a similar gendered trend emerges amongst Filipinos. For 2002, 1.1% of males and 2.8% of females are classified as obese (WHO 2008). Estimates for the next 13 years show almost no changes in obesity rates for males, increasing only to 1.2% by 2015, while the prevalence of obese females increases from 3.7% in 2005, to 5.5% in 2010, and, finally, to 7.8% in 2015 (ibid.). Clearly, the above figures suggest that the Philippines' health profile is undergoing changes brought on by spreading "globesity." These changes are more readily evident in females compared to males.

So far, public and private health agencies have been slow to recognize, much less actively respond, to the challenges of rising weight gains.

At best, their efforts at addressing overnutrition and related trends entail raising awareness about healthy lifestyle choices via select public education initiatives (Sy 2008). In 1994, a group of concerned physicians formed the Philippine Association for the Study of Overweight and Obesity (PASOO) to deal with growing problems of aggregate weight gains amongst Filipinos. Notably, PASOO has implemented a nationwide project aimed at publicizing obesity concerns among healthcare providers. PASOO has published some weight management guidelines for physicians interested in treating affected patients (ibid.). Given that such strategies these have only recently taken affect, it still may be too early to assess their effectiveness at positively influencing local dietary and lifestyle habits.

Presently, it appears that females and urbanites are at most risk to the ill effects of rising weight gains in the Philippines (Mydans 2003; WHO 2008). It is worth noting, however, that these health changes affect nearly all segments of society (FAO 2001:15). Of particular concern is the growing impact of obesity and obesity-related conditions on the health and well-being of children and young adults (FAO 2001; Lobstein, Baur, & Uauy 2004; Mydans 2003). Clearly, these groups stand vulnerable to the long term health repercussions of being overweight and obese. The fact that the country's demographic profile reflects a relatively young population, with some 35% of Filipinos aged 14 years old or younger, makes these figures all the more troubling.

While empirically based studies seeking to establish corporate fast food's role in rising obesity in the Philippines remain hard to come by, it is not difficult to dismiss the notion that fast food's increased availability has played only a minor role in this emerging trend. Significantly, PASOO head, Dr. Augusto D. Litonjua, alludes to this as he blames rising obesity in the Philippines on "malling," a practice he defines as "spending the day in shopping malls and eating at fast-food restaurants" (Mydans 2003).

FAST FOOD SURVEY—DAGUPAN CITY, PANGASINAN

The underlying dynamics of fast food consumption amongst key segments of Philippine society can be elucidated through various research approaches. For the purposes of this article, an intensive consumer survey is utilized as the primary methodology for teasing out general attitudes and practices now defining aspects of the country's fast food scene in the Philippine hinterland. Collected data from a comprehensive questionnaire applied to over 160 college students in July 2005 in Dagupan City, Pangasinan provide fresh insights into the ways provincial Filipinos in their late teens and early twenties conceive of corporate fast food, utilize its products, and adapt to the contexts it creates.

A tertiary city with a vibrant, if sometimes chaotic, urban life, Dagupan stands as one of the most populous and important commercial, educational, and financial centers in the northern Philippines. Nestled along the Lingayen Gulf some 210 kilometers north of Metro-Manila, the city comprises around 130,000 residents living in approximately 25,000 households spread across 31 municipal precincts. Over the years, numerous quick-service eateries have emerged and prospered locally, thanks to a consumer population increasingly exposed to fast food marketing and mass consumption (Dannhaeuser 2004:139–145).

Corporate fast food first appeared in Dagupan during the early 1980s with the launch of a few small multinational eateries, most notably Dunkin' Donuts and Shakey's Pizza, in or around the city center. Over subsequent years several other national and transnational chains opened franchise or branch outlets in downtown, including Dagupan's inaugural Jollibee restaurant. Fast food expansion accelerated considerably following a major earthquake in July 1990 and the opening of three large-scale shopping malls in greater Dagupan during the mid-to-late 1990s. These modern facilities housed popular eateries such as Chowking, Greenwich Pizza, McDonald's, KFC, and Jollibee. In 2005, around 40 fast food restaurants—representing 13 distinct national and transnational brands—were operating in the Dagupan area. Among these were four Jollibee restaurants and two McDonald's outlets, all located within short traveling distance of the city's three major universities: the University of Pangasinan, the University of Luzon, and the Colegio de Dagupan.

Men and women undergraduates between the ages of 18 and 23, from mainly low- and medium-income backgrounds, and enrolled at these three institutes of higher learning comprise the primary pool of informants from which survey data are drawn. After receiving permission from school administrators at the respective universities, my IRB-approved questionnaire was administered in classrooms under my supervision with the help of a Filipino research assistant and the course instructors. The questionnaire's written and oral instructions were provided in English with my research assistant addressing student questions in the local dialect of Pangasinan in a small number of instances. The basis for most survey questions comes from my previous research experience studying the variegated impact of retail globalization in the Philippines beginning in 1994 and continuing through 1997, 1998, 2005, and 2006, although a few of the survey questions are influenced by ones asked by Yan to Chinese college students in the early 1990s (1997:454–457). With few exceptions, it took no longer than 30 minutes for students to complete and return their survey forms at each university. Once all of the questionnaires were collected, student responses underwent rigorous statistical analysis through the software program Statistical Package for the Social Sciences (SPSS). Emerging patterns and trends were carefully scrutinized and organized into tables (see below).

College students are utilized as research participants for three primary reasons: (1) the university classrooms where surveys were applied greatly expedite questionnaire distribution and collection; (2) students are highly exposed to fast food influences, especially given the close proximity of quick-service eateries to their respective campuses; and finally, (3) few segments of Philippine society are arguably more brand conscious and knowledgeable about the latest consumer trends and fashions than young adults.

When considered altogether, the student survey responses that are summarized in the tables below contribute a deeper understanding about corporate fast food's influence over young adults living in towns and cities across the provincial Philippines. Moreover, they help delineate some of the prevailing consumption patterns, brand preferences, and perceptions of corporate fast food cuisine's substantiality and nutritional value within developing contexts.

CONSUMPTION PATTERNS AND BRAND PREFERENCES

Research findings establish rather conclusively just how pervasive fast food consumption is amongst college students in today's Philippines. Results indicate that nearly nine out of ten research participants currently eat fast food at least one or two times per month (see Table 1). Almost half of undergraduates report consuming this style of cuisine more frequently; that is, around three or more times monthly.

Approximately 86 per cent of respondents dine at Jollibee at least once or twice each month, with more than one-third of students eating there no less than three times per month. Somewhat less favored is McDonald's, with roughly 70 per cent of those surveyed patronizing the Golden Arches one or two times monthly. Not as many, approximately one-quarter of research participants, visit McDonald's more than three times each month.

TABLE 1 Frequency of Fast Food Consumption—"How often do you eat fast food?"—Dagupan City 2005. (N = 161)*

	Fast food	Jollibee	McDonald's
Never	0% (0)	0.6 (1)	3.3 (5)
3 or fewer times per year	10.1 (16)	13.7 (22)	27.2 (41)
1–2 times per month	42.4 (67)	52.8 (85)	45.7 (69)
3–4 times per month	19.6 (31)	22.4 (36)	13.9 (21)
More than 4 times per month	27.8 (44)	10.6 (17)	9.9 (15)
Total	99.9 (158)	100.1 (161)	100 (151)

*Marginal totals can be less than 161 due to missing values. Data from the "Fast Food" column define corporate fast food in a very broad sense. Thus, it does not directly relate to any particular restaurant chain nor does it narrowly focus on national and multinational brands. Likewise, it is not limited to one specific genre of fast food. Data presented in the "Jollibee" and "McDonald's" columns pertain only to the respective chains.

Interestingly, however, McDonald's is more favored than Jollibee amongst those students who eat fast food only three or fewer times per year. Comparative figures for both restaurant chains reveal that the Golden Arches attracts a slightly larger, albeit statistically significant ($p \leq .0015$), number of these infrequent fast food patrons relative to Jollibee. If anything, this preference may indicate that occasional fast food diners attach a type of novelty value to McDonald's, possibly related to its longstanding global appeal, which is not presently associated with Jollibee's more homegrown brand image.

Notwithstanding findings from this subset of research participants, practically all of the survey data presented in Table 1 suggests that Jollibee is more well-liked and frequently patronized by college students than McDonald's. Beyond matters of taste, Jollibee's popularity over McDonald's amongst young adult provincial Filipinos is likely informed by subtle expressions of neo-patriotism or post-colonial resistance against the real and perceived hegemony of American retail forms (Matejowsky 2008:320–322).

Significantly, even as conditions of poverty remain prevalent across much of Philippine society, the popularity of quick-service eateries amongst Filipinos appears more than just narrowly focused on those with discretionary income (AC Nielsen 2004). Its broad appeal apparently dates back some years, based on the responses of those surveyed.

Most students report first eating fast food sometime during childhood (see Table 2). In fact, nearly half of undergraduate Dagupeños state that their earliest experience with this cuisine took place before the age of five. At the very least, the survey data suggest that research participants have fast food histories that measure in years, if not decades. Surely, these findings should come as not altogether surprising, especially given ongoing industry efforts at marketing fast food to families and children. With kid-friendly corporate mascots, on-site playgrounds, birthday parties, and simple menu options, Jollibee, McDonald's, and other leading restaurant chains in the Philippines

TABLE 2 Age at First Fast Food Consumption—"How old were you when you first tried fast food?" —Dagupan City 2005. (N = 160)

Age	
Never ate fast food	1.3% (2)
1–5 years	45.6 (73)
6–10 years	28.1 (45)
11–15 years	18.1 (29)
16–18 years	5.0 (8)
19 years or older	1.9 (3)
Total	100 (160)

Chi square = 149.99 ($p \leq .001$).

have done much towards building a loyal base of young consumers (Conde 2005).

FAST FOOD STATUS AND SUBSTANTIALITY

When attention shifts to questions of how undergraduate Dagupeños characterize the status and substantiality of corporate fast food, in general, and McDonald's and Jollibee, specifically, several notable patterns arise (see Table 3). Probably most conspicuous is the fact that only about one in ten research participants define this style of cuisine exclusively in terms of a formal meal. With the Philippines' main staple item of steamed rice playing little more than a secondary role on the menu boards of most quick-service eateries, Chowking being the notable exception, such responses become more easily understandable.

Rice has long served as the foundation for agricultural and culinary practices in the Philippines and other parts of East and Southeast Asia, (Ohnuki-Tierney 1997:166–169). So integral is this cereal grain to local dietary habits and culture that it is rarely, if ever, omitted from daily meals (Kittler & Soucher 2007:314). Certainly, it becomes difficult for provincial Filipinos in their late teens and early twenties to conceptualize notions of what can or does constitute a proper meal within the context of corporate fast food when McDonald's, Jollibee, and other top-selling brands continually emphasize their versions of Western standbys like hamburgers and French fries, and steamed rice appears not as widely promoted on restaurant menus.

Given the centrality of rice to Filipino foodways and its general marginalization at most national and multinational fast food chains, rationales for understanding why so many survey participants equate fast food with the casual fare eaten between standard meals, and not the more filling and ample-sized selections of breakfast, lunch, or dinner assume sharper clarity. Over 40% of undergraduate Dagupeños characterize fast food solely in terms of snacks, while some 50% classify it within a broader framework,

TABLE 3 Perceptions of Fast Food/Jollibee/McDonald's as Snack Food or Proper Meal—"Is fast food/Jollibee food/McDonald's food a snack or meal?"—Dagupan City 2005. (N = 161)*

	Fast food	Jollibee	McDonald's
Proper Meal	9.4% (15)	7.1 (11)	6.8 (10)
Snack	40.9 (65)	41.3 (64)	43.2 (64)
Both	49.7 (79)	51.6 (80)	50 (74)
Total	100 (159)	100 (155)	100 (148)

*Marginal totals can be less than 161 due to missing values. Data from the "Fast Food" column define corporate fast food in a very broad sense. Thus, it does not directly relate to any particular restaurant chain nor does it narrowly focus on national and multinational brands. Likewise, it is not limited to one specific genre of fast food. Data presented in the "Jollibee" and "McDonald's" columns pertain only to the respective chains.

TABLE 4 Time(s) of Fast Food Consumption—"What time(s) do you eat at Jollibee/McDonald's?"—Dagupan City 2005.*

	Jollibee	McDonald's	
Breakfast	21.4% (33)	12.4 (19)	$p \leq .0177$
Lunch	61.9 (96)	52.9 (81)	$p \leq .0551$
Merienda	81.9 (127)	82.4 (126)	$p \leq .04544$
Dinner	20.6 (32)	15 (23)	$p \leq .0996$

*Students could answer as many dining that personally apply.

comprising both proper meals and snack food. These findings remain consistent when the survey focus narrows and only considers the respective bills of fare of Jollibee and McDonald's.

Notions of fast food as snack food are also evident when students are asked to indicate what meal(s) or time(s) during the day that they typically dine at Jollibee or McDonald's (see Table 4). Significantly, the most popular response was not breakfast, lunch, or dinner but rather *merienda*. As Table 4 demonstrates, research participants are almost four times as likely to eat *merienda* rather than breakfast or dinner at Jollibee. These same patterns are slightly more pronounced though not statistically significant ($p \leq .0177$) when related to McDonald's.

As a traditional afternoon snack or "fourth meal," *merienda* is somewhat analogous to British afternoon tea in that it offers Filipinos opportunities for consuming something light and often sweet a few hours before dinnertime. *Merienda* not only helps stave off hunger into the late afternoon and evening, it also provides a short downtime for friends and peers to get together and casually socialize. With all three universities located within close proximity to a McDonald's or Jollibee, it stands to reason that the time students most frequently patronize these eateries coincides with *merienda*. The fact that both restaurant chains offer diners clean surroundings and modern amenities away from the sometimes harsh realities of Dagupan's urban life only enhances their allure for this daily social gathering.

Beyond questions of fast food as snacks or proper meals, how survey participants regard this type of cuisine in terms of hunger satisfaction offers some revealing, if sometimes contradictory, insights into prevailing dietary and nutritional regimes (see Table 5). Indeed, almost seven out of ten students report that consuming fast food leaves them feeling full. Even though a majority of survey respondents view selections from Jollibee, McDonald's, and other quick-service eateries more as snacks than proper meals (see Table 3), only about one-third characterize menu items from these chain restaurants as not filling. Curiously, these findings stand in marked contrast to similar inquiries into fast food and hunger satisfaction among Asian college students in developing urban contexts (Yan 1997:45–46). In a very real sense, menu offerings at both Jollibee and McDonald's are considered

TABLE 5 Substantiality of Fast Food Consumption—"Does fast food/Jollibee food/McDonald's food make you feel full?"—Dagupan City 2005. (N = 161)*

	Fast food	Jollibee	McDonald's
Full	65.8% (102)	69.7 (106)	61.4 (89)
Not Full	34.2 (53)	30.3 (46)	38.6 (56)
Total	100 (155)	100 (152)	100 (145)

*Marginal totals can be less than 161 due to missing values. Data from the "Fast Food" column define corporate fast food in a very broad sense. Thus, it does not directly relate to any particular restaurant chain nor does it narrowly focus on national and multinational brands. Likewise, it is not limited to one specific genre of fast food. Data presented in the "Jollibee" and "McDonald's" columns pertain only to the respective chains.

substantial fare by undergraduate Dagupeños even as most survey participants do not feel fast food sufficiently comprises a formal meal.

NUTRITIONAL PERCEPTIONS

Possibly more relevant to the overall aims of this article is how students perceive the nutritional or health status of corporate fast food cuisine. Whether this style of cuisine is considered "good for you," "bad for you," or "neither good nor bad," it is essential that local perspectives on this topic receive proper consideration, inasmuch as corporate fast food's influence over Filipino eating habits appears to have now firmly taken root (AC Nielsen 2004). In this way, a more accurate understanding of the interplay between increased fast food consumption and local health and health behaviors emerges. Such findings hold important implications as the need for realigning components of the state's health apparatus more towards obesity and obesity-related conditions intensifies.

Surprisingly, when asked to characterize the dietary value of fast food in terms of its overall health benefits, less than 6% of those surveyed view it negatively (see Table 6). Many more, some 83%, consider it either positively or neutrally with regard to its impact on bodily health. That so few respondents view corporate fast food cuisine as unhealthy may possibly stem from beliefs similar to those highlighted by Yan (1997:44–45; 2000:211) about fast food's "scientific design" *vis-à-vis* more traditional cuisine in urban China. The underlying reasons as to why so many undergraduate Dagupeños perceive fast food in this manner is something that clearly warrants further consideration in future research efforts. At this stage, it seems that public notions that corporate fast food cuisine is, if not beneficial, then certainly not harmful, seem difficult to dislodge, especially given the industry's modern image and standardized preparation scheme.

TABLE 6 Nutritional Perceptions of Fast Food—"In terms of nutrition, fast food is":—Dagupan City 2005. (N = 160)

Response	
Good for you	38.8% (62)
Bad for you	5.6 (9)
Neither good nor bad	43.8 (70)
Don't know	11.9 (19)
Total	100.1 (160)

Chi square = 69.65 ($p \leq .001$). In Table 6 corporate fast food is defined in a very broad sense. Thus, it does not directly relate to any particular restaurant chain nor does it narrowly focus on national and multinational brands. Likewise, it is not limited to one specific genre of fast food.

No less significant is the fact that Jollibee, McDonald's, and other leading chains do not place a high priority on publicizing the nutrition information of their products. Unlike recent developments in the U.S. and Europe, there has been no comparable push in the Philippines by consumers, policymakers, or health advocates calling for increased scrutiny of fast food's nutritional value. Far from secretively withholding data on calories, fat content, and daily recommended dietary allowances, industry players have received almost no encouragement to actively disseminate this kind of information. At the local level, this means that quick-service eateries typically do not provide the nutrition tables or labeling that are increasingly standard features of Western fast food operations.

The lack of public and/or corporate engagement on this matter may simply reflect the fact that up until recently, problems of overnutrition were generally recognized as peripheral to the nation's basic health needs. As a developing country, the Philippines faces myriad social, economic, and political issues that clearly have a more immediate impact on the lives of everyday citizens. With few Filipinos now visibly suffering from obesity and obesity-related conditions, the need to actively publicize nutrition information has not been injected with any real sense of urgency. Of course, just how much local eating habits would change if fast food nutrition information was more readily available is still open to question. Strictly speaking, it would be a good first step in creating a more informed consumer population given the now widespread popularity of corporate fast food cuisine (AC Nielsen 2004).

NUTRITIONAL PERCEPTIONS—FILIPINO VS. AMERICAN BRANDS

Delving deeper into local perceptions of corporate fast food and nutrition amongst undergraduate Dagupeños, research findings also reveal how the

TABLE 7 Dining Preference Rankings of Filipino and American Fast Food Brands*—Dagupan City 2005. (N = 161)

	Filipino fast food brands	American fast food brands	
First	61% (99)	30 (49)	$p \leq .000$
Second	44 (71)	48 (78)	$p \leq .764$
Third	45 (73)	47 (76)	$p \leq .64$
Fourth	47 (76)	43 (69)	$p \leq .235$
Fifth	40 (64)	51 (82)	$p \leq .024$
Sixth	34 (55)	55 (88)	$p \leq .0001$

*Students are asked to individually rank six fast food brands, three American (McDonald's, Shakey's Pizza, and Kentucky Fried Chicken) and three Filipino (Jollibee, Chowking, and Greenwich Pizza) in terms of dining preference. "First" ranking entails what respondents view as the most preferred brands while "Sixth" ranking denotes what respondents view as the least preferred brand.

nationality of restaurant operations influences local consumption patterns in key ways. Whether a chain is identified as Filipino or non-Filipino (i.e., American) appears to shape consumer practices and attitudes towards fast food. As Tables 7 and 8 demonstrate, out of six possible restaurant choices (three Filipino brands and three American brands), survey participants generally rank Jollibee and other domestic outfits as not only more favorable in terms of dining preference compared to their U.S. counterparts, they also categorize their menu items as more nutritious.

Clearly, homegrown chains hold a competitive advantage over their American rivals in terms of creating and promoting products that appeal to Filipino sensibilities (Conde 2005; Wilson 2004). Rather than relying on core menu concepts developed overseas to fit the established tastes of Western appetites, indigenous companies have thrived by designing food items with Filipino consumers specifically in mind. This ability to effectively

TABLE 8 Nutritional Rankings of Filipino and American Fast Food Brands*—Dagupan City 2005. (N = 161)

	Filipino fast food brands	American fast food brands	
First	64.6% (104)	28 (45)	$p \leq .000$
Second	53.4 (86)	39.1 (63)	$p \leq .005$
Third	46.6 (75)	47.2 (76)	$p \leq .544$
Fourth	34.8 (56)	56.5 (91)	$p \leq .000$
Fifth	36.7 (59)	54 (87)	$p \leq .001$
Sixth	34.8 (56)	54 (87)	$p \leq .0003$

*Students are asked to individually rank six fast food brands, three American (McDonald's, Shakey's Pizza, and Kentucky Fried Chicken) and three Filipino (Jollibee, Chowking, and Greenwich Pizza) in terms of nutritional value. "First" ranking entails what respondents view as the most nutritious brand while "Sixth" ranking denotes what respondents view as the least nutritious brand.

incorporate local predilections for sweet and juicy fare into their respective menus is largely born out of a more intimate understanding of traditional foodways. Indeed, McDonald's and other American fast food operators have struggled to compete with indigenous companies, especially Jollibee, in the production of dishes better suited to local tastes (ibid.). While the Golden Arches has experienced some success with distinctly localized products like Mango Shakes and McSpaghetti (pasta noodles with sweet tomato sauce and chopped frankfurter bits), their core menu essentially revolves around the hamburgers (i.e., Big Mac and Quarter Pounder with Cheese) and French fries that have been served at their U.S. outlets for decades (Business Asia 2000; Economist 2002).

That the cuisine of Filipino fast food brands is considered more nutritious than its American counterparts is, perhaps, not altogether surprising (see Table 8). The familiarity that consumers have with the flavors and ingredients favored by homegrown chains arguably does much to influence local perceptions of their menus' overall wholesomeness. No less important is the fact that steamed rice is more readily available at the domestic quick-service eateries. Significantly, leading Chinese fast food chain and Jollibee subsidiary Chowking serves this staple item with many, if not most, of its entrées. It seems to follow then, that students would perceive Filipino brands, especially Chowking, as higher in nutritional value compared to McDonald's and other U.S. chains, given the centrality of rice to traditional foodways and its near-absence at these latter eateries.

QUESTIONS AND DISCUSSION

So what general inferences can be drawn from the responses of those surveyed? Should research findings be approached primarily as the isolated experience of undergraduate Dagupeños, or should they be considered as representative of a broader national trend whereby everyday young adult Filipinos stand poised to experience significant weight gains in the near and distant future thanks in part to the adverse influence of corporate fast food? Implicit in this latter perspective is the idea that the Philippines is now in the incipient stages of a "Jollibesity" epidemic: a burgeoning public health crisis involving a major shift towards overnutrition and obesity that is driven primarily by the insidious spread of quick-service eateries and Western nutritional regimes across local communities.

Slightly less ominous, but no less important, does the collected data tend to reflect a consumer population significantly or only somewhat misinformed about the negative health consequences of fast food and diets rich calories and saturated fats? Are these provincial fast food patrons failing to grasp many of this cuisine's ill effects simply because relevant nutritional information remains largely unavailable?

If fast food consumers and producers in the Philippines are increasingly confronting these types of questions, it appears that the country's fast food industry has not yet felt sufficient pressure to change operating practices in any major way. Unlike the recent experience of leading fast food operators in U.S. and Europe, Jollibee, McDonald's, and other popular chains in the Philippines have yet to incorporate healthy menu items into their signature bills of fare, much less adequately provide consumers with nutrition information about their signature products. To date, the salads, fruit selections, and other light fare now available at many Western quick-service eateries have failed to make a real appearance on the menu boards of national and multinational chains throughout the Philippines.

CONCLUSION

Although fast food consumption may be only one factor helping to drive up obesity and obesity-related conditions worldwide, it remains a dynamic agent in the popularization of Western culinary systems, especially in advanced less developed countries like the Philippines (Hawkes 2002; Mydans 2003; Pingali 2007). The adoption of new dietary practices and nutritional regimes in what was once called the Third World has paralleled an increased incidence of chronic medical disorders among indigenous populations that until recently were mainly associated with developed societies (Nugent 2005; Popkin & Gordon-Larsen 2004). Misconceptions about fast food's nutritional value currently present serious obstacles for governments and health agencies learning to combat the growing implications of populations increasingly subject to the ill effects of globesity.

If survey results from college students in Dagupan City are any indication, it appears that young adult provincial Filipinos are susceptible to the effects of aggregate weight gains and their ancillary outcomes, thanks in part to the widespread availability and consumption of corporate fast food. Compounding this vulnerability is a consumer population that is largely misinformed about fast food's overall nutritional value. The fact that public health services remain largely oriented towards problems of hunger and undernutrition and not obesity only serves to exacerbate matters (FAO 2001).

When considered altogether, the collected survey data provide a new level of insight into local perceptions of corporate fast food cuisine amongst young adults within developing contexts. As provincial Filipinos in their late teens and early twenties adopt certain Western dietary practices, it is apparent from the responses of those surveyed that local notions of fast food relating to diet, nutrition, and hunger satisfaction do not always conform to prevailing views in the industrialized West. If anything, they foreshadow a new and more complex global health paradigm in which, ironically, problems of obesity and overnutrition are no longer exclusive to developed countries.

REFERENCES

"A Busy Bee in the Hamburger Hive. If McDonald's is the Goliath of Fast Food, Tony Tan's Jollibee is its Filipino David." *Economist* February 28, 2002.

Adair, L. S. 2004. Dramatic Rise in Overweight and Obesity in Adult Filipino Women and Risk of Hypertension. *Obesity Research* 12.8: 1335–1341.

"Cashed-up Filipinos Feast on Fast Food." *Business Asia* February 11, 2000.

Conde, C. H. Jollibee Stings McDonald's in Philippines. *International Herald Tribune* May 31, 2005.

"Consumers in Asia-Pacific—Our Fast Food/Take Away 2nd Half, 2004." *AC Nielsen*. September 18, 2008. http://www2.acnielsen.com/reports/index_confidence.shtm

Cuevas, L. C. Jollibee's 2006 Earnings Jump on Strong Sales. *Manila Times International* February 15, 2007.

Dannhaeuser, N. 2004. *Chinese Traders in a Philippine Town. From Daily Competition to Urban Transformation*: Ateneo de Manila University Press.

Food and Agriculture Organization of the United Nations. "Nutrition Country Profiles—Philippines." August 2001. FAO, Rome. http://www.fao.org/ ag/agn/nutrition/phi-e.stm

Gibson, R. S. 2005. *Principles of Nutritional Assessment*: Oxford University Press.

Gill, T. 2006. "Epidemiology and Health Impact of Obesity: An Asian Perspective." *Asia Pacific Journal of Clinical Nutrition*. 15: 3–14.

Hawkes, C. 2002. Marketing Practices of Fast Food and Soft Drink Multinationals: A Review. *Globalization, Diets, and Noncommunicable Diseases*. Geneva, World Health Organization.

International Obesity Task Force. "The Developing World's New Burden: Obesity." September 3, 2008. http://www.iotf.org/popout.asp?linkto= http://www.fao.org/FOCUS/E/obesity/obes1.htm

Kim, S. & Barry M. Popkin. 2006. Commentary: Understanding the Epidemiology of Overweight and Obesity—a Real Global Public Health Concern. *International Journal of Epidemiology* 35.1: 60–67.

Kittler, P. G. & Kathryn P. Soucher. 2007. *Food and Culture*. New York: Wadsworth Publishing.

Lobstein, T., L. Baur, & R. Uauy. 2004. Obesity in Children and Young People: a Crisis in Public Health. *Obesity Reviews* 5: 4–85.

Matejowsky, T. 2006. Global Tastes/Local Contexts: An Ethnographic Account of Fast Food in San Fernando City, the Philippines. *Fast Food/Slow Food: The Economic Anthropology of the Global Food System. Society for Economic Anthropology Monograph Series 24*. Richard Wilk (ed.). Walnut Creek: Altimira Press, pp. 145–159.

Matejowsky, T. 2007. SPAM and Fast Food "Glocalization" in the Philippines. *Food Culture and Society* 10.1: 23–41.

Matejowsky, T. 2008. Jolly Dogs and McSpaghetti: Anthropological Reflections on Global/Local Fast Food Competition in the Philippines. *Journal of Asia-Pacific Business* 9.4: 311–328.

Mydans, S. "Clustering in Cities, Asians are Becoming Obese." *New York Times*. March 13, 2003. http://query.nytimes.com/gst/fullpage.html?res=9C0CE2DF133EF930A25750C0A9659C8B63

Nugent, R. 2005. Obesity Creeping up on Less Developed Countries. *Population Reference Bureau*. September 10, 2008. http://www.prb.org/Articles/2005/Obesity CreepingUponLessDevelopedCountries.aspx

Ohnuki-Tierney, E. 1997. McDonald's in Japan. Changing Manners and Etiquette. *Golden Arches East: McDonald's in East Asia*. James L. Watson (ed.). Stanford: Stanford University Press, pp. 161–182.

Pingali, P. 2007. Westernization of Asian Diets and the Transformation of Food Systems: Implications for Research and Policy. *Food Policy* 32.3: 281–298.

Popkin, B. M., Bing Lu, & Fengying Zhai. 2002. Understanding the Nutrition Transition: Measuring Rapid Dietary Changes in Transition Countries. *Public Health Nutrition* 5.6: 947–953.

Popkin, B. M. & Penny Gordon-Larsen. 2004. The Nutrition Transition: Worldwide Obesity Dynamics and Their Determinants. *International Journal of Obesity & Related Metabolic Disorders* 28.11: S2–S9.

Prentice, A. M. 2006. The Emerging Epidemic of Obesity in Developing Countries. *International Journal of Epidemiology* 35.1: 93–99.

Rosenthal, E. Fast Food Hits the Mediterranean; a Diet Succumbs. *New York Times*. September 24, 2008, A1, 12.

Schlosser, E. 2001. *Fast Food Nation: The Dark Side of the All-American Meal*. Boston: Houghton Mifflin Co.

Smith, A. F. 2006. *Encyclopedia of Junk Food and Fast Food*. Westport, CT. Greenwood Press.

Stein, J. 2007. The Hungry American. Foreign Fast Food Chains are Moving into the U.S. and Showing How the World Really Sees Us. *Time* 116.

Stix, G. 2007. A Question of Sustenance. *Scientific American* 297.3: 54–58.

Sy, R. A. G. Prevalence of Obesity in Medical Practice in the Philippines. September 17, 2008. http://www.iotf.org/oonet/philippines.htm

Ulijaszek, S. J. 2007. Obesity: a Disorder of Convenience. *Obesity Reviews* 8, Supplement 1: 183–187.

Virola, R. A. 2007. Anti-Poverty? How about Pro-Middle Class? *Statistically Speaking*. National Statistical Coordination Board. December 10, 2007. www.nscb.gov.ph.

Watson, J. L. 1997. *Golden Arches East: McDonald's in East Asia*. Stanford: Stanford University Press.

Yan, Y. 1997. McDonald's in Beijing: The Localization of Americana. *Golden Arches East: McDonald's in East Asia*. James L. Watson (ed.). Stanford: Stanford University Press, pp. 39–76.

Yan, Y. 2000. Of Hamburger and Social Space: Consuming McDonald's in Beijing. *The Consumer Revolution in Urban China*. Deborah S. Davis (ed.). Berkeley: University of California Press, pp. 201–225.

Wilson, K. 2004. RP Fast-Food Chain Beats McDonald's at its Own Game Philippine Daily Inquirer, June 27, 2004. http://money.inquirer.net breakingnews/view_breakingnews.php?yyyy=2004&mon=06&dd=27&file=2

World Health Organization. 2008. BMI/Overweight/Obesity prevalence. Country Comparable Data. June 18, 2008. http://www.who.int/ncd_surveillance/infobase/web/InfoBaseCommon/

World Health Organization. 2002. *Globalization, Diets, and Noncommunicable Diseases*. Geneva, WHO. http://whqlibdoc.who.int/publications/ 9241590416.pdf

World Health Organization. Obesity and Overweight. September 3, 2008. http://www.who.int/mediacentre/factsheets/fs311/en/index.html

ACKNOWLEDGMENTS

The author wishes to thank Josie Gonzalez, Mario Granada, Martha Heine, Dr. Barbara Kinsey, Dr. Leslie Sue Lieberman, Lorena Matejowsky, Dr. Michael Newlin, and Andrew Todd for their valued contributions to this work. Moreover, gratitude is extended to the University of Central Florida (UCF)'s Department of Anthropology, UCF's Office of Commercialization and Research, and the UCF Southern Region for their support during this research endeavor.

APPENDICES

APPENDIX 1 McDonald's Stationary Menu*—Dagupan City 2005

Big Mac	Chicken McDo with Rice (fried chicken)
Burger McDo (small hamburger)	Burger McDo Steak (burger steak with gravy)
French Fries	Mini Apple Pie
Filet-O-Fish	Mini Taro Pie
Chicken McNuggets	McFloat (frozen dessert)
McSpaghetti	McFlurry (frozen dessert)
Happy Meal	

*Listed items represent McDonald's core menu in the Philippines during summer 2005. Not included are seasonal items or promotions that are periodically made available for short periods of time.

APPENDIX 2 Jollibee Stationary Menu*—Dagupan City 2005

Champ Hamburger (large hamburger)	Shanghai-Rolls (small egg rolls)
Yum! Hamburger (small hamburger)	Palabok-Fiesta (traditional Filipino pasta)
Jolly Crispy Fries	Burger Steak (burger steak with gravy)
Jolly Hot Dog	Peach Mango Pie
Chickenjoy (fried chicken)	Swirl Bitz (frozen dessert)
Jolly Spaghetti	

*Listed items represent Jollibee's core menu in the Philippines during summer 2005. Not included are seasonal items or promotions that are periodically made available for short periods of time.

A House of Honey: White Sugar, Brown Sugar, and the Taste for Modernity in Colonial and Postcolonial Indonesia[1]

G. ROGER KNIGHT

School of History and Politics, University of Adelaide, South Australia

This article sets out to review aspects of the history of a key world food commodity, and particularly to review the historical trajectory of white sugar and its links to ideas about "modernity." It argues that the idea of white sugar, in tandem with the manufacture of this form of the commodity, was taken up by new elites in the new states of the ex-colonial world during the middle decades of the twentieth century, and (following Sidney Mintz) that white sugar became literally the taste of modernity for elites and masses alike. It explores the ramifications of this argument in the context of the Netherlands Indies/Indonesia during a period of time extending from the 1930s through the 1950s.

In the 1980s, in coffeeshops in Jakarta, unless you offered precise requests to the contrary, your drink would arrive dosed with a very heavy load of sweetener. That sweetener, moreover, would almost invariably have been in the form of white, crystalline, factory-made sugar. The extensive use of sweetener in the diet of the mass of the Indonesian population, and, most certainly, the marked preference for white, factory-made sugar, were twentieth century developments. They took place, moreover, in a country which, although it had once been host to one of the world's greatest colonial "white" sugar industries, had been far more familiar historically to indigenously produced brown sugar than with the white form of the commodity. Indeed, until quite late in Indonesia's colonial past, its massive output of white sugar had been almost entirely produced for export. The domestic market had been catered for—very largely—by "native" Indonesian producers using "traditional" methods quite alien to the large Dutch-owned factories in which

Indonesia's white sugar was produced. White sugar only began to dominate the Indonesian market for sweetener in the second half of the twentieth century. In the existing account, this Indonesian taste for sweetener and the shift in consumer preferences from brown to white, appear as merely incidental concerns.[2] Yet, from the standpoint of the history of one of the world's iconic foodstuffs—and of food and foodways in general—these matters are anything but marginal, all the more so because they evoke themes that are of global as well as local significance. Based on unpublished archival sources as well as on the existing published literature on Java sugar, and working from a historian's perspective, the discussion that follows attempts an initial outline, therefore, of a hitherto somewhat neglected but important topic.

Sugar is not only of the world's key food commodities but also one whose appearance and sensation on the palate have long been subject to radical change. "Sugar" as we know it—a relatively stable, storable, and tradable commodity made from boiling down the sweet juices of grass-originated canes—was invented in Asia and subsequently made its way westward, via the Levant and the Mediterranean, into the Atlantic World. This was a centuries-long development.[3] In both East and West, however, sugar only became an item of cheap mass consumption in the nineteenth and early twentieth centuries. The history of that consumption, up to and including the present day, has always been closely bound to questions of color—and associated issues of taste and texture. Sugar is not a naturally white product. Indeed, its "natural" color, when manufactured from cane juice in the fairly rudimentary fashion that held good in both Asia and the New World until quite late in the eighteenth century, was an infinitely varied shade of brown. It might even be black. Since that time, the prevailing global fashion in sugar has switched from brown to white—and now seems in the process of returning to brown, at least among some categories of consumers.

It should be emphasized that there is nothing in the least trivial or inconsequent about these changes in consumer preference. On the contrary, the political economy of the switch from brown to white sugar (and back again) was one of great import for both producers and consumers. The process was one intimately bound up not only with issues of fashion, purity, hygiene, and modernity but also with ones of who controlled production and benefited from distribution.[4] From the mid-nineteenth century onward, there existed a fundamental division in the international sugar economy between centrifugal and non-centrifugal sugar. The former was the product of industrialized manufacture, spun into white crystalline form in machines which, in their earliest form at least, looked like nothing so much as top-loading washing machines (and which operated in a similar manner). Non-centrifugal sugar, on the other hand, was typically the brown product of "traditional," pre-industrial manufacturing techniques, in which boiled cane juice was set to solidify in vats or pots.

Nor was technique the only difference between the two. Generalizing broadly, by the late nineteenth century, centrifugal sugar was the product of large, heavily capitalized, industrial plants and was likewise distributed worldwide through capitalist commodity circuits, characterized by the presence of big, often international businesses. In contrast, non-centrifugal sugar manufacture tended to be carried out by relatively small-scale operators—indeed, in some contexts, it was a "backyard" industry—and to be sold through locally based trading networks. In short, the switch from brown to white involved far more than color and taste alone.

This article explores some of the ramifications of these several dimensions of shifts in consumer preference, and begins by outlining, in a global context, how mass-produced white sugar passed from Imperial origins into the diets of (ex-) imperial subjects, in the process displacing older brown sugars in popular esteem. It then examines this general theme in the particular context of the displacement of brown sugar by white in Indonesia (the erstwhile Netherlands Indies) during the mid-twentieth century decades that saw the country's transition from colonialism to independence. Briefly stated, in respect to consumer preferences, Indonesia shared in a global trend to equate white sugar—and the plethora of soft drinks closely associated with it—with all that was up-to-date, fashionable, and desirable. This article, however, is also concerned with the locally specific. It argues that the switch from brown to white was strongly promoted as part of a nationalist project to modernize Indonesia, promoted by the elites who took over the country from the Dutch at the end of the 1940s. This was strikingly manifested in mid-twentieth century Indonesia by the construction, under government patronage, of a vast new white sugar factory—the "House of Honey" of the article's title—in one of the most densely populated parts of the new Republic in the mid-1950s. Based on an examination of published and unpublished data drawn from a variety of contemporary archives, however, the article also argues for need to establish a historian's perspective. Underpinning the modernizing project of the elites—and local responses to global trends in patterns of consumption—was a situation, virtually unique to colonial Indonesia. This was one in which, during the interwar decades, locally established white and brown sugar producers began to vie for a share of the Indonesian domestic market—and continued to do so long after colonial rule came to an end in 1949. Accordingly, the latter half of the article is given over to an analysis of the dynamics of this ongoing situation—and the eventual victory of Indonesia's white sugar manufacturers—in which it is argued that domestic cultural preferences in matters relating to sweetness were closely bound up with, and to an extent dependent upon, the political economy of white sugar's local production.

In respect to all three facets of this argument, the case of Indonesia is of very special interest. As a Dutch colony, the archipelago was home to one of the world's largest cane sugar industries. Indeed, for more than half a century, it was second only to Cuba in respect to the quantities of cane sugar with which it supplied the world market. Based exclusively on the island of Java, and controlled largely by Dutch interests, it exported its output of centrifugally manufactured white sugar to all quarters of the globe—though by the early twentieth century the great bulk of its overseas markets were in Asia itself. At the same time, however, Java was also possessed of a large and growing brown sugar industry, largely run by native Indonesian producers. Hence, the scene was set for a potent interaction as the two different industries sought to accommodate themselves to—and at the same time to influence—changing mid-twentieth century patterns of consumer demand.

THE RISE OF WHITE SUGAR: FROM IMPERIALISM TO MODERNITY

The nineteenth century saw the development in Western Europe and North America of industrialized refining dependent on the steam, steel, and applied science to re-work the crude, raw brown sugars, generally produced in tropical and sub-tropical colonies, into a white, dry, and granular commodity. Prior to this, true white sugar was a (relatively) expensive rarity. Its bulk manufacture in the new breed of refineries was initially geared to markets in the West, where whiteness in sugar became part of a larger, late imperial discourse in which the question of color became central. Its large-scale manufacture initially took place, that is to say, in a context not only of mass production but also of "hygiene" and "purity" that had larger associations with contemporary imperialism, racism, and control over colonized peoples. Specifically, the introduction of an advanced technology of white sugar refining served to purge the commodity of both of its inherent color and of its association with an "impure" raw material, produced by "inferior" black, brown, or yellow labor. The latter-day slogan of "Untouched by Human Hand" had, it might be suggested, a particular resonance for the Imperial discourses to which sugar came to belong.[5]

Nonetheless, white sugar did not remain the exclusive preserve of western consumers. From the late nineteenth century onward, it found a large and growing market among the elites—and subsequently the masses—of Asia, Africa, and the southern Americas. From its origins in a distinctively imperial ethos, that is to say, white sugar took on a life of its own. An integral part of this development, moreover, was that it ceased to be the exclusive preserve of sugar refineries. So-called Factory White (aka "plantation white" or *blanco* in the terminology of the New World producers) became available for direct consumption by purchasers prepared to accept a certain dilution of quality in return for a lower price. Made in the same (or similar) factories that produced crude white sugar for sale to refineries, it resulted from a variety of techniques (involving chemical treatment of cane juice during the process of its manufacture into sugar) practiced fairly widely across the international sugar economy during the course of the nineteenth century. By the end of the century it was being mass-produced, above all by the beet sugar manufacturers of Central Europe, in sufficient quantities to rival the output of sugar refineries and became the mainstay of exports to "third world" markets.[6] Meanwhile, industrialized refineries made their appearance outside Europe and North America, primarily in East Asia, and "Factory White" began to be manufactured, c. 1900 onward, in huge quantities in Dutch Java, primarily for sale in the Indian subcontinent and China.

In short, by the early twentieth century, sugar—whitened in one way or another—was beginning to become widely available to "third world" consumers, and by the mid-century was well on the way to displacing such local traditionally made sugars as had once dominated the market. White sugar became emblematic globally, not of colonialism but of a modernity that was perceived as the very antithesis of colonial subjugation and its purportedly attendant backwardness. Why was this so? Global trends were clearly involved, and we can turn most usefully here to Sidney Mintz's classic discussion of the occasions and forms in which sucrose "penetrates the food preferences" of ordinary people, and in which, in particular, whiteness in sugar came to constitute a critical mark of distinction.[7] In such a context, as Mintz has insisted, ". . . the difference between old-fashioned and indigenous, and modern and more acculturated, was not between the absence and presence of sugar *but between which form of sugar was deemed necessary,* and how much of a household's budget one was willing to spend upon it."[8] More generally, anthropologists have drawn our attention to the idea that "sugar seems not only good to eat, but good to think, not only metabolic but metaphoric; not only sucrose but symbol," and that it embodied "a set of at least implied meanings: white sugar was a more refined product, and those who consumed it, more advanced; brown . . . sugar, and those who consumed it, less so."[9] As Mintz himself has remarked, brown sugar now became a hallmark of all that was old-fashioned rather than modern, rural rather urban, primitive rather than advanced. In contrast, white sugar and the sugar-rich beverages whose manufacture was predicated on the availability of this form of the sucrose ("tasteless except for its sweetness") succeeded in gaining the vital "cachet of youth and modernity."[10]

Yet, there was very evidently a further dimension to the switch from white to brown among the (former) subjects of empire. In whichever form (refined or "Factory White"), white sugar *manufacture* per se came to be prized by national elites throughout the new states of the emergent "third world" as a hallmark of modernity. It was a commodity in which national self-sufficiency became just as important a national priority as was the case, say, with steel or cement. Sugar, at least until around the middle of the twentieth century was a high-tech industry, still near the cutting edge of technological advance that it had occupied for much of the nineteenth century. To this extent, its espousal by national elites in the third world reflected an idolatry of modern technology that was, it might be suggested, particularly characteristic of states that otherwise shared very unequally in the economic benefits of the world capitalism that such technology was developed to serve.[11]

THE "HOUSE OF HONEY" AND THE QUEST FOR MODERNITY IN MID-CENTURY INDONESIA

We can best begin the story in the 1950s, in the first decade of Indonesian independence. It was during this decade that the young Sultan of Yogyakarta, a staunch supporter of the nationalist cause and de facto ruler of several million subjects in Central Java, embarked on one of his most important—and certainly the most expensive—projects. This was the building of a new sugar factory—named *Madukismo* or "House of Honey"—to replace those destroyed in Yogyakarta during the final phase of the national revolution against the Dutch. For his new factory, the Sultan obtained capital from the Indonesian government and turned to East German (rather than Dutch) engineers to execute the project.[12] The upshot was the creation of what was proudly described by one of the Sultan's key aides as "the largest and most modern" factory of its kind anywhere in Southeast Asia.

"Modern" was the key word. Located a few kilometers south of the city of Yogyakarta itself, the House of Honey was ceremonially opened in 1958 by no less a figure than the president of the republic himself, Ir. Sukarno. The president—trained as an engineer—was no mere titular figurehead; revered as the father of his people, he was widely perceived as the personification of the Indonesian national project, whose inspiration he had been since the 1920s. No matter that the House of Honey closed down almost immediately after it began operations, due to unanticipated difficulties with its "semi-automatic" machinery, and did not reopen for another twelve months or more. It remained as a powerful *symbol* of the intent of the national project in relation to the production of the sugar.

Madukismo was designed to supply industrially manufactured white sugar to a rapidly growing number of Indonesian consumers, for whom this form of the commodity was now judged—at least by their leaders—as inseparable from the modernity that was one of the national project's key promises. Brown sugar, at the time widely manufactured in Yogyakarta and other parts of Central and East Java, simply would not do. As was the case with other emergent nations in the third world, sugar had to be white, pure, and granular. Anything less would have comprised the state's modernity. In neighboring Papua New Guinea a decade or later, it was to be much the same story: suggestions that decentralized manufacture of soft brown sugar might best fill the needs of the territory's taste for sweetness were rejected in a favor of a single, huge industrial plant, unambiguously designed to produce centrifugal white sugar.[13]

As far as the national elites who ran Indonesia after the departure of the Dutch were concerned, the modernity exemplified by a taste for white rather than brown was also bound quite closely to the national project's romance with technology. Idolatry was the other side of the same coin. Rudolph Mrazek has drawn attention to the intimate links between technology and national identity, and to the indigenous *Engineers of Happy Land*, who so readily took their cue from their colonialist counterparts and contemporaries.[14] Technology mattered enormously to the engineers of the Indonesian national project, and this concern could not help but include sugar, both in its form and its methods of manufacture. For people such as this, the succession of great state-of-the-art sugar factories built in the colony in the 1910s and 1920s—vast buildings full of gleaming machinery—represented the apogee of the Dutch colonial achievement, insofar as it could be measured in technological terms.

THE PRODUCTION AND CONSUMPTION OF SUGAR IN COLONIAL INDONESIA

The argument so far has been that white sugar's mid-twentieth century history revolved around the evolution of a *global* taste for, and association of modernity with, the white crystalline form of the commodity that had originally been created under the aegis of colonialism with Western consumers in mind. At the same time, this quest for modernity was also bound up with a fascination for modern technology among the governing elites of the newly independent states of the "third" and the reflection of this in the espousal of large, scale, high-tech manufacture of white sugar. In newly independent Indonesia, unlike the other examples cited, this espousal did not require the setting up of a wholly new industry. Indeed, quite the contrary was the case. Brand new factories such as *Madukismo*, though highly charged with symbolism, were an exceptional development. A network of highly industrialized factories, turning out substantial amounts of white sugar, continued to exist from colonial times. Even more to the point, well before the Dutch left at the end of the 1940s, the output of that network of factories had already begun to infiltrate colonial Indonesia's domestic market.

That market was potentially a very large one. By the 1930s, the island of Java, by far the mostly densely settled part of the Indonesian archipelago, had had a population in excess of forty million. Even so, the prospect of substantial domestic sales was one that the industry's Dutch executives were slow to grasp. Their efforts were geared almost exclusively on the export market, and by the early century on sales in the Indian subcontinent, China and Japan. It was only after 1930, *in extremis* in consequence of the collapse of overseas sales in the wake of the interwar depression, that the island's colonial sugar companies discovered the domestic consumer. Prior to that, they kept no formal record of their domestic sales. There was irony here, for what made this neglect all the more curious, was that the Java industry had long thrived on supplying the native market elsewhere in Asia with cheap, "Factory White" sugar. Indeed, by the 1920s, "Factory White" had become the mainstay of the industry, with around sixty percent of factories geared to this kind of production.[15]

Yet, this neglect of the potential of the domestic market was not just the consequence of commercial myopia. The industry was also encouraged in its indifference to domestic sales by what was widely perceived in colonial circles as a matter of taste. The mass of the population was not indifferent to sucrose sweetness.[16] On the contrary, there are indications that they reveled in it. Rather, the problem in the early twentieth century was perceived in terms of the extent to which the Indies' domestic market for sugar was provisioned with *gula Jawa* or Java sugar, manufactured extensively throughout the island.[17] From a colonial standpoint, the industry's leading savant neatly described the situation early in the twentieth century, when he wrote, "the consumption of cane sugar of European standard is not great. . . . The sugar produced in the European sugar works is chiefly consumed by the Europeans, [locally resident] Chinese and wealthy natives, *while the bulk of the inhabitants . . . prefer evaporated juice to crystals*."[18]

By the late nineteenth century, the production of sugar of this latter, evaporated kind was clearly an expanding industry, located primarily in the East Java, the part of the island that extends through the valley of the great Brantas river to the strait that separates Java from Bali.[19] Beginning in the 1920s, moreover, these producers were beginning to discard traditional wooden or wood-and-stone cane mills and replacing them with much more efficient iron ones, most of them imported from the United States. By 1924, there were around 130 such mills in the Brantas valley alone, and by the end of the colonial era there were said to be hundreds of them in use.[20] Faced during the 1930s by growing competition for a share of the market by the island's big, industrialized white sugar factories, moreover, Java's brown sugar producers were not without resource. Among other things, they set about mimicking the "Factory White" with which their rivals sought to flood the market.

Briefly stated, what happened was this.[21] Around 1934, some relatively large-scale *gula Jawa* producers in East Java developed what would now be termed value-added techniques for improving the profitability of their product. They did so by inventing or (more probably) evolving methods of working up crude *gula Jawa* into something that resembled "Factory White" to an extent that thoroughly alarmed the colonial manufacturers of the latter commodity. Working up *gula Jawa* in this way was a highly labor-intensive process, made possible, it might be suspected, by the very low level of wages prevalent during the Depression. Using manual labor, ordinary, pre-industrial brown sugar was beaten free of much of the molasses content from which it acquired its distinctive character. What was left was a fine-grained, so-called sand sugar, whose Javanese name, *gula tanjung,* indicated its yellowish tint. Illicitly mixed with industrially manufactured sugar—at least this was what Dutch sources asserted—it could easily be passed as "Factory White"—and as such was sold to local Chinese traders for sale on the domestic market. Indeed, on some occasions it was produced at the direct instigation such traders.

POSTCOLONIAL RIVALRIES: BROWN AND WHITE FROM THE 1930S TO THE END OF THE CENTURY

In the discussion so far, two factors have been emphasized. One was the extent to which the cause of white sugar was espoused by the country's nationalist elites as a key dimension of the search for modernity that lay at the heart of their project. The second is the extent to which the infiltration of the Indonesian market by white sugar took place against a background of the long-standing and persistent production of various forms of native brown sugar. Far from being moribund, as we have just seen, in the interwar decades brown sugar production of this kind was both expanding and adaptive, so that the developing contest between the two forms of the commodity was by no means an unequal or short-term one.

As we have already seen, the big Dutch-owned combines that dominated the Java's colonial-era white sugar producers only began to investigate the possibilities of domestic sales following the downturn of the international market at the end of the 1920s. Their newfound interest initially met with only limited success. Despite innovations such as the packaging of sugar into small bags for direct sale in Java's myriad of rural villages, sales were disappointing. The sales drive coincided with a severe downturn in economic conditions in the Javanese countryside. Indeed, they could hardly have chosen a worse time. According, for instance, to reports from the manager of the railway that ran through the sugar belt of the north coast of Central and West Java, and whose freight business heavily dependent on the transport of sugar, attempts at direct sales ran up against declining buying power—and the opposition of the Indonesian–Chinese middlemen who usually handled the trade. He reckoned that in the area serviced by his lines, only a couple of factories had much success in selling their output locally.[22]

Much depended, of course, on price. Thanks to government regulations that prohibited the import of sugar from overseas,[23] the Java factories were able to sell their sugar within the Netherlands Indies at prices twenty percent or more higher than those for which they disposed of it overseas.[24] This degree of protection also meant, however, that throughout the 1930s factory sugar was almost always more expensive than its "native-made" counterpart, and significantly outsold by it.[25]

Meanwhile, insofar as can be statistically determined, the production of "native" brown sugar—*gula Jawa* in short—appears to have increased significantly during the interwar decades. The area recorded as planted with cane for the manufacture of *gula Jawa* rose from a little over ten and half thousand hectares in 1934 to more than eighteen thousand hectares in 1940—an increase of nearly forty percent. It was estimated that while around one quarter of the cane thus grown was sold for direct consumption (Dutch: *kauwriet* or chewing cane), the remainder went into the production of *gula Jawa*.[26] Given the nature of the product, however, and the variety of names with which it appeared on the market in different localities, only very broad approximation is possible of the amount of "native" sugar that reached Indonesian consumers. Insofar as it was made from cane, Dutch estimates were that by the late 1930s it was something shy of 100,000 tons annually (less than a tenth of what the island's big industrial factories produced at the time).[27] The figure is potentially deceptive, however, since it only relates to brown sugar made from cane, and takes no account of palm sugar—made, that is to say, from the boiled-down sap of various kinds of palm tree indigenous to Southeast Asia.[28] Its manufacture was an archetypal backyard industry, and not even assiduous Dutch officials managed to collect data on its production. However, a colonial estimate—made c. 1918—was that twice as much "native" sugar was made from palm sap as from cane juice.[29] If this approximate ratio continued to hold for the interwar decades, it might be roughly estimated that, at the end of the 1930s, the "native" sugar industry was producing in total perhaps as much as 300,000 tons annually of cane and palm sugar. This came near to matching the quantity of industrially manufactured white sugar that was sold in Indonesia immediately prior to the Second World War. On the eve of the war, that is to say, brown sugar accounted for more than fifty percent of Indonesian domestic sales—and for very much more than that among Indonesian consumers themselves, since an unquantifiable but substantial amount of the white sugar sold on the domestic market went to the Dutch colonial population, numbering around a quarter of a million souls c. 1940. As we shall see, brown sugar continued to account for a considerable share of the Indonesian market in the early decades of independence. One contemporary estimate was that as late as the mid-1960s, it amounted to around one-third of all the sugar consumed in Indonesia.[30]

Nonetheless, the long-term trend, already in evidence by the 1930s and greatly accentuated by the 1950s, was for the big, industrial factories of Java to find an increasing proportion of their sales in Indonesia itself, and in so doing displace brown sugar manufacturers as the country's prime suppliers of sucrose. Eventually indeed, the white sugar producers stopped exporting altogether, and concentrated exclusively, c. 1960 onward, on the home market. It is worth emphasizing, however, that this represented the culmination of developments that had begun much earlier, during the final decades of Dutch rule. Between 1914 and 1940 there was an almost eight-fold increase in the amount of white sugar that was sold on the Indonesian domestic market. Whereas at the beginning of the period, domestic sales amounted to no more five percent of total production, by its end they accounted for almost twenty-five percent.[31] Moreover, these sales were profitable, at a time when the industry was struggling to recover from the effects of the interwar depression. The upshot, as was remarked by executives of the biggest of the Dutch companies involved in the sugar business, was that domestic sales were "of great influence on the ultimate financial results" of the industry.[32] Moreover, although (as we have just seen) white sugar made only limited inroads in Java itself, its prewar sales in other parts of the Indonesian archipelago were altogether more promising—and pointed to significant future developments. By the late 1930s, white sugar, manufactured in Java, began to find a ready market in the so-called Outer Islands—notably Sumatra, Kalimantan, and Sulawesi—where cash-crop smallholders and traders were growing in prosperity.[33] The development was suggestive, as it was elsewhere, of the way in which white sugar was taken up by the better off elements in the "third world," as a mark of distinction signifying their modernity.

POSTCOLONIAL TRENDS

The trend toward the increased uptake of white sugar was consolidated after the Second World War and the winning of independence in 1949. As the directors of one of the big ex-colonial sugar companies remarked early in the '50s, domestic sugar consumption within Indonesia demonstrated a continually upward trend, and "demand on the domestic market is ever increasingly for white sugar."[34] The upshot was that between the beginning of the 1950s and 1958 annual domestic consumption of factory-produced white sugar in Indonesia increased by almost two hundred and fifty percent, from around 277,000 tons to over 692,000 tons.[35]

The decade of the 1940s had been one of great difficulty for Java's big industrialized factories. Colonial Indonesia was invaded by the Japanese in 1942, and though the conquerors had their own sugar empire in East Asia, based on a network of big refineries in Japan itself, they had no use at this time for Java's output. Moreover, the exigencies of war virtually prohibited shipping. When the war ended, the Java producers became caught up in the national struggle for independence, and when that became violent—as it did twice between 1945 and Dutch acceptance of the Indonesian Republic at the end of 1949—factories were put to the torch as Republican troops and guerillas adopted a scorched-earth policy in the face of Dutch military advance. Such cane as was planted in these circumstances was also burnt or—rather more significantly—cut down and used for making brown sugar, something that continued to happen after independence had been achieved.[36] In the circumstances, it might have looked as if Java's white sugar industry had reached the end of the road. Yet, it had not done so—and survived for a variety of reasons that are inextricably intertwined with global trends and elite responses (and self-interest) in a unique political economy of postcolonial white sugar, which saw Java disappear totally from the ranks of world producers, but remain as a considerable producer for the Indonesian domestic market, albeit on a scale that never matched that of the colonial era.

Independence came at the end of 1949, and though Dutch economic power in the New Republic only outlasted the departure of Dutch administrators and Dutch military by less than a decade, it was significant insofar as it enabled a core of (ex-) colonial firms to rebuild their factories. They were encouraged in this by some financial support from the Indonesian government and—perhaps crucially—by the fact that increasing sales within the Republic were a great deal more lucrative than anything that was to be gained from exports. As one keen-eyed oversees observer noticed in 1956, the industry benefited from the "very high internal price for sugar...which is very substantially above the world price."[37]

The sudden nationalization of the industry in 1958 caught the Dutch by surprise. It proved, however, to be a vital phase in the white sugar's rise to hegemony in the domestic market. On nationalization, most factories passed into the hands of the Indonesian army—and not long after that, so too did the Indonesian Republic. The army had already been feeling its way toward controlling Indonesia since the mid-1950s, and in an incremental coup in 1965–1967 it succeeded in doing so, under the leadership of General Suharto, who supplanted Sukarno as head of state. In short, the white sugar industry found itself with powerful friends. Immediately after nationalization took effect in 1958, the army had used its martial law powers to prevent labor unrest within the industry, which was declared to be one of national importance.[38] Subsequently, the destruction of Indonesia's Communist party and its workers' affiliates in a series of army-inspired or sanctioned communal massacres in 1965–1966—many sugar districts were very hard hit—made it clear, in the most brutal way, that the white sugar producers had the full backing of the state.[39] Under Suharto (1966–1998), the sugar industry, like most Indonesian businesses, was heavily infiltrated by military officers and their Indonesian–Chinese business associates, who were the vital economic sinews of the regime. International support for the Suharto—in Cold War terms he was a pro-Western, anti-communist, and hence "friendly" dictator—also meant, moreover, that money was available for the rehabilitation of factories that had fallen into disrepair.[40] Against a background of what must surely have been a growing (but as yet little documented) preference for this form of the commodity among Indonesian consumers, the future of white sugar production appeared assured.

Some of the explanation for this was to be found in the way in which the regime—and its allies in the countryside—manipulated the supply of cane in support of the white sugar producers. Prior to this, there is evidence that they were being starved of raw material, in part at least through its diversion into brown sugar manufacture.[41] Until the mid-1970s, Java's white sugar factories had remained largely dependent for their cane on plantation-style agriculture devised by the Dutch in the late nineteenth century and carried out by hired laborers under the direct management of industry personnel. By the end of the decade, however, the regime had begun to promote the smallholder production of cane, in the obvious expectation that this would provide the industry with a better supply of raw material than seemed to be possible under existing arrangements.[42] During the 1980s, smallholder cane, organized through local middlemen and under the auspices of an "Intensified Smallholder Cane Programme" inaugurated by the Indonesian government came to predominate.

The upshot was that the finite supplies of cane that could be produced in tightly packed rural Java were diverted away from brown sugar producers.[43] The precise dynamics of the situation are difficult to untangle, but, however broadly conceived, they serve very effectively to underline the nexus between political economy and a far from autonomous cultural preference for white over brown. A growing taste for white, industrially manufactured sugar undermined the market for *gula Jawa* of the traditional kind, thereby making possible the diversion of smallholder cane into the production of factory sugar. Simultaneously, however, the extent to which smallholder cane was drawn into the orbit of factory sugar presumably helped foster a taste for white sugar by virtue of the extent to which it dried up the supply of raw material to brown sugar producers and thereby diminished the supply of *gula Jawa*.

A PYRRHIC VICTORY

Nonetheless, the white sugar industry, once so prominent, had moved in the second half of the twentieth century to the sidelines of the Indonesian economy, and its victory was a Pyrrhic one. Java's industrial manufacturers of white sugar proved incapable of matching supply to ever-increasing local demand, and Indonesia became one of the world's largest *importers* of the commodity. Attempts—the first time in its long history—to expand the industrialized production of white sugar beyond the confines of Java itself met with some success. In Java, meanwhile, smallholder cane growing was increasingly confined to unirrigated land that the colonial-era factories would never have given a second glance to. The upshot was that cane yields overall were around half those enjoyed in colonial times, with commensurate modest levels of sugar productivity. Meanwhile, consumption in Indonesia as a whole continued to far outstrip domestic output, and had to be fed by massive imports. By 1980, for example, imports of sugar were more than four times greater than they had been a decade earlier. Allowing for considerable variations over time, the trend continued for the remainder of the twentieth century—and into the twenty-first.[44] The penultimate stage of postcolonial developments in the white sugar industry appeared to have been reached, at the very end of the century. In the wake of the Asian Meltdown of 1997–8 (its impact was particularly severe and enduring in Indonesia), a slow wave of factory closures took place that seemed to foreshadow the final end of Java sugar as a large-scale industry. But sugar seems to have escaped extinction yet again, not least because of the vested interests with which, as always, it has been surrounded.[45]

The necessary postscript, however, concerns consumption. This article began with the loading of white refined sugar into a cup of coffee in the Indonesia of almost a generation ago. It is not a scene that would be repeated so commonly today, at least not in the coffeehouses in the shopping malls patronized by the country's expanding middle classes. The sheer volume of sugar might still be there—but now it might well be raw and brown, and packaged accordingly. As Mintz has observed, in sugar as in other foodways, we now see a familiar process repeated in the case of the brown and white forms of the commodity: "Soon enough, the old supposedly impure foods will reappear in attractive modern and expensive packages, whereupon they will be touted as 'natural' . . . The first buyers of these 'natural' foods will surely be among those who first gave them up in order to eat a more refined version."[46]

What this article has also sought to demonstrate, moreover, is a point that is, at the very least, implicit in Mintz's entire oeuvre. This is that shifts in consumer preferences—in this particular case from brown to white sugar, and now, so it would seem, back again—need to be contextualized in terms of the political economy of both consumption and production. To be sure, in relation to the sugar that people ate in Indonesia during the second half of the twentieth century, shifts in taste reflected global trends. At the same time, however, those trends were articulated locally—their realization made possible, one is tempted to say—by a very particular historical course of events.

This began in the 1930s, when Java's colonial white sugar producers began to look round for domestic markets to replace those that they had just lost overseas, and continued through a series of mid-century developments—invasion, revolution, and the departure of the Dutch—that might well have also seen the end of white sugar manufacture in the newly independent Indonesia. That this did not happen, and that, instead, it was the country's indigenous, traditional brown sugar producers who appeared to face annihilation, is something which this article has sought to explain. But fashions, and the political economy so closely interwoven with them, are indeed fickle, as Mintz indicates. Globally, the refined has now indeed become the impure—and in local circumstances in which the production of white sugar has itself become as marginalized in both economic and political terms, as was the case with the brown version of the commodity in preceding decades. And of this second shift, from white back to brown again, the full history has yet to be written.

NOTES

1. In preparing this paper for publication, I am particularly grateful to the editor of *Food and Foodways*, and to two anonymous reviewers, whose keenness pointed me (I hope) the right way for revisions.

2. For the extensive historiography of the Indonesian sugar industry (with a heavy emphasis on the colonial era), see e.g., Peter Boomgaard, "Treacherous cane: The Java sugar industry" in Bill Albert and Adrian Graves (eds.), *The world sugar economy in war and depression*, London: Routledge, 1988, pp. 157–69; Robert E. Elson, *Javanese peasants and the colonial sugar industry: Impact and change in an East Java Residency, 1830–1940*, Singapore: Oxford University Press, 1984; M.R. Fernando, "Peasants and plantation economy. The social impact of the European plantation economy in Cirebon Residency from the cultivation system to the end of the first decade of the twentieth century" (Ph.D. diss., Monash University, Melbourne, 1982); G. Roger Knight, *Colonial production in provincial Java: The sugar industry in Pekalongan-Tegal, 1800–1942*, Amsterdam: V.U. Press, 1993; G. Roger Knight, "The Sugar Industry of Colonial Java and its Global Trajectory," *South East Asia Research* 8, 3 (2000), pp. 249–274; Djoko Suryo, "Social and economic life in rural Semarang under colonial rule in the later nineteenth century" (Ph.D. diss., Monash University, 1982.)

3. For a general introduction, see G.H. Galloway, *The Cane Sugar Industry. An Historical Geography to 1914*, Cambridge: Cambridge University Press, 1989.

4. The classic text is that of Sidney W. Mintz, *Sweetness and Power. The Place of Sugar in Modern History*, New York: Viking, 1985 (and, for a succinct commentary, see Mintz, "Sweet Polychrest," *Social Research* 66,1 (Spring 1999), pp. 85–101). See also, e.g., Sidney and Michael Cantor, "Socio-Economic Factors in Fat and Sugar Consumption" in M. Kare and O. Maller (eds.), *The Chemical Senses and Nutrition*. New York: Academic Press, 1977, pp. 429–46; Woodruffe D. Smith, "Complications of the Commonplace: Tea, Sugar, and Imperialism," *Journal of Interdisciplinary History*, 23 (2), 1992; Paul Rozin, "Sweetness, Sensuality, Sin, Safety, and Socialisation: Some Speculations," in J. Dobbing (ed.), *Sweetness*. London: Springer, 1987.

5. For a development of these and kindred themes, see G. Roger Knight, "Paradoxical White: Imperial and Postcolonial Sugar," in Leigh Boucher, Jane Carey, and Katherine Ellinghaus (eds.), *Historicising Whiteness: Transnational Perspectives on the Construction of Identity*, Melbourne: RMIT Publishing in Association with the School of Historical Studies, University of Melbourne, 2007, pp. 346–354.

6. For a brief introduction to "Factory White," see, e.g., John Perkins and Roger Munting, "Science versus Nature: The Cane–Beet Sugar Rivalry," in Pal Ahluwahlia, Bill Ashcroft, and Roger Knight (eds.), *White and Deadly: Sugar and Colonialism*, New York: Nova Science Publishers, 1999.

7. Famously, a critical dimension of Mintz's argument is that sugar both compliments complex carbohydrates in the popular diet and partly supplants them. See Mintz, *Sweetness and Power*, p. 127 and pp. 133–145.

8. S. W. Mintz and M. Weismantel, "Sweet Interloper," in L. Plotnicov and R. Scaglion (eds.), *Consequences of Cultivar Diffusion*, Ethnology, Monographs 17 (Pittsburgh: Department of Anthropology, University of Pittsburgh, 1999), 55–74.

9. For this particular formulation, see Frederick Errington and Deborah Gewertz, *Yali's Question: Sugar, Culture, and History*, Chicago: Chicago University Press, 2004, pp. 54 and 63–68, pp. 63–64, to which I am also indebted for the second quotation, which is from Lévi-Strauss (1962).

10. Mintz, "Sweet Interloper," passim.

11. The author is grateful for this point to one of the anonymous reviewers of an earlier draft of this article submitted to *Food and Foodways*.

12. For this and for what follows about Madukismo, see Selosoemardjan, *Social Changes in Jogjakarta*, Ithaca, NY: Cornell University Press, 1962, pp. 296–7.

13. Errington and Gewertz, *Yali's Question*, pp. 54 and 63–68. These were not isolated instances. Indeed, at the very moment that the Sultan was employing East German engineers to creating his own House of Honey, the biggest of the Dutch sugar companies still operating in newly independent Indonesia was also engaged in Ethiopia, creating for emperor Haile Selassi a grand sugar factory to supply *his* people with white industrially manufactured sugar. See J. P. van de Kerkhof, "'Defeatism Is Our Worst Enemy.' Rehabilitation, Re-Orientation and *Indonesianisasi* at Internatio and HVA, 1945–1958," *Lebaran Sejarah* 8 (2), 2005, pp. 116–7; M. Teklemariam, "Sugar Industry Development in Ethiopia," *ISHS Acta Horticulturae*, vol. 270, pp. 49–58. The establishment of the Wonji sugar factory in northeastern Ethiopia dated from an agreement between the emperor and the Amsterdam-based HVA sugar company in 1951.

14. Rudolf Mrazek, *Engineers of Happy Land. Technology and Nationalism in a Colony*, Princeton, NJ: Princeton University Press, 2002, passim.

15. Calculated from statistics of "*Suikerproduct der fabrieken, naar de suikersoort verdeeld*" in *Archief voor de Suikerindustrie in Nederlandsch Indie* [Surabaya], Algemeen Syndicaat van Suikerfabriekanten, vol. 34 (1927): 3: 4–8. For an extended contemporary description of the carbonation process by which "Factory White" was processed in early twentieth-century Java, see H. C. Prinsen Geerligs, *De Fabricatie van Suiker uit Suikerriet op Java. Handboek ten Dienste van de Suikerriet-Cultuur en de Rietsuiker-Fabricage op Java*, vol. 3, Amsterdam: De Bussy, 1911, p. 160ff.

16. Pioneering colonial-era work on the Indonesian diet is reported in A. M. P. Scheltema, *The Food Consumption of the the Native Population of Java and Madura (Done into English by Dr. A. H. Hamilton)* Batavia: National Council for the Netherlands and the Netherlands Indies of the Institute of Pacific Relations, 1936.

17. Indigenous sweeteners ranged through the many varieties. These were brown rather than white sugars, produced by evaporation rather than through the action of the centrifuge, and soft rather than crystalline in texture. There are several terms in use here, including *gula merah* ("red" sugar), *gula mangkok* (the reference being to the cup-like shape in which the sugar, as the result of having been molded in the half-shell of a coconut, is presented for sale), *gula tebu* (cane sugar), and *gula aren* or arenga-sugar, at one time regarded as the best, hence the most expensive, of sweeteners made from palm sap rather than from cane. In colonial parlance, at least, sugars of this kind were generally referred to as *gula Jawa* or Java(nese) sugar. See H. Deinum, *Bevolkingssuiker* in C. J. J. van Hall and C. van de Koppel, *De Landbouw in de Indische Archipel (II a)*, The Hague: Van Hoeve, 1948, pp. 405–426; *Encyclopaedie van Nederlandsch-Indie*, Tweede Druk, vol. 6, The Hague, Nijhoff, 1932, pp. 380–383.

18. H. C. Prinsen Geerligs, *The World's Cane Sugar Industry*, Altricham, Norman Rodger, 1912, p. 139. Emphasis added.

19. For a detailed account, see G. H. van der Kolff, *Bevolkingsrietcultuur in Nederlandsch-Indie*, Batavia: Kolff, 1925, passim.

20. Van der Kolff, *Bevolkingsrietcultuur*, pp. 106–8; H. Deinum, *Bevolkingssuiker* in C. J. J. van Hall and C. van de Koppel, *De Landbouw in de Indische Archipel (II a)*,The Hague, Van Hoeve, 1948. p. 414. The American imports initially came from the Cincinnati-based Blymyer Iron Works.

21. This and the other information in the paragraphs relating to *gula tanjung* comes from contemporary documents preserved in the files of the Dutch organization (NIVAS) that oversaw the sales of Java sugar during the 1930s. See, in particular, the file labeled *Inlandse Suiker* 1934–1940 in NA, Archief Nederlandsch Indisch Vereniging tot Afzet van Suiker [hereafter NIVAS] 2.20.09.03/548.

22. Jaarverslag [hereafter JV] Semarang-Cheribon Stroomtram Mij, 1930: 27–29; 1931: 30–31; 1932: 22, NA Archief Semarang-Cheribon Stroomtram Mij, 2.20.17/013/191VIII.

23. "Suikerinvoer Ordonnantie 1934," *Indisch Verslag*, Batavia, Landsdrukkerij, 1935(1): 45.

24. In 1934, for example, when the price of Java sugar on the Amsterdam market ranged from 3.37 to 4.87 guilders per quintal (i.e., 100 kilo), the state-regulated wholesale sugar price on the Java domestic market was between 5.40 and 5.80 guilders. See *Indisch Verslag* 1935 (1:) 57.

25. JV NHM Agentschap Sourabaya 1935: 21, NA NHM 5193.

26. JV NIVAS 1939–40: 47–48 NA NIVAS 2.20.09.03/14.

27. There are various estimates, none of them too disparate. Java's "single seller" sugar organization NIVAS's, estimate was that in 1939 rather less *gula Jawa* (87,975 tons) had been produced than in 1938 (91,193 tons). It offered no estimate for 1940. See JV NIVAS 1938–9: 38–9; 1939–40:47 and 1940–41:70 in

NA NIVAS 2.20.09.03/14 and 15. According to the colonial government's figures, the output of what was designated as *gula mangkok*—the form of the sweetener made from cane and deriving its name from the half coconut shells in which it was set after boiling down—amounted to 71,584 tons in 1929 and 90,765 in 1940. See P. Creutzberg, *Changing Economy of Indonesia (1): Indonesia's Export Crops 1816–1940,* The Hague: Nijhoff, 1975, pp. 75–76.

28. According to Deinum ["Bevolkingssuiker," p. 419], there are in Indonesia/Southeast Asia three kinds of palm tree from which sugar is produced on a commercial scale. These are the Arenga Palm (*Arenga saccharifera*), the "Siwilan" or "Lontar" Palm *(Borassus flabillifer)* and Coco Palm (*Cocos nucifera*).

29. Cited in Creutzberg, *Indonesia's Export Crops*, pp. 63–64.

30. According to the data for the period 1939–1967 assembled by the distinguished Indonesian sugar expert, Mubyarto ("The Sugar Industry," *Bulletin of Indonesian Economic Studies,* 5 (2), 1969, pp. 52–4), in the year 1965–6 recorded brown sugar production amounted to some 330,000 tons, as compared with the 601,000 tons of white, industrially manufactured sugar produced in 1966.

31. The earlier figure was in the region of 50,000 tons, the later one 370,000 tons. See Prinsen Geerligs, *The World's Cane*, p. 13; Creutzberg, *Indonesia's Export Crops*, p. 64.

32. Jaarverslag [hereafter JV] NHM Factorij Batavia 1934:206, NA NHM 4566.

33. See, e.g., *Indisch Verslag,* Batavia, Landsdrukkerij, 1937(1):154.

34. *JV Koloniale Bank* 1953:7, Amsterdam: Koninklijk Instituut voor de Tropen, no. L1116; JV Cultuurmij Gending 1956: 6, NA Archief Koloniale Bank 2.20.04/1149.

35. JV NHM Factorij Djakarta 1958:2: 1, NA NHM 4572.

36. In 1956, for example, the expatriate manager at Bandjaratma sugar factory on the north coast of Central Java was convinced that some, at least, of the substantial amount of cane stolen from the factory's plantations—it amounted in that year to around twenty percent of the total harvest—was being used for the preparation of *gula Jawa*. See "Bandjaratma. Rapport 12/4/1957 and 11/8/1956," Rapporten Bandjaratma, NA Archief Koloniale Bank 2.20.05/116.

37. D. W. Fryer, "Recovery of the Sugar Industry in Indonesia," *Economic Geography,* 33, 2 (1957), pp. 181 [Fryer had spent some months in Indonesia in 1956]: "There is undoubtedly scope for a very substantial increase in domestic consumption. This largely arises from the very high internal price of sugar in Indonesia, 3.3 Rp. per kg. (about 15 cents per pound), which is very substantially above the world price; a reduction on the various taxes on sugar could bring about a substantial increase in local demand."

38. JV NHM Factorij Djakarta 1958:2: 1, NA NHM 4572.

39. For a first-hand account of what happened in the sugar area of the Brantas valley in East Java, see Pipit Rochijat, "Am I P.K.I. or Non P.K.I.?," *Indonesia,* 40 (1985) pp. 37–47. On the massacres in general, see Robert Cribb (ed.), *The Indonesian Killings 1965–1966,* Clayton, Vic., Monash University, Monash Papers on Southeast Asia no. 21.

40. During the 1970s, a number of its factories took on a new lease of life when the state financed rehabilitation, either through direct loans or by standing guarantor for loans from international agencies. One such operation in North Java, for example, direct heir to a legacy of colonial-era production extending back into the 1830s, remained in production at the very end of the twentieth century, thanks to its extensive reconstruction in the 1970s. See Rudolf Solindungan Sinaga, *A normative sugarcane supply function and optimum land rental plan for a proposed expansion of the Sragi sugar factory in central Java, Indonesia*, Bozman, Mont., Montana State University, 1975.

41. Early in the 1960s, for example, one acute observer noted (albeit in a manner richly redolent of industry orthodoxy on the score of brown versus white) that: "mills have been working below capacity for lack of cane, yet in some regions a crude sugar product (*gula mangkok*), inefficiently refined in the villages from peasant cane, is able to sell profitably, and even to find export outlets." See Jamie Mackie, "Indonesian Government Estates," p. 347.

42. Key work on the Java sugar industry during the second half the twentieth century is reported in: Colin Brown "The Intensified Smallholder Cane Programme: First Five Years," *Bulletin of Indonesian Economic Studies*, 18 (1) 1982, pp. 39–60; Colin Brown, "Land Use Policy in the Java Sugar Industry, 1945–1957," Paper prepared for the ASAA/CAS/ISEAS Conference, Singapore, 1–3 February 1989; Aard J. Hartveld, "Raising Cane. Linkages, Organisations and Negotiations in Malang's Sugar Industry, East Java," Ph.D. diss., Landbouwuniversiteit Wageningen, 1996; Ernst Spaan and Aard Hartveld, "Socio-economic change and rural entrepreneurs in pre-crisis East Java, Indonesia: Case study of a Madurese upland community," *Sojourn: Social Issues in Southeast Asia*, 17 (2), 2002, pp. 274–300; Mubyarto, "The

Sugar Industry: From Estate to Smallholder Cane," *Bulletin of Indonesian Economic Studies*, 13(2) 1977, pp. 29–44; Frans Husken, "Cycles of Commercialisation and Accumulation in a Central Javanese Village," in G. Hart et al. (eds.), *Agrarian Transformations. Local Processes and the State in Southeast Asia*, Berkeley: University of California Press, 1989, pp. 303–331; Hiroyoshi Kano, Frans Husken and Djoko Suryo (eds.), *Beneath the Smoke of the Sugar Mill*, Yogyarta, Gadjah Mada University Press, 2001.

43. E.g., Hartveld, *Raising Cane* (p. 59), describes a situation in which, under inflationary conditions, peasant farmers "preferred to cultivate food crops or to process the cane into brown sugar. Consequently, the mills were operating below capacity and asked the assistance of the administrative or military authorities to force the landowners to lease their land or the out-growers to sell them their cane."

44. Colin Brown, "The Intensified Smallholder Cane Programme," p. 45, Table Three. For developments in late twentieth and early twenty-first centuries, see Tim Stapleton, *The Political Economy of Indonesian Trade Policy: The Case of Sugar*, Readings in International Development Economics, Asia Pacific School of Economics and Government, Australian National University, November 2005, pp. 34–53; Tim Stapleton, "Institutional Determination of Indonesian Sugar Trade Policy," *Bulletin of Indonesian Economic Studies*, 42, 1 (2006), pp. 95–103.

45. For an extended analysis, see Stapleton, *The Case of Sugar*, passim.

46. Mintz, "Sweet Polychrest," p. 96.

Afterword

Rachel Laudan

In this anthology we have an impressive series of cross-national studies stretching over three centuries and much of the earth's surface. In their introduction, Carolyn de la Peña and Benjamin Lawrance ask: What do they add up to? What big questions in the study of food itself do they address (as opposed to questions in the disciplines in which the authors have been trained)? And is there some more general story to which they contribute? The editors end their introduction by inviting us to consider these as involving the multiple collisions between foods and peoples, both of them in transit, and how this transforms food and eaters into cuisine.

I am grateful to them for giving me an opening to talk about why I believe that cuisine is a useful way of thinking about food. It is a topic that I explore more fully in my world food history, *Cuisine and Empire*, to appear with the University of California Press. Here I shall use certain key concepts – cuisine, culinary philosophy, culinary determinism, and culinary geography – to engage with the authors and editors of this volume, indicating points of coincidence, areas of disagreement, and ways to move forward.

First, though, let me review what de la Peña and Lawrance have to say about the history and future of food studies. Taking as their starting point late twentieth-century work on economic world systems and global trade narratives, the editors suggest that the essays offer a way to move beyond the studies of commodities and their paths from producer to consumer that have filled library shelves in the past ten or fifteen years. Such studies, argue the editors, although they have enormously enriched our understanding of beans, bananas, chocolate, tea, vanilla, potatoes and a host of other foodstuffs, suffer from three shortcomings.

First, commodity tracing is deceptive because, as Nemser's chapter on Spanish attitudes to the pre-Hispanic beverage *pulque*, Knight's discussion of sugar, and Russek's chapter on the appeal of ethnic restaurants in 1930s America show, food is global in ways that go far beyond the simple movement of commodities from one spot to another. Second, the essays reveal that the widely-held assumption that local food is what grows locally, an assumption encapsulated in the word 'locavore,' is also too narrow because local is defined as much by culture as by geography, as evidenced by Edward's discussion of Virginia ham. Bobrow-Strain makes it clear that the rest of the world thinks of sliced white bread as the quintessential local American food. Wiley reveals how milk-drinking had to be promoted by appeal to local Indian and Chinese values before it was acceptable. Third, the editors use Maroney's history of curry's journey to England, Matejowsky's analysis of fast-food trends in the Philippines, and Goldstein's exploration of how cuppers in Rwanda learn what Americans like about their coffee to attack the thesis that globalization means homogenization, or the McDonaldization of Everything.

The time has come, the editors say, to talk of things other than commodities and focus on global foodways, exploring local cases in a trans-national context. They congratulate the authors of the chapters for asking questions that advance that agenda, particularly questions about how taste is created, about the relations of taste and value, and about the links between taste, value, global and local.

Just as de la Peña and Lawrance have worried about the reduction of food studies to commodity studies, my starting point was a parallel concern about the widespread tendency to elide farming and food. Jared Diamond, for example, in his best seller, *Guns, Germs and Steel*, which devotes one quarter of its pages to harnessing agriculture, mentions cooking only once. Yet we do not eat wheat and we do not eat cattle. We eat bread and beef stew or roast. To run together food and farming misses all the complex processing and cooking that turns farm products into dishes that we put in our mouths. It's a widespread practice. Food aid, in popular parlance, all too often means the delivery of farm products, food politics often ends up being farm politics. All of these usages divorce food from the meals that we actually consume.

To see how limiting it is to think of food studies only in terms of farming or commodities, just consider that no one researching clothing would limit themselves to the history of sheep herding, silkworms, and cotton plantations, nor would those studying architecture think it comprised the understanding of quarrying, brick making and lumbering. Yet again, no one would think trade in these commodities exhausted the scope of clothing studies or architecture. Yet farming and, as the editors remind us, trade and the life story of commodities, dominate talk about food. The articles in *Food and Foodways*, from whence this anthology sprung, have since the journal's inception been a shining exception to this rule, as are the chapters in this volume. They demonstrate the potential gains when those of us who do food studies put our own agenda first, not an agenda inherited from other disciplines.

I suggest, therefore that we begin by thinking about food as an artifact, something that humans make in the kitchen and the processing plant, food as something that has been cooked. Thinking of food as an artifact, the product of cooking, is not the only way to look at food: how we dine, how we are nourished, and many other questions are legitimate, and, more than legitimate, important. I would argue, however, that using cooking as a starting point enables us to bring useful perspectives to bear on food studies.

Human food differs from that of other living beings just because it has been cooked, that is to say that it has been transformed after slaughtering or harvesting. While we may grant that from time to time we enjoy uncooked fruit or even raw meat or fish, the fact remains that all human societies rely for the bulk of their calories on cooked food, and that no human societies live successfully on raw food. Cooking, in this sense, includes not only heating (and cooling) but also the multiple other manipulations – mechanical, chemical and biochemical, chopping, grinding, acidifying, soaking, and fermenting, in home, institutional, and industrial kitchens and processing plants – to which we subject our foodstuffs. Food is the result of millennia of experimentation. Cooking is quite likely one of our oldest techniques, turning natural products into what we are willing or happy to put in our mouths. It remains one of the most important, without which we could not survive.

I want to pursue some of the consequences of food as something cooked, particularly those with bearing on the questions raised by authors and editors. I shall do so in three steps: first, why we cook, what a culinary philosophy is, and how the movement of foods from raw to cooked creates taste and value; second, moving to the geographical movement of food, the concepts of culinary politics and culinary determinism; and third, cuisines and their encounters as a way of undermining the distinction between the global and the local.

So first, why do we cook? We cook to bring the natural world in line with our cultural values, with our culinary philosophy. When I first ran across the term "culinary philosophy" I thought it one more bit of pretentiousness. It was in a cookbook by Camellia Panjabi, *50 Great Curries of India*, and she related how the distinguished chef Anton Mosiman asked her to include a section on the culinary philosophy of India without which, he said, he would not know how to interpret the recipes.[1] As I read on, the light dawned. Panjabi described how the Hindu housewife thought about planning the meal. She thought about how much money she had, what was in season, whether there were guests, what the family astrologer said about foods to be avoided in light of planets in ascendance, and what heating or cooling foods (in the humoral sense) were needed to balance the temperament of different family members. As the passage moved from the familiar to the unfamiliar, I had a shock of recognition. This was culinary philosophy, the values the cook sought to enhance. The Hindu housewife's values only overlapped partially with my own, but the strategy of cooking to advance or achieve values was exactly the same.

The values are the most basic ones: the society and economy we think is desirable, the relation with the gods, if we believe in them, that we want to achieve, the ways we think we should interact with nature including our own bodies. Naturally these are often implicit, learned and internalized, coming to the surface only when we encounter others like the Hindu housewife with different values. As a modern American, I tend to value inexpensive meals available to all (not the vast feasts designed to accentuate social difference that were common through most of history). I don't choose my foods according to the rules of feasting and fasting of many of the world's religions, but I do pay great attention to cooking to enhance the health of my family and the well-being of the planet.

The example I have given is of the individual cook in the domestic kitchen. But because we live in society, we share many values with the rest of society, we consume many foods that are produced not in the home kitchen but in the industrial kitchen. And, I might add, tensions between different culinary philosophies are one of the most important sources of culinary change.

What the preceding discussion does shed light on, I suggest, are the editors' questions about what makes foods tasty and what gives them value. I would argue that as commodities, the raw materials of the food we put in our mouths, are transformed by cooking, they acquire good or bad taste, high or low value depending on the culinary philosophy of the diner or observer.

Take, for example, the Virginia ham discussed by Megan Edwards. Pork was not as prestigious as beef (large, red and masculine) or game (aristocratic), say, in early modern Europe. On the other hand, ham was regarded as both tasty and of high economic value. Salted foods were valued in part because they were 'cured', that is the natural cycle of corruption and decay had been stopped, creating products that held the promise of long life. Because salt stimulated the appetite, they were appropriate as 'appetizers' for high-class meals. Curing turned highly perishable meat into a commodity that could be safely shipped long distances. As it was cured (cooked), pork became tastier and more valuable.

Again, consider the *pulque* of seventeenth-century Mexico described by Nemser. Here we have two sets of values in conflict. The poor, often mixed-race people in Mexico

City liked the taste of *pulque* mixed with herbs, roots, and fruits. The rulers of the city, Spaniards with residual suspicions of *pulque*'s role in "witchcraft" as they often characterized native religion, thought that mixing *pulque* reduced its whiteness and purity, so that *pulque mesclado* like the mixed-race consumers had lower value. In fact it was not only of low value, it destroyed the virtue of the poor, making them shiftless, undependable and liable to revolt. (Interestingly, when Spanish colonists drank *pulque* with additives, they called it *curado*, or cured, and saw it as higher value than plain *pulque*).

White bread, as Bobrow-Strain shows, was thought to endow and embody the strength of the American nation during the Cold War. Culminating a tradition going back centuries, and particularly important in the late nineteenth century, the search for health and strength was believed to be satisfied by white bread because baking maximized the protein-like gluten in wheat flour. Noodles, spaghetti, or – heaven forbid – rice or maize, simply did not deliver the same health benefits, or hence, the same value.

Knight's analysis of the shifting fortunes of brown and white sugar in twentieth-century Indonesia neatly complements the previous discussions of whiteness as something produced by transforming raw materials, such as the milky *pulque* created fermenting the sap of the maguey plant and the white bread created by milling and sieving wheat. Following independence from the Dutch, Indonesians keen to express their identity as citizens of a modern nation, shifted from brown sugar produced on a small scale by indigenous techniques, to the pure white sugar produced in large refineries that the Dutch had produced for export. Then, just as American tastes had begun to shift from white to brown bread in the 1970s with the reaction against the complex comprising agribusiness, industrial food, and the Cold War, so Indonesian taste shifted back to the more "natural" and "local" brown sugar.

Coffee washing, as Goldstein shows, creates the taste of coffee that Americans prefer and thus allows the coffee to be sold at a premium price, but in specific markets. Milk, which might seem to be a natural, uncooked food, is regarded by Hindus as having been cooked by Mother Cow, bringing it to the highest point of perfection, locating it in a culinary philosophy that had to be brushed under the rug, as Wiley points out, before milk could be re-conceptualized as a health food for Muslims as well as Hindus.

To summarize, good tastes and bad are created by cooking, both in the sense of changing chemical composition and in the sense of moving foods closer to (or farther from) fulfilling the culinary philosophy of the individual, group, or society. Because these values vary from group to group, tastes are not universal (except possibly in the case of high calorie items like sugar and fat, though even these have society-specific manifestations; fluffy cake versus dense sweets for example). Transfer of foods from one society to another, then, means adjustments of processing to fit different values, or of values to fit the product.

Second, we turn to how the movement of foods has been shaped by culinary politics and that in turn by culinary determinism. Connected to the belief that food had to be cooked to conform to cultural values or culinary philosophy was a belief held widely, perhaps almost universally, in the past in culinary determinism or "you are what you eat." When we use this now-hackneyed phrase, we usually link it with identity rather than physical characteristics. Your Italian or Jewish grandmother's cooking is part of your heritage, your identity.

For most of human history, though, it was meant quite literally. What you ate you assimilated and it turned into you. What you ate made you stronger or weaker, smarter or duller, more or less virtuous, even wicked. At the moment, such beliefs seem archaic, even dangerous, though they continue to underpin discussions of obesity, childhood malnutrition, and the like. Whether or not we agree, though, we have to take them seriously if we are to understand culinary politics.

Central to culinary politics is deciding when to eat food other than your own, decisions that are rooted in power relations and culinary determinism. As de la Peña and Lawrance suggest, eating the global may function as "a culinary imaginary with which individuals can affiliate for enhanced prestige by altering consumption." And this certainly happens, as is clear in Bobrow-Strain's chapter on white bread and Wiley's on milk. In both cases prestige follows from the fact that white bread and milk had been since about the beginning of the twentieth century privileged foods of the economic and military powerhouses, Great Britain and the United States. If you were a culinary determinist, it was natural to conclude that eating white bread and milk made strong individuals and that these made strong states. In the late nineteenth century, states that wished to emulate the performance of Britain or the US, including Italy, Japan, Mexico, and Brazil, prudently embarked on programs to induce their citizens to give up polenta, steamed rice, tortillas or manioc and shift to white bread. When, following World War II, the United States began shipping its surplus wheat worldwide, it went to consumers who had been exposed for a century to the idea that white bread made strong individuals and strong nations. The same was true of milk a few decades later.

Culinary politics can also provide a framework for the complex history of curry described by Maroney, one that leads me to somewhat different emphases. In the eighteenth century, the British of the East India Company who went to India saw themselves as taking on the mantle of the ruling Mughal class, as a successor set of "high caste" rulers. At a time when social status was more important than, say, ethnicity, in deciding what you ate, eating Mughal dishes was unthreatening, indeed it was the natural thing to do if you could not transfer your own diet to the foreign country. It was food for rulers, and thus according to culinary determinism, good for Mughals and British alike. The earliest British recipes for curry in Hannah Glasse are striking for their fidelity to the Indian dishes from which they were derived, with freshly ground, lightly used spices.

Only later, when the British as a whole began to see themselves as superior to the Indians, were curry recipes re-worked: the sauce changed from the traditional Indian product, to one based on a "strong" white-flour roux. Following independence in 1947, power relations changed again, and Indian migrants to Britain could denounce roux-based curry as having nothing to do with the dishes of their native land. Setting up restaurants, they reintroduced techniques of thickening sauces with onions, garlic, ginger and spices.

The culinary politics of the seventeenth-century Spanish conquerors with the indigenous was different from that of the British and the Mughals. The Spanish, as conquerors rather than successors, had at all costs to avoid foods that would lower their moral status to that of the poor in Mexico City, including those mixed-blood individuals who drank mixed *pulque*. Hence here the "culinary imaginary" far from being an entry into the prestige of a global world, caused them, as it would the British in nineteenth-century India, to avoid at all costs "going native."

In the case of ethnic restaurants, outlined by Russek, the culinary politics is different again. Migrants to the United States from southern or eastern Europe brought with them their cuisines that, so the Americans believed, were those of weaker nations or empires, such as the Greek food of the Ottoman Empire, and thus, according to culinary determinism, should not be incorporated into the American diet. The migrants were, however, becoming American citizens, and native-born Americans were beginning the tricky project of coming to terms with their new fellow citizens or citizens-to-be. Restaurants offered a way that Americans could briefly and safely experience these foods without running the danger of being weakened by eating them regularly. And doubtless, the proprietors of the restaurants apart from using English emphasized the dishes with meat so important to strong nations.

The preceding discussion suggests that talking about globalization of foodstuffs cannot ignore the calculations that cooks and diners make about how new foods and cooking methods will affect them, calculations frequently based in culinary determinism but differing in their outcomes depending on specific power relations.

Third, I move from talking of individual foods and the cultural values attributed to them to cuisines as a whole. Foods – white bread, milk, coffee, sugar, ham, or *pulque*, for example – do not stand alone but are part of larger structures, systems or styles of cooking. Since English lacks a good single word for style or system of cooking, I shall call these different styles "cuisines," which, in Latin and Romance languages means at once the kitchen and the style of cooking. It is important to stress that as I use it (and as I increasingly see it used in cookbook titles for example) cuisine carries no overtones of "high" or "elite," unless so specified.

A cuisine is held together by its culinary philosophy. It depends on techniques that are used over and again, a preferred set of foodstuffs that can be processed and cooked by these techniques, to make dishes and meals that satisfy the culinary philosophy of the diners, the consumers of the food. Because it is not easy to invent a cuisine, because it is such a tight structure, cuisines tend to persist over long periods of time and to resist fusing with cuisines based on radically different philosophies.

Although cuisines can be subdivided indefinitely down to the level of the individual household, if we want to understand the history and politics of food on the grand scale we can see it as the creation, spread and eventual disappearance of large families of cuisine, going back millennia. Already by 1000 BC, at the moment the earliest date when we can use a combination of history, archaeology and plant genetics to define and distinguish cuisines, the globe was dominated by about eight major cuisines, all of which had originated in one or a small number of places and spread across continents and oceans. The globalization of cuisines (unless you insist that globalization means circumnavigation) is an ancient phenomenon. When migrants, the military, missionaries, or other agents transferred a cuisine from one place to another, they invariably had to adjust it to the new natural and cultural environment, all the while maintaining its essential features.

What happens in culinary transfer is well illustrated by Edwards' study of Virginia ham. The culinary aim of the settlers in Virginia was to transfer the Anglo version of Modern Western Cuisine, including its bread, beef, and other preferred foodstuffs, including ham, to the Americas as intact as possible. Already in England and Europe, small differences in circumstances had resulted in a variety of different techniques for making ham: air-dried in Cumbria, smoked in Devon, and unsmoked in Wiltshire and Cumberland. Virginia, as Edwards show, had one more set of particularities: excellent quality pork thanks to the plentiful forests, hardwood for smoking, and a paucity of salt and saltpeter that tilted the settlers in the direction of a dry cured smoked ham that was able to compete on equal terms with the diverse hams of Europe. Although, as she also suggests, the settlers may also have benefitted from the preserving knowledge of Native Americans and Africans, the case of Virginia ham is one element in the expansion of Anglo Cuisine.

What happens, though, when two cuisines (or cuisine families) come in contact? Almost all the chapters in this volume deal with aspects of the grand set of encounters of the last three hundred and fifty years. This is the encounter between the great families of Traditional Cuisine, which for convenience I will call Buddhist, Hindu, Islamic and Christian (as well as a number of less articulated, more local cuisines) on the one hand, and Modern Cuisines, particularly Anglo cuisines on the other. The expansion of Anglo Cuisines went hand in hand first with the British Empire and then with the global economic and military power of the United States. To say this is neither to exalt nor to apologize for the phenomenon. It is simply to recognize that at the end of the eighteenth century there were perhaps twelve million people who ate Anglo cuisine worldwide, while by the 1930s there were 200 million. Thus, although those who ate other cuisines also increased (the Chinese and Indian populations each roughly doubling from 200 million to 4-500 million and the Spanish empire with its Catholic Cuisine increasing from 25 million to 90 million) no other cuisine increased as rapidly, grew so fast worldwide, or altered commerce and agriculture over such wide swathes of the earth's surface as Anglo cuisine.[2]

The result of the massive expansion of Anglo Cuisines was the creation of a complex pattern of external and internal borders with the cuisines encountered. The relations between cuisines across these borders depended on the particular culinary politics of the border. For example, migrants brought the Christian Cuisines and Islamic-influenced Cuisines of the Mediterranean with them to the United States while governments in the Buddhist-shaped cuisine of post-Mao China and the Hindu-Islamic Cuisine of India contemplated incorporating the milk-drinking of Anglo Cuisines into their traditional practices, situations examined by Russek and Wiley respectively. Wiley, for example, shows that the Chinese, most of whom still accepted a culinary philosophy in which health was dealt with in humoral terms, were open to milk as promoting growth and with references to calcium and protein, so important in Anglo culinary philosophy, dropped. Also of interest is that milk stands as a surrogate for Anglo Cuisine as a whole, conferring its benefits without involving the Herculean task (undertaken by the Japanese before World War II) of transforming the nation's cuisine in the Anglo image. And furthermore, children, both the cosseted hope for the future and relatively unfixed in their culturally-induced tastes, were the target audience.

Nothing summed up Anglo Cuisine better than the McDonald's hamburger, with its white bread, beef, and a gesture at a healthy fresh vegetable, accompanied by a cold milky or fizzy drink, eaten in bright, clean surroundings. As Matejowsky points out, when McDonald's opened in the Philippines in the 1970s, the idea was an instant success with middle class Filipinos who under colonialism had long been exposed to the idea that consuming beef and bread prepared and consumed in clean modern surroundings was prestigious, healthy and appropriate for citizens of a modern nation. Able to adjust the basic concept to specifically Filipino tastes, local chains, particularly Jollibee's, were able to outdo McDonald's in fast food retailing. The ironic result was that the success of the Philippines in competing with the United States in this economic arena reinforced and accentuated eating habits that were already known to be associated with the diseases of abundance in the United States, driving home the point that cuisines are transferred as packages.

In short, within the general pattern of the expansion and encounter between cuisines, encounters shaped by culinary politics, culinary determinism, and culinary philosophy, are a host of different negotiations and different outcomes. What is transferred or rejected (whole cuisines, particular dishes, individual foodstuffs), how they are used (at the same or different meals, as prestige items or for the poor, with the same or different accompaniments), who does the transferring and to whom (merchants, missionaries, bureaucrats, diplomats, women, children etc), and where the transfer takes place (retail, homes, restaurants) is different in every case. The complexity of this multitude of patterns of encounter, I believe, makes finding analytic concepts that are widely applicable, such as the ones that I tentatively suggest here, all the more important if we are not to throw up our hands in despair at the complexity of it all.

Finally, and to conclude, this afterword is a plea for placing culture at the center of food studies, whether histories, sociologies, anthropologies, or any other specific approach. Cuisines, far from being an epiphenomenon perched on a pinnacle whose base is food production and trade in commodities, come first. When culinary philosophy changes, cuisine changes, when cuisine changes, patterns of commerce and types of farming change in response.

Coming to the question of what is local from the history of cuisines, I arrive at exactly the same conclusion as the editors. What makes a food or a cuisine local is culture, not geography or agriculture or the "rich bounty" of the region. As the authors in this volume reveal in their different studies, the rich and various layering of different cultural influences at different spots on the earth's surface, not nature, has given us local foods or local cuisines. Indeed I would go further. As the complex pattern of expanding and encountering cuisines continues over time, the local becomes more diverse, more specific, not one homogenous whole as the despairing theory of the McDonaldization of everything supposes.

Notes

1. C. Panjabi, *50 Great Curries of India* (1994), 1518, 185.
2. J. Belich, *Replenishing the Earth: The Settler Revolution and the Rise of the Anglo World, 1783-1939* (2009), 4.

Index

Page numbers in *Italics* represent tables.